Spine Rehabilitation in 2022 and Beyond

Spine Rehabilitation in 2022 and Beyond

Editors

Deed E. Harrison
Ibrahim M. Moustafa
Paul A. Oakley

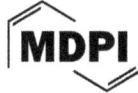

Basel • Beijing • Wuhan • Barcelona • Belgrade • Novi Sad • Cluj • Manchester

Editors
Deed E. Harrison
CBP NonProfit, Inc.
Eagle
USA

Ibrahim M. Moustafa
University of Sharjah
Sharjah
United Arab Emirates

Paul A. Oakley
York University
Toronto
Canada

Editorial Office
MDPI
St. Alban-Anlage 66
4052 Basel, Switzerland

This is a reprint of articles from the Special Issue published online in the open access journal *Journal of Clinical Medicine* (ISSN 2077-0383) (available at: https://www.mdpi.com/journal/jcm/special_issues/WB57SSGGE8).

For citation purposes, cite each article independently as indicated on the article page online and as indicated below:

Lastname, A.A.; Lastname, B.B. Article Title. *Journal Name* **Year**, *Volume Number*, Page Range.

ISBN 978-3-0365-8812-4 (Hbk)
ISBN 978-3-0365-8813-1 (PDF)
doi.org/10.3390/books978-3-0365-8813-1

© 2023 by the authors. Articles in this book are Open Access and distributed under the Creative Commons Attribution (CC BY) license. The book as a whole is distributed by MDPI under the terms and conditions of the Creative Commons Attribution-NonCommercial-NoDerivs (CC BY-NC-ND) license.

Contents

About the Editors vii

Preface ix

Deed E. Harrison, Paul A. Oakley and Ibrahim M. Moustafa
Don't Throw the 'Bio' out of the Bio-Psycho-Social Model: Editorial for Spine Rehabilitation in 2022 and Beyond
Reprinted from: *J. Clin. Med.* **2023**, *12*, 5602, doi:10.3390/jcm12175602 1

Philip A. Arnone, Steven J. Kraus, Derek Farmen, Douglas F. Lightstone, Jason Jaeger and Christine Theodossis
Examining Clinical Opinion and Experience Regarding Utilization of Plain Radiography of the Spine: Evidence from Surveying the Chiropractic Profession
Reprinted from: *J. Clin. Med.* **2023**, *12*, 2169, doi:10.3390/jcm12062169 11

Fabio Zaina, Rosemary Marchese, Sabrina Donzelli, Claudio Cordani, Carmelo Pulici, Jeb McAviney, et al.
Current Knowledge on the Different Characteristics of Back Pain in Adults with and without Scoliosis: A Systematic Review
Reprinted from: *J. Clin. Med.* **2023**, *12*, 5182, doi:10.3390/jcm12165182 37

Fabio Zaina, Irene Ferrario, Antonio Caronni, Stefano Scarano, Sabrina Donzelli and Stefano Negrini
Measuring Quality of Life in Adults with Scoliosis: A Cross-Sectional Study Comparing SRS-22 and ISYQOL Questionnaires
Reprinted from: *J. Clin. Med.* **2023**, *12*, 5071, doi:10.3390/jcm12155071 53

Martina Marsiolo, Silvia Careri, Diletta Bandinelli, Renato Maria Toniolo and Angelo Gabriele Aulisa
Vertebral Rotation in Functional Scoliosis Caused by Limb-Length Inequality: Correlation between Rotation, Limb Length Inequality, and Obliquity of the Sacral Shelf
Reprinted from: *J. Clin. Med.* **2023**, *12*, 5571, doi:10.3390/jcm12175571 75

Ibrahim M. Moustafa, Tamer Shousha, Ashokan Arumugam and Deed E. Harrison
Is Thoracic Kyphosis Relevant to Pain, Autonomic Nervous System Function, Disability, and Cervical Sensorimotor Control in Patients with Chronic Nonspecific Neck Pain?
Reprinted from: *J. Clin. Med.* **2023**, *12*, 3707, doi:10.3390/jcm12113707 87

Amal Ahbouch, Ibrahim M. Moustafa, Tamer Shousha, Ashokan Arumugam, Paul Oakley and Deed E. Harrison
An Investigation of the Association between 3D Spinal Alignment and Fibromyalgia
Reprinted from: *J. Clin. Med.* **2023**, *12*, 218, doi:10.3390/jcm12010218 109

Ibrahim M. Moustafa, Aliaa Attiah Mohamed Diab and Deed E. Harrison
Does Forward Head Posture Influence Somatosensory Evoked Potentials and Somatosensory Processing in Asymptomatic Young Adults?
Reprinted from: *J. Clin. Med.* **2023**, *12*, 3217, doi:10.3390/jcm12093217 121

Maryam Kamel, Ibrahim M. Moustafa, Meeyoung Kim, Paul A. Oakley and Deed E. Harrison
Alterations in Cervical Nerve Root Function during Different Sitting Positions in Adults with and without Forward Head Posture: A Cross-Sectional Study
Reprinted from: *J. Clin. Med.* **2023**, *12*, 1780, doi:10.3390/jcm12051780 137

Aisha Salim Al Suwaidi, Ibrahim M. Moustafa, Meeyoung Kim, Paul A. Oakley and Deed E. Harrison
A Comparison of Two Forward Head Posture Corrective Approaches in Elderly with Chronic Non-Specific Neck Pain: A Randomized Controlled Study
Reprinted from: *J. Clin. Med.* **2023**, *12*, 542, doi:10.3390/jcm12020542 153

Ibrahim M. Moustafa, Aliaa A. Diab and Deed E. Harrison
The Efficacy of Cervical Lordosis Rehabilitation for Nerve Root Function and Pain in Cervical Spondylotic Radiculopathy: A Randomized Trial with 2-Year Follow-Up
Reprinted from: *J. Clin. Med.* **2022**, *11*, 6515, doi:10.3390/jcm11216515 173

Ibrahim Moustafa Moustafa, Aliaa Attiah Mohamed Diab and Deed Eric Harrison
Does Improvement towards a Normal Cervical Sagittal Configuration Aid in the Management of Lumbosacral Radiculopathy: A Randomized Controlled Trial
Reprinted from: *J. Clin. Med.* **2022**, *11*, 5768, doi:10.3390/jcm11195768 193

Ahmed S. A. Youssef, Ibrahim M. Moustafa, Ahmed M. El Melhat, Xiaolin Huang, Paul A. Oakley and Deed E. Harrison
Randomized Feasibility Pilot Trial of Adding a New Three-Dimensional Adjustable Posture-Corrective Orthotic to a Multi-Modal Program for the Treatment of Nonspecific Neck Pain
Reprinted from: *J. Clin. Med.* **2022**, *11*, 7028, doi:10.3390/jcm11237028 209

Ibrahim Moustafa Moustafa, Tamer Mohamed Shousha, Lori M. Walton, Veena Raigangar and Deed E. Harrison
Reduction of Thoracic Hyper-Kyphosis Improves Short and Long Term Outcomes in Patients with Chronic Nonspecific Neck Pain: A Randomized Controlled Trial
Reprinted from: *J. Clin. Med.* **2022**, *11*, 6028, doi:10.3390/jcm11206028 229

Bertel Rune Kaale, Tony J. McArthur, Maria H. Barbosa and Michael D. Freeman
Post-Traumatic Atlanto-Axial Instability: A Combined Clinical and Radiological Approach for the Diagnosis of Pathological Rotational Movement in the Upper Cervical Spine
Reprinted from: *J. Clin. Med.* **2023**, *12*, 1469, doi:10.3390/jcm12041469 245

Evan A. Katz, Seana B. Katz and Michael D. Freeman
Non-Surgical Management of Upper Cervical Instability via Improved Cervical Lordosis: A Case Series of Adult Patients
Reprinted from: *J. Clin. Med.* **2023**, *12*, 1797, doi:10.3390/jcm12051797 253

About the Editors

Deed E. Harrison

Deed E. Harrison, D.C., graduated from Life Chiropractic College West in 1996. Dr. Harrison has developed and researched original spinal rehabilitation procedures and has lectured thousands of Chiropractors at nearly 1000 educational conferences around the world. He has authored (co-authored) approximately 234 peer-reviewed spine-related publications, seven spine textbooks, and numerous conference proceedings. He is a highly respected chiropractic researcher and authority in today's profession. Dr. Harrison is a manuscript reviewer for several top-tier peer-reviewed Spine journals, including Spine, Journal of Clinical Medicine, PloS One, Clinical Biomechanics, Clinical Anatomy, Archives of Physical Medicine and Rehabilitation, the European Spine Journal, European Journal of Physical Medicine and Rehabilitation, BMC Complimentary Alternative Medicine, and BMC Musculoskeletal Disorders. Dr. Harrison is a Guest Editor for two Special Issues on spine rehabilitation for the Journal of Clinical Medicine. Additionally, Dr. Harrison is a past member of the International Society for the Study of the Lumbar Spine (ISSLS), a former International Chiropractors Association's (ICA) Nevada State Assembly Representative member, and the acting Chair of the PCCRP Chiropractic Radiography Guidelines. He formerly held a position on the Chiropractic Physicians Board of Nevada. Currently, Dr. Harrison is the President/CEO of Chiropractic BioPhysics® (CBP®) Technique and President of CBP NonProfit, Inc., a spinal research foundation. Lastly, he directs and owns a large chiropractic rehabilitation and education facility in Eagle, ID, USA, called the Ideal Spine Health Center.

Ibrahim M. Moustafa

Ibrahim M. Moustafa is an academic and physiotherapy expert with a remarkable career spanning over a decade. He earned his doctoral degree in physical therapy from Cairo University in 2009 and has since made significant contributions to the field. In 2014, Dr. Moustafa achieved the rank of Associate Professor, solidifying his expertise in physiotherapy. In 2022, he reached the pinnacle of his academic career, earning the title of Full Professor. His dedication to research and innovation in spinal rehabilitation and the neurophysiological underpinnings of posture correction has resulted in numerous publications in esteemed international journals and conferences. Dr. Moustafa's outstanding achievements have not gone unnoticed. He was honored with the Mediterranean Regional Research Award and has also received other prestigious regional accolades. His commitment to advancing the field of physiotherapy is further evidenced by his role as a dedicated reviewer for several renowned international journals. Dr. Moustafa serves as an Editorial Board Member for the *Journal of Pain Management and Medicine* and *Austin Spine Journal*. Furthermore, he is Managing Editor for the *Bulletin of Faculty of Physical Therapy* at Cairo University, demonstrating his commitment to fostering academic excellence and research. Since 2018, Dr. Moustafa has been entrusted with the esteemed position of Chairperson of the Physiotherapy Department at the University of Sharjah, a testament to his leadership and dedication to education. Dr. Moustafa's visionary approach to research and his role as the founder and coordinator of the Neuromusculoskeletal Research Group underscore his enduring commitment to advancing the field of physiotherapy, making him a respected figure in academia and research.

Paul A. Oakley

    Dr. Oakley maintains a busy spine clinic, consults for Chiropractic BioPhysics Non-Profit (a Spine Research Foundation), and is pursuing his Ph.D. on postural steadiness and spinal deformity. He has published well over 100 scientific papers, conference abstracts, and book chapters, and has presented research at numerous scientific conferences, including the International Society of Biomechanics, the North American Conference on Biomechanics, the International Chiropractic Pediatric Association, the Association of Chiropractic Colleges, the Canadian Society of Biomechanics, and the World Federation of Chiropractic. Dr. Oakley is advanced certified and an instructor for CBP techniques, and he has participated in creating chiropractic guidelines for both the practice of Chiropractic and the use of X-rays in the profession. He has a B.Sc. in Kinesiology (Laurentian University, Sudbury, Ontario), an M.Sc. (Queen's University, Kingston, Ontario), and a Doctor of Chiropractic degree (Palmer College of Chiropractic, Davenport, Iowa).

Preface

Spinal disorders and disabilities are among the leading causes of work loss, suffering, and healthcare expenditures throughout the industrialized world. Spine disorders' psychosocial and economic impact demands continued research into the most effective preventative and interventional treatment strategies. In the past two decades, the role that sagittal plane alignment of the spine and posture has on human performance, health, pain, disability, and disease has been a primary research focus among spine surgical and rehabilitation specialists. It has been extensively demonstrated that sagittal plane alignment of the cervical and lumbar spines impacts human health and well-being. Limits of normality for various sagittal spine alignment parameters have been documented, providing chiropractors, physical therapists, surgeons, and other spine specialists with standardized goals to compare patients to in both pre- and post-treatment decision-making strategies. High-quality evidence points to spine corrective rehabilitative methods offering superior long-term outcomes for treating patients with various spine disorders. The economic impact, health benefits, generalized awareness of posture and spine deformities, and newer sagittal spine rehabilitation treatments demand continued attention from clinicians and researchers alike. These are the purposes of this collection of publications in this Special Issue.

Deed E. Harrison, Ibrahim M. Moustafa, and Paul A. Oakley
Editors

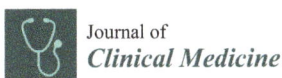

Editorial

Don't Throw the 'Bio' out of the Bio-Psycho-Social Model: Editorial for Spine Rehabilitation in 2022 and Beyond

Deed E. Harrison [1,*], Paul A. Oakley [2,3] and Ibrahim M. Moustafa [4,5]

1. CBP Nonprofit (a Spine Research Foundation), Eagle, ID 83616, USA
2. Independent Researcher, Newmarket, ON L3Y 8Y8, Canada; docoakley.icc@gmail.com
3. Kinesiology and Health Science, York University, Toronto, ON M3J 1P3, Canada
4. Neuromusculoskeletal Rehabilitation Research Group, RIMHS–Research Institute of Medical and Health Sciences, University of Sharjah, Sharjah 27272, United Arab Emirates; iabuamr@sharjah.ac.ae
5. Department of Physiotherapy, College of Health Sciences, University of Sharjah, Sharjah 27272, United Arab Emirates
* Correspondence: drdeed@idealspine.com or drdeedharrison@gmail.com

1. Introduction

Spinal injuries, disorders and disabilities are among the leading causes for work loss, suffering, and health care expenditures throughout the industrialized world [1–6]. The psycho-social and economic impact of general and specific spine disorders demands continued research into the most effective types of preventative and interventional treatment strategies. Specifically, low-back-pain (LBP)- and neck-pain-related disorders are the 1st and 4th leading causes of work loss and disability in the world [1–6]. Though billions are spent annually in experimental, epidemiology, and interventional strategies, precise treatment regimens aimed towards improving, resolving, and preventing these spinal disorders are highly varied and have limited and/or only short-term efficacy [1–6]. Thus, spinal disorders and related disabilities remain a high priority research avenue within the health sciences; in particular, there is an urgent need to increase the knowledge related to the manual rehabilitation disciplines [5,6].

Pain and disability with a spinal origin have several proposed psycho-social [1–9] and biomechanical contributing factors [10,11] which has given rise to the well-known 'bio-psycho-social' model of understanding injury mechanisms leading to the development of chronic pain and disabilities. Problematically, in recent decades, many authors have begun to minimize the 'bio' (tissue injury, damage, anatomical disorder, etc.) component of the problem, thus favoring the 'psycho-social' aspects such as catastrophizing, fear/anxiety and avoidance behavior components in the development of chronic pain in the patient [1–9], as some authors are quite adamant that the 'tissue injury' component plays a rather limited role [6]. It can be argued, though, that the lack of appreciation for the tissue component of spine pain/disorders is shortsighted, based on an incomplete review of recent systematic reviews, and based on limitations with early analytical methods, whereas today's technology and more detailed investigations have identified a significant role for the tissue component as contributing to the presence and development of chronic spine pain and disability [12–15]. Furthermore, proponents of the stronger role that the 'psycho-social' part of the equation plays in spine conditions often fail to acknowledge that recent systematic literature reviews with meta-analysis have identified a clear controversy regarding the quality and true impact that fear-avoidance, pain-catastrophizing (PC), and 'psycho-social' model elements play in individuals with chronic musculoskeletal pain (CMP) disorders [7–9]; for example, the following has been stated: *"Despite the very low quality of the available evidence, the general consistency of the findings highlights the potential role that PC may play in delaying recovery from CMP. Research that uses higher quality study designs and procedures would allow for more definitive conclusions regarding the impact of PC on pain and*

Citation: Harrison, D.E.; Oakley, P.A.; Moustafa, I.M. Don't Throw the 'Bio' out of the Bio-Psycho-Social Model: Editorial for Spine Rehabilitation in 2022 and Beyond. *J. Clin. Med.* **2023**, *12*, 5602. https://doi.org/10.3390/jcm12175602

Received: 21 August 2023
Accepted: 23 August 2023
Published: 28 August 2023

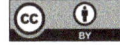

Copyright: © 2023 by the authors. Licensee MDPI, Basel, Switzerland. This article is an open access article distributed under the terms and conditions of the Creative Commons Attribution (CC BY) license (https://creativecommons.org/licenses/by/4.0/).

function." [7]. The current authors of this Editorial offer this perspective for context and not to dismiss the role that the psycho-social component plays in initiating and developing chronic spine related disorders.

It is often understood but understated that the 'bio' component in the 'bio-psycho-social' model also stands for biomechanics (not just biology) either segmentally or globally of the whole spine–body system [10,11]. While the mechanical causes of musculo-skeletal pain are not completely understood, they are thought to be linked to the interconnected functions of anatomical components (soft and hard tissues) of the spine where injury and pain can be caused by any incident that alters joint mechanics (kinematics, kinetics, alignment), tissue integrity, and muscle function via alterations and increases in general loading and load sharing of the various tissues [10,11]. Of interest, several authors have attempted to completely dismiss or minimize the role that biomechanics (alignment and loading) plays in the onset and development of musculoskeletal disorders [16–20]. For example, in a systematic review, it was concluded that *"Evidence from epidemiological studies does not support an association between sagittal spinal curves and health including spinal pain."* [16]. Complicating the matter, in each of the reviews that proposed a minimization of the role that biomechanics (alignment and loading) plays in chronic spine disorders [16–20], serious flaws in the study design and literature reviews were identified [19–24] highlighting the controversy and confusing the situation further.

Importantly, in the past two decades, the role that biomechanics of the sagittal plane alignment of the spine and three-dimensional posture has on human performance, health, pain, disability, and diseases has been a primary research focus among spine surgical and rehabilitation specialists across the scientific literature [25–37]. It has been quite extensively demonstrated that sagittal plane alignment and biomechanics of the lumbo-pelvic [25–32], thoracic hyper-kyphosis [33–35], and cervical [36,37] spines have clear impacts on human health and well-being, musculoskeletal disorders, and chronic pain disorders. Limits of normality for a variety of sagittal spine alignment parameters have been documented, providing chiropractors, physical therapists, surgeons, and other spine specialists with standardized goals to compare patients to in both pre- and post-treatment decision-making strategies [25–40]. Furthermore, conservative interventional methods have been developed and tested for their effects on improving altered sagittal plane alignment and preliminary and promising results have been found for a multi-modal program including lumbar extension traction (LET) [38], cervical extension traction (CET) [39], thoracic extension traction (TET) [40], bracing for thoracic hyper-kyphosis [41], and various specific exercise regimens for thoracic-kyphosis [41,42]. Problematically, some authors continue to ignore the evidence for these new types of sagittal plane curve-inducing (LET and CET) and curve-reducing (TET) traction methods and spinal bracing and their role in improving the sagittal plane alignment of the spine and improving chronic musculoskeletal disorders [4].

2. Purposes of Special Issue on Spine Rehabilitation

All too familiar are approaches to spine care involving functional rehabilitation programs including exercises for strength gains, range of motion increases, generalized stretching and strengthening procedures, massage, and soft tissue manipulation techniques, as well as physiotherapeutic modalities such as ultrasound and muscle stimulation, etc. An alternative to the traditional and popular functional approaches is a structural rehabilitation approach. Structural rehabilitation involves some aspects of functional rehabilitation methods but focuses on unique types of posture and spine correction methods for the primary purpose to realign and 'over-correct' the spine and altered postures [43].

Although spinal bracing and postural exercise techniques have shown preliminary evidence for providing structural spine and posture realignment [41,42], one evolved technique that has laid a substantial foundation towards the structural approach to spine care is the Chiropractic Biophysics® technique group [43]. From the mid-1990s to the mid-2000s, the Harrison research team performed a series of spine modeling studies of the sagittal spinal curves (Figure 1) [43]. This has formed the foundational spinal model to which patient comparison can be made for initial assessment of alignment abnormality and follow-up assessment to monitor treatment effects. Further, elaborate assessment and corrective treatment methods are based on the fundamental assessment of posture in terms of translations and rotations of the separate body segments in relation to each other (Figures 2 and 3) [43].

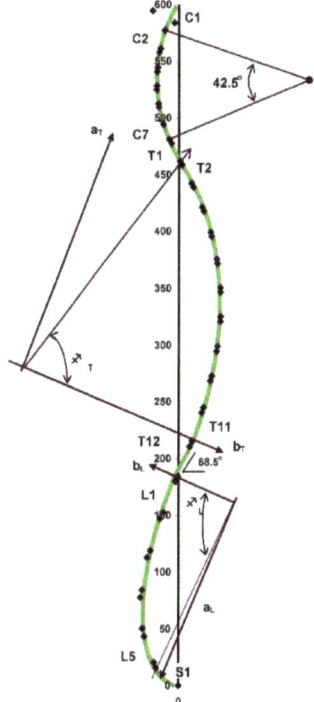

Figure 1. This diagram is the CBP® Full spine Normal Model. It documents the proper path of the spine from a side view. Ideally, the back of your vertebra should align along this mathematical model. It is composed of specific ellipses as shown in the following regions on the left: • C1-T1: cervical (neck) • T1-T12: thoracic (rib cage) • T12-S1 lumbar (low back). The ideal spine has near perfect vertical balance of the upper- and lower-most vertebra for each of these three spinal regions. Each region has points of inflection—the mathematical term for change in direction from concavity to convexity with which to compare your six spinal X-rays against. Along the entire spine, each vertebra has a graphed mathematical point to correspond to. Such a spinal analysis helps determine proper (or improper) posture and alignment and how much correction may be required.

Beginning in approximately 2010, Moustafa and colleagues (teaming up with Harrison and later Oakley) spearheaded the fundamental missing randomized controlled trials (RCTs) seeking to understand the efficacy and clinical utility of CET and LET methods [38,39,44,45]. These RCTs demonstrated that patients with cervical, thoracic, and lumbo-pelvic sagittal plane abnormality-related symptoms receiving spine correction via CET and LET methods achieved greater long-term health outcomes (pain, disability, mobility, etc.) versus patients who only received conventional functional based treatments that do not consistently improve spinal alignment [38,39,44,45]. Though today there are reliable and predictable means to restore the natural curvatures of the spine and improve sagittal balance and generalized posture alignment [38–42], the evidence is still preliminary and there are many areas for further research including the need for randomized trials on TET methods, an understanding of which sub-groups of populations with spine disorders might benefit the most, what is the ideal dose–response of treatment frequency and durations versus outcomes for different patient populations, and many other areas. Furthermore, more information from better quality case–control designs and cohort populations are needed to identify what type of effects (if any) that specific spine displacements have on musculoskeletal function, neurophysiology, and performance; in other words, more than just pain and disability outcome measures must be looked at and understood for a comprehensive understanding of the impact that altered spine/posture alignment has on spine related disorders and in improving human health and well-being. Additionally, there is a lack of information on non-sagittal spine displacements, and how these spine and posture displacements impact human health and disease needs to be comprehensively investigated. Finally, the economic impact, health benefits, and generalized awareness of full spine displacements and the newer 'structural rehabilitation' spine treatment methods demand continued attention from clinicians and researchers alike; the topics outlined above are the purposes of this collection of studies.

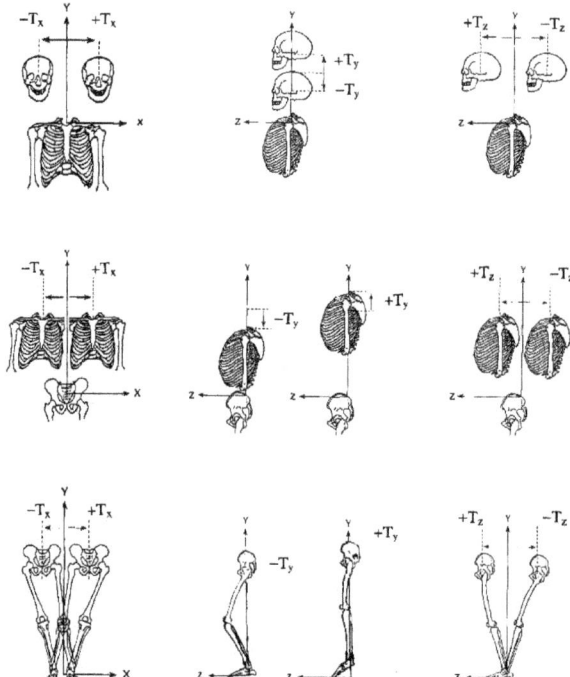

Figure 2. Translational Components of Abnormal Body Postures. In each region (head, ribcage, and pelvis), six distinct translation displacements are shown with "engineering" lines. Thus, 18 postural abnormalities as single postures are shown.

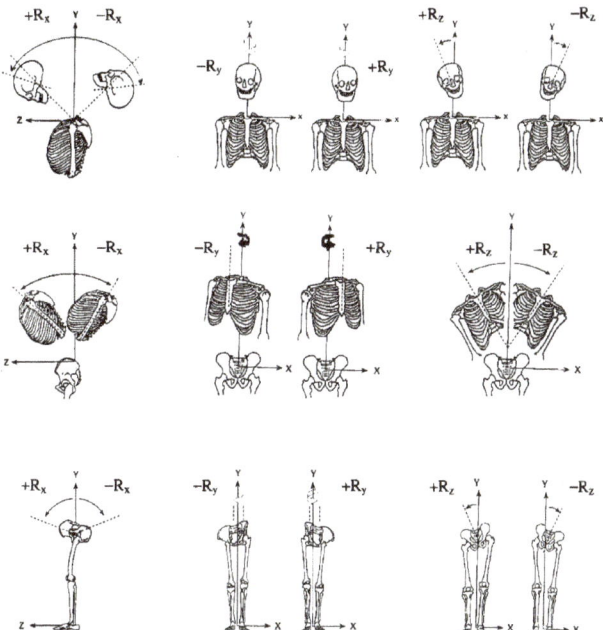

Figure 3. Rotational Components of Abnormal Body Postures. In each region (head, ribcage, and pelvis), six distinct rotation displacements are shown with "engineering" lines. Thus, 18 postural abnormalities as single postures are shown.

3. Special Issue Main Accepted Articles

At the time of the writing of this Editorial, there were 15 unique manuscripts accepted for publication in the Special Issue: *Spine Rehabilitation in 2022 and Beyond*. These manuscripts include the following categories of articles: a cross-sectional survey comparing two distinct quality of life questionnaires in adults with scoliosis [46]; a retrospective consecutive cohort investigation examining the relationship of vertebral y-axis rotation of the lumbar spine in functional scoliosis with leg length inequality to sacral shelf lateral tilt angles [47]; a profession wide survey of the chiropractic profession regarding spine radiography utilization examining clinical opinions and experience [48]; a novel clinical manual method comparing manual palpation and motion vs. diagnostic imaging to determine pathological rotational instability movement of the upper cervical spine [49]; four case–control investigations seeking to identify any correlations between spine and posture displacements and patient pain, disability, neurophysiology, and sensory–motor control variables [50–53]; one case series looking at the relationship between non-surgical sagittal plane cervical spine correction and the improvement in upper cervical spine rotational instability [54]; five randomized trials examining the relationship between correction/reduction of cervical and thoracic posture deformities and spine displacements and improvements of a variety of clinical outcome measures including pain, disability, neurophysiology, range of motion, and sensory–motor control measures [55–59]; and, lastly, one systematic literature review that sought to understand the differences in low back pain and disability characteristics in adults with and without scoliotic spine deformities [60].

Importantly, each one of these 15 accepted manuscripts offers unique and succinct relevant data that provide further evidence that the 'bio' (biology and biomechanics) component of the 'bio-psycho-social' model of spine care is extremely important to understanding patient pain, disability, and dysfunction and to providing enhanced treatment procedures that improve the outcomes of patient care [46–60]. As such, this Special Issue on spine rehabilitation provides useful, cutting-edge, relevant information that should prove to be useful to improve patient care and outcomes in populations suffering from a wide variety of spine related disorders. We thank all the authors of each of these manuscripts for their work, dedication, and insights they provided to bring their team's data together in an effective scientific manner. We are confident that each of the manuscripts contained in this collection will be well cited and used by future clinicians from many disciplines and researchers to treat patients around the globe and to improve upon the information presented [46–60].

4. Conclusions

Good quality data currently exist and continue to evolve to support the 'bio' element in the biopsychosocial model of chronic pain disorders. This Special Issue, dedicated to 'spine rehabilitation in 2022', features highlights of several research avenues taking place, such as the link between altered posture and physical performance, altered posture and pathological conditions, as well as the therapeutic improvement in spine alignment and posture correlating with positive patient outcomes. These lines of research are desperately needed and, unfortunately, continue to be underrecognized. We believe a tidal wave of 'bio' evidence is mounting, and a better of the understanding of the biomechanics in spine care will lead to more effective treatments. We hope for the biomechanical spine literature to continue to gain a wider acknowledgement and acceptance by the chronic spine pain community.

Author Contributions: Conceptualization, I.M.M., P.A.O. and D.E.H.; writing—I.M.M., P.A.O. and D.E.H. All authors have read and agreed to the published version of the manuscript.

Conflicts of Interest: Dr. Deed Harrison (DEH) lectures to health care providers on rehabilitation methods and is the CEO of a company which sells products to physicians for patient care to aid in improvement of postural and spine ailments as described in this manuscript. PAO is a paid consultant for CBP NonProfit, Inc. IMM declares no conflict of interest.

References

1. Cohen, S.P. Epidemiology, diagnosis, and treatment of neck pain. *Mayo Clin. Proc.* **2015**, *90*, 284–299. [CrossRef] [PubMed]
2. Cohen, S.P.; Hooten, W.M. Advances in the diagnosis and management of neck pain. *BMJ* **2017**, *358*, j3221. [CrossRef] [PubMed]
3. Kondo, Y.; Ota, R.; Fujita, H.; Miki, T.; Watanabe, Y.; Takebayashi, T. Quality of Japanese Online Information on Causes of Neck Pain: A Biopsychosocial Analysis. *Cureus* **2023**, *15*, e41353. [CrossRef] [PubMed]
4. Chou, R.; Côté, P.; Randhawa, K.; Torres, P.; Yu, H.; Nordin, M.; Hurwitz, E.L.; Haldeman, S.; Cedraschi, C. The Global Spine Care Initiative: Applying evidence-based guidelines on the non-invasive management of back and neck pain to low- and middle-income communities. *Eur. Spine J.* **2018**, *27* (Suppl. S6), 851–860. [CrossRef]
5. Liew, B.X.W.; Hartvigsen, J.; Scutari, M.; Kongsted, A. Data-driven network analysis identified subgroup-specific low back pain pathways: A cross-sectional GLA:D Back study. *J. Clin. Epidemiol.* **2023**, *153*, 66–77. [CrossRef]
6. Buchbinder, R.; van Tulder, M.; Öberg, B.; Costa, L.M.; Woolf, A.; Schoene, M.; Croft, P.; Lancet Low Back Pain Series Working Group. Low back pain: A call for action. *Lancet* **2018**, *391*, 2384–2388. [CrossRef]
7. Martinez-Calderon, J.; Flores-Cortes, M.; Morales-Asencio, J.M.; Luque-Suarez, A. Pain-related fear, pain intensity and function in individuals with chronic musculoskeletal pain: A systematic review and meta-analysis. *J. Pain* **2019**, *20*, 1394–1415. [CrossRef]
8. Martinez-Calderon, J.; Jensen, M.P.; Morales-Asencio, J.M.; Luque-Suarez, A. Pain Catastrophizing and Function In Individuals With Chronic Musculoskeletal Pain: A Systematic Review and Meta-Analysis. *Clin. J. Pain* **2019**, *35*, 279–293. [CrossRef] [PubMed]
9. Luque-Suarez, A.; Falla, D.; Morales-Asencio, J.M.; Martinez-Calderon, J. Is kinesiophobia and pain catastrophising at baseline associated with chronic pain and disability in whiplash-associated disorders? A systematic review. *Br. J. Sports Med.* **2020**, *54*, 892–897. [CrossRef]
10. Oxland, T.R. Fundamental biomechanics of the spine—What we have learned in the past 25 years and future directions. *J. Biomech.* **2016**, *49*, 817–832. [CrossRef]
11. Patwardhan, A.G.; Khayatzadeh, S.; Havey, R.M.; Voronov, L.I.; Smith, Z.A.; Kalmanson, O.; Ghanayem, A.J.; Sears, W. Cervical sagittal balance: A biomechanical perspective can help clinical practice. *Eur. Spine J.* **2018**, *27* (Suppl. S1), 25–38. [CrossRef] [PubMed]
12. Brinjikji, W.; Diehn, F.E.; Jarvik, J.G.; Carr, C.M.; Kallmes, D.F.; Murad, M.H.; Luetmer, P.H. MRI Findings of Disc Degeneration are More Prevalent in Adults with Low Back Pain than in Asymptomatic Controls: A Systematic Review and Meta-Analysis. *AJNR Am. J. Neuroradiol.* **2015**, *36*, 2394–2399. [CrossRef] [PubMed]

13. Raastad, J.; Reiman, M.; Coeytaux, R.; Ledbetter, L.; Goode, A.P. The association between lumbar spine radiographic features and low back pain: A systematic review and meta-analysis. *Semin. Arthritis Rheum.* **2015**, *44*, 571–585. [CrossRef] [PubMed]
14. Din, R.U.; Cheng, X.; Yang, H. Diagnostic Role of Magnetic Resonance Imaging in Low Back Pain Caused by Vertebral Endplate Degeneration. *J. Magn. Reson. Imaging* **2022**, *55*, 755–771. [CrossRef]
15. Jamaludin, A.; Kadir, T.; Zisserman, A.; McCall, I.; Williams, F.M.K.; Lang, H.; Buchanan, E.; Urban, J.P.G.; Fairbank, J.C.T. ISSLS PRIZE in Clinical Science 2023: Comparison of degenerative MRI features of the intervertebral disc between those with and without chronic low back pain. An exploratory study of two large female populations using automated annotation. *Eur. Spine J.* **2023**, *32*, 1504–1516. [CrossRef]
16. Christensen, S.T.; Hartvigsen, J. Spinal curves and health: A systematic critical review of the epidemiological literature dealing with associations between sagittal spinal curves and health. *J. Manip. Physiol. Ther.* **2008**, *31*, 690–714. [CrossRef]
17. Jenkins, H.J.; Downie, A.S.; Moore, C.S.; French, S.D. Current evidence for spinal X-ray use in the chiropractic profession: A narrative review. *Chiropr. Man. Therap.* **2018**, *26*, 48. [CrossRef]
18. Corso, M.; Cancelliere, C.; Mior, S.; Kumar, V.; Smith, A.; Côté, P. The clinical utility of routine spinal radiographs by chiropractors: A rapid review of the literature. *Chiropr. Man. Therap.* **2020**, *28*, 33. [CrossRef]
19. Oakley, P.A.; Betz, J.W.; Harrison, D.E.; Siskin, L.A.; Hirsh, D.W.; International Chiropractors Association Rapid Response Research Review Subcommittee. Smoke Screen to Distract from Flawed Science: A Response to Côté et al. Over Criticisms to Their Deficient 'Rapid Review' on Chiropractic X-Ray Utility. *Dose Response* **2021**, *19*, 15593258211058341. [CrossRef]
20. Oakley, P.A.; Cuttler, J.M.; Harrison, D.E. Response to Letters from Anderson and Kawchuk et al.: X-Ray Imaging Is Essential for Contemporary Chiropractic and Manual Therapy Spinal Rehabilitation: Radiography Increases Benefits and Reduces Risks. *Dose Response* **2018**, *16*, 1559325818809584. [CrossRef]
21. Harrison, D.E.; Betz, J.; Ferrantelli, J.F. Sagittal spinal curves and health. *J. Vertebr. Sublux. Res.* **2009**, *2009*, 1–8.
22. Oakley, P.A.; Harrison, D.E. Selective usage of medical practice data, misrepresentations, and omission of conflicting data to support the 'red flag only' agenda for chiropractic radiography guidelines: A critical assessment of the Jenkins et al. article: "Current evidence for spinal X-ray use in the chiropractic profession". *Ann. Vert. Sublux. Res.* **2019**, *2019*, 141–157.
23. Oakley, P.A.; Harrison, D.E. Are Restrictive Medical Radiation Imaging Campaigns Misguided? It Seems So: A Case Example of the American Chiropractic Association's Adoption of "Choosing Wisely". *Dose Response* **2020**, *18*, 1559325820919321. [CrossRef] [PubMed]
24. Oakley, P.A.; Betz, J.W.; Harrison, D.E.; Siskin, L.A.; Hirsh, D.W.; International Chiropractors Association Rapid Response Research Review Subcommittee. Radiophobia Overreaction: College of Chiropractors of British Columbia Revoke Full X-Ray Rights Based on Flawed Study and Radiation Fear-Mongering. *Dose Response* **2021**, *19*, 15593258211033142. [CrossRef]
25. Mekhael, E.; El Rachkidi, R.; Saliby, R.M.; Nassim, N.; Semaan, K.; Massaad, A.; Karam, M.; Saade, M.; Ayoub, E.; Rteil, A.; et al. Functional assessment using 3D movement analysis can better predict health-related quality of life outcomes in patients with adult spinal deformity: A machine learning approach. *Front. Surg.* **2023**, *10*, 1166734. [CrossRef] [PubMed]
26. Terran, J.; Schwab, F.; Shaffrey, C.I.; Smith, J.S.; Devos, P.; Ames, C.P.; Fu, K.M.; Burton, D.; Hostin, R.; Klineberg, E.; et al. The SRS-Schwab adult spinal deformity classification: Assessment and clinical correlations based on a prospective operative and nonoperative cohort. *Neurosurgery* **2013**, *73*, 559–568. [CrossRef]
27. Pellisé, F.; Vila-Casademunt, A.; Ferrer, M.; Domingo-Sàbat, M.; Bagó, J.; Pérez-Grueso, F.J.; Alanay, A.; Mannion, A.F.; Acaroglu, E.; European Spine Study Group (ESSG). Impact on health related quality of life of adult spinal deformity (ASD) compared with other chronic conditions. *Eur. Spine J.* **2015**, *24*, 3–11. [CrossRef] [PubMed]
28. Kyrölä, K.; Repo, J.; Mecklin, J.P.; Ylinen, J.; Kautiainen, H.; Häkkinen, A. Spinopelvic Changes Based on the Simplified SRS-Schwab Adult Spinal Deformity Classification: Relationships with Disability and Health-Related Quality of Life in Adult Patients With Prolonged Degenerative Spinal Disorders. *Spine* **2018**, *43*, 497–502. [CrossRef]
29. Kim, H.J.; Yang, J.H.; Chang, D.G.; Lenke, L.G.; Suh, S.W.; Nam, Y.; Park, S.C.; Suk, S.I. Adult Spinal Deformity: A Comprehensive Review of Current Advances and Future Directions. *Asian Spine J.* **2022**, *16*, 776–788. [CrossRef]
30. Yahata, M.; Watanabe, K.; Tashi, H.; Ohashi, M.; Yoda, T.; Nawata, A.; Nakamura, K.; Kawashima, H. Impact of spinal sagittal malalignment on locomotive syndrome and physical function in community-dwelling middle aged and older women. *BMC Musculoskelet. Disord.* **2023**, *24*, 620. [CrossRef]
31. Chun, S.W.; Lim, C.Y.; Kim, K.; Hwang, J.; Chung, S.G. The relationships between low back pain and lumbar lordosis: A systematic review and meta-analysis. *Spine J.* **2017**, *17*, 1180–1191. [CrossRef] [PubMed]
32. Sadler, S.G.; Spink, M.J.; Ho, A.; De Jonge, X.J.; Chuter, V.H. Restriction in lateral bending range of motion, lumbar lordosis, and hamstring flexibility predicts the development of low back pain: A systematic review of prospective cohort studies. *BMC Musculoskelet. Disord.* **2017**, *18*, 179. [CrossRef] [PubMed]
33. Roghani, T.; Allen, D.D.; Gladin, A.; Rahimi, A.; Mehrabi, M.; Rezaeian, Z.S.; Farajzadegan, Z.; Katzman, W.B. The Association Between Physical Function and Hyperkyphosis in Older Females: A Systematic Review and Meta-analysis. *J. Geriatr. Phys. Ther.* **2023**; *ahead of print*. [CrossRef]
34. Petcharaporn, M.; Pawelek, J.; Bastrom, T.; Lonner, B.; Newton, P.O. The relationship between thoracic hyperkyphosis and the Scoliosis Research Society outcomes instrument. *Spine* **2007**, *32*, 2226–2231. [CrossRef]
35. Garrido, E.; Roberts, S.B.; Duckworth, A.; Fournier, J. Long-term follow-up of untreated Scheuermann's kyphosis. *Spine Deform.* **2021**, *9*, 1633–1639. [CrossRef]

36. Ling, F.P.; Chevillotte, T.; Leglise, A.; Thompson, W.; Bouthors, C.; Le Huec, J.C. Which parameters are relevant in sagittal balance analysis of the cervical spine? A literature review. *Eur. Spine J.* **2018**, *27* (Suppl. S1), 8–15. [CrossRef]
37. Protopsaltis, T.S.; Scheer, J.K.; Terran, J.S.; Smith, J.S.; Hamilton, D.K.; Kim, H.J.; Mundis GMJr Hart, R.A.; McCarthy, I.M.; Klineberg, E.; Lafage, V.; et al. How the neck affects the back: Changes in regional cervical sagittal alignment correlate to HRQOL improvement in adult thoracolumbar deformity patients at 2-year follow-up. *J. Neurosurg. Spine* **2015**, *23*, 153–158. [CrossRef]
38. Oakley, P.A.; Ehsani, N.N.; Moustafa, I.M.; Harrison, D.E. Restoring lumbar lordosis: A systematic review of controlled trials utilizing Chiropractic Bio Physics® (CBP®) non-surgical approach to increasing lumbar lordosis in the treatment of low back disorders. *J. Phys. Ther. Sci.* **2020**, *32*, 601–610. [CrossRef]
39. Oakley, P.A.; Ehsani, N.N.; Moustafa, I.M.; Harrison, D.E. Restoring cervical lordosis by cervical extension traction methods in the treatment of cervical spine disorders: A systematic review of controlled trials. *J. Phys. Ther. Sci.* **2021**, *33*, 784–794. [CrossRef]
40. Oakley, P.A.; Harrison, D.E. Reducing Thoracic Hyperkyphosis Subluxation Deformity: A Systematic Review of Chiropractic BioPhysics® Methods Employed in its Structural Improvement. *J. Contemp. Chiropr.* **2018**, *1*, 59–66.
41. Jenkins, H.J.; Downie, A.S.; Fernandez, M.; Hancock, M.J. Decreasing thoracic hyperkyphosis—Which treatments are most effective? A systematic literature review and meta-analysis. *Musculoskelet. Sci. Pract.* **2021**, *56*, 102438. [CrossRef] [PubMed]
42. Ponzano, M.; Tibert, N.; Bansal, S.; Katzman, W.; Giangregorio, L. Exercise for improving age-related hyperkyphosis: A systematic review and meta-analysis with GRADE assessment. *Arch. Osteoporos.* **2021**, *16*, 140. [CrossRef] [PubMed]
43. Harrison, D.E.; Oakley, P.A. An introduction to Chiropractic BioPhysics® (CBP®) technique: A full spine rehabilitation approach to reducing spine deformities. In *Complementary Therapies*; Bernardo-Filho, M., Ed.; IntechOpen: London, UK, 2022; pp. 1–35. [CrossRef]
44. Oakley, P.A.; Moustafa, I.M.; Harrison, D.E. Restoration of cervical and lumbar lordosis: CBP® methods overview. In *Spinal Deformities in Adolescents, Adults and Older Adults*; Bettany-Saltikov, J., Ed.; IntechOpen Publishers: London, UK, 2019; pp. 1–19.
45. Oakley, P.A.; Moustafa, I.M.; Harrison, D.E. The Influence of Sagittal Plane Spine Alignment on Neurophysiology and Sensorimotor Control Measures: Optimization of Function through Structural Correction. In *Therapy Approaches in Neurological Disorders*; Bernardo-Filho, M., Ed.; [Online First]; IntechOpen: London, UK, 2021. [CrossRef]
46. Zaina, F.; Ferrario, I.; Caronni, A.; Scarano, S.; Donzelli, S.; Negrini, S. Measuring Quality of Life in Adults with Scoliosis: A Cross-Sectional Study Comparing SRS-22 and ISYQOL Questionnaires. *J. Clin. Med.* **2023**, *12*, 5071. [CrossRef] [PubMed]
47. Marsiolo, M.; Careri, S.; Bandinelli, D.; Toniolo, R.M.; Aulisa, A.G. Vertebral rotation in functional scoliosis caused by limb-length inequality: Correlation between rotation, limb length inequality, and obliquity of the sacral shelf. *J. Clin. Med.* **2023**, *12*, 5571.
48. Arnone, P.A.; Kraus, S.J.; Farmen, D.; Lightstone, D.F.; Jaeger, J.; Theodossis, C. Examining Clinical Opinion and Experience Regarding Utilization of Plain Radiography of the Spine: Evidence from Surveying the Chiropractic Profession. *J. Clin. Med.* **2023**, *12*, 2169. [CrossRef]
49. Kaale, B.R.; McArthur, T.J.; Barbosa, M.H.; Freeman, M.D. Post-Traumatic Atlanto-Axial Instability: A Combined Clinical and Radiological Approach for the Diagnosis of Pathological Rotational Movement in the Upper Cervical Spine. *J. Clin. Med.* **2023**, *12*, 1469. [CrossRef]
50. Moustafa, I.M.; Shousha, T.; Arumugam, A.; Harrison, D.E. Is Thoracic Kyphosis Relevant to Pain, Autonomic Nervous System Function, Disability, and Cervical Sensorimotor Control in Patients with Chronic Nonspecific Neck Pain? *J. Clin. Med.* **2023**, *12*, 3707. [CrossRef] [PubMed]
51. Moustafa, I.M.; Diab, A.A.M.; Harrison, D.E. Does Forward Head Posture Influence Somatosensory Evoked Potentials and Somatosensory Processing in Asymptomatic Young Adults? *J. Clin. Med.* **2023**, *12*, 3217. [CrossRef]
52. Kamel, M.; Moustafa, I.M.; Kim, M.; Oakley, P.A.; Harrison, D.E. Alterations in Cervical Nerve Root Function during Different Sitting Positions in Adults with and without Forward Head Posture: A Cross-Sectional Study. *J. Clin. Med.* **2023**, *12*, 1780. [CrossRef]
53. Ahbouch, A.; Moustafa, I.M.; Shousha, T.; Arumugam, A.; Oakley, P.; Harrison, D.E. An Investigation of the Association between 3D Spinal Alignment and Fibromyalgia. *J. Clin. Med.* **2023**, *12*, 218. [CrossRef]
54. Katz, E.A.; Katz, S.B.; Freeman, M.D. Non-Surgical Management of Upper Cervical Instability via Improved Cervical Lordosis: A Case Series of Adult Patients. *J. Clin. Med.* **2023**, *12*, 1797. [CrossRef] [PubMed]
55. Suwaidi, A.S.A.; Moustafa, I.M.; Kim, M.; Oakley, P.A.; Harrison, D.E. A Comparison of Two Forward Head Posture Corrective Approaches in Elderly with Chronic Non-Specific Neck Pain: A Randomized Controlled Study. *J. Clin. Med.* **2023**, *12*, 542. [CrossRef]
56. Youssef, A.S.A.; Moustafa, I.M.; El Melhat, A.M.; Huang, X.; Oakley, P.A.; Harrison, D.E. Randomized Feasibility Pilot Trial of Adding a New Three-Dimensional Adjustable Posture-Corrective Orthotic to a Multi-Modal Program for the Treatment of Nonspecific Neck Pain. *J. Clin. Med.* **2022**, *11*, 7028. [CrossRef] [PubMed]
57. Moustafa, I.M.; Diab, A.A.; Harrison, D.E. The Efficacy of Cervical Lordosis Rehabilitation for Nerve Root Function and Pain in Cervical Spondylotic Radiculopathy: A Randomized Trial with 2-Year Follow-Up. *J. Clin. Med.* **2022**, *11*, 6515. [CrossRef]
58. Moustafa, I.M.; Shousha, T.M.; Walton, L.M.; Raigangar, V.; Harrison, D.E. Reduction of Thoracic Hyper-Kyphosis Improves Short and Long Term Outcomes in Patients with Chronic Nonspecific Neck Pain: A Randomized Controlled Trial. *J. Clin. Med.* **2022**, *11*, 6028. [CrossRef] [PubMed]

59. Moustafa, I.M.; Diab, A.A.M.; Harrison, D.E. Does Improvement towards a Normal Cervical Sagittal Configuration Aid in the Management of Lumbosacral Radiculopathy: A Randomized Controlled Trial. *J. Clin. Med.* **2022**, *11*, 5768. [CrossRef] [PubMed]
60. Zaina, F.; Marchese, R.; Donzelli, S.; Cordani, C.; Pulici, C.; McAviney, J.; Negrini, S. Current Knowledge on the Different Characteristics of Back Pain in Adults with and without Scoliosis: A Systematic Review. *J. Clin. Med.* **2023**, *12*, 5182. [CrossRef]

Disclaimer/Publisher's Note: The statements, opinions and data contained in all publications are solely those of the individual author(s) and contributor(s) and not of MDPI and/or the editor(s). MDPI and/or the editor(s) disclaim responsibility for any injury to people or property resulting from any ideas, methods, instructions or products referred to in the content.

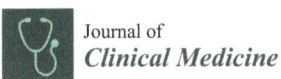

Article

Examining Clinical Opinion and Experience Regarding Utilization of Plain Radiography of the Spine: Evidence from Surveying the Chiropractic Profession

Philip A. Arnone [1,*], Steven J. Kraus [2], Derek Farmen [1], Douglas F. Lightstone [3], Jason Jaeger [4] and Christine Theodossis [5]

1. The Balanced Body Center, Matthews, NC 28105, USA
2. Biokinemetrics, Inc., Carroll, IA 51401, USA
3. Institute for Spinal Health and Performance, Folsom, CA 95630, USA
4. Community Based Internship Program, Associate Faculty, Southern California University of Health Sciences, Whittier, CA 90604, USA
5. Chair, Radiology Department, Sherman College of Chiropractic, Boiling Springs, SC 29316, USA
* Correspondence: drphilarnone@gmail.com

Abstract: Plain Radiography of the spine (PROTS) is utilized in many forms of healthcare including the chiropractic profession; however, the literature reflects conflicting opinions regarding utilization and value. Despite being an essential part of Evidence-Based Practice (EBP), few studies assess Doctors of Chiropractic (DCs) clinical opinions and experience regarding the utilization of (PROTS) in practice. In this study, DCs were surveyed regarding utilization of PROTS in practice. The survey was administered to an estimated 50,000 licensed DCs by email. A total of 4301 surveys were completed, of which 3641 were United States (US) DCs. The Clinician Opinion and Experience on Chiropractic Radiography (COECR) scale was designed to analyze survey responses. This valid and reliable scale demonstrated good internal consistency using confirmatory factor analysis and the Rasch model. Survey responses show that 73.3% of respondents utilize PROTS in practice and 26.7% refer patients out for PROTS. Survey responses show that, among US DCs, 91.9% indicate PROTS has value beyond identification of pathology, 86.7% indicate that PROTS is important regarding biomechanical analysis of the spine, 82.9% indicate that PROTS is vital to practice, 67.4% indicate that PROTS aids in measuring outcomes, 98.6% indicate the opinion that PROTS presents very low to no risk to patients, and 93.0% indicate that sharing clinical findings from PROTS studies with patients is beneficial to clinical outcomes. The results of the study indicated that based on clinical experience, the majority of DCs find PROTS to be vital to practice and valuable beyond the identification of red flags.

Keywords: X-ray utilization; Evidence-Based Practice (EBP); chiropractic practice; clinical opinion; chiropractic survey; radiographs

1. Introduction

Doctors of Chiropractic (DCs) are portal of entry healthcare providers trained in the diagnosis and management of spinal related conditions, with an emphasis on biomechanical dysfunction, in addition to screening for pathology. Interestingly, an estimated 85% of chronic low back pain cases are diagnosed as "non-specific low back pain", not as a result of injury, but as a result of an unknown cause, typically from spinal biomechanical dysfunction [1]. DCs offer safe [2–4], non-pharmaceutical, non-surgical approaches to musculoskeletal conditions that have been shown to reduce opioid usage [5–8] and decrease surgical intervention [9,10] and disability [11–13] when compared to other therapies. Research shows that when a patient sees a DC first after a low back injury, surgical intervention is reduced to 1.5% compared to 42.7% when initially evaluated by a surgeon even after considering other important variables [9]. Additionally, chiropractic intervention

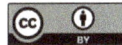

has been shown to reduce opioid usage by 56% [8], and a survey taken in 2012 found "over 96% respondents with spine-related problems who reported the use of chiropractic manipulation stated that the therapy helped them with their condition" [14]. While there are many different methodologies utilized within chiropractic to determine care, plain radiography has a long history of utilization by the profession as a viable tool in assessing spinal dysfunction [15]. Current chiropractic scope of practice, while varied from state to state, allows DCs to order, perform, and interpret radiographs for various reasons including the evaluation of musculoskeletal disorders, red flags, biomechanical analysis and to aid in patient management [16].

Plain radiography of the spine (PROTS) is utilized in healthcare to help practitioners identify suspected red flags, is easily accessible, quick, and is valuable in the diagnosis of various conditions; however, there are limitations [17]. PROTS has limited ability to detect soft tissue injury, may lead to unnecessary procedures due to incidental findings and only produces single, flat images that lack detailed views of three-dimensional structures [18]. Despite recognized value, there is debate within the literature regarding red flags [19,20], pathology, safety [21], and spinal biomechanical analysis [22–27]. These debates have led to diametrically opposing viewpoints within the chiropractic profession on the risks, ethics and economics of ionizing radiation exposure, as well as the value PROTS provides in cases of mechanical spine pain. As a result, there are efforts to alter clinical guidelines regarding PROTS suggesting plain radiography be limited to only red flags (history of recent trauma, infection, cancer, failure to respond to treatment, neurological deficits, chronicity, etc.) [28], as well as guidelines suggesting PROTS should be expanded for the qualitative and quantitative assessment of the biomechanical components of the spine in addition to red flags [29]. Currently, individual interpretation and implementation of clinical research have created diversity in clinical opinions regarding PROTS, leading to different clinical experiences throughout the chiropractic profession, which to date have not been explored.

Clinical opinion and experience are important components of Evidenced-Based Practice (EBP). EBP was implemented with the goal of improving and evaluating patient care [30] and has rapidly gained acceptance in the developed world [31]. The EBP model requires the integration of three factors: robust research evidence, clinical expertise, and patient values [32,33]. A doctor's clinical opinion, experience, and expertise, including the knowledge, judgment, and critical reasoning acquired through training and professional experience, are essential for implementing evidence-based practices [32,33]. Despite evidence supporting chiropractic care for mechanical spine pain, there is limited research regarding DCs' clinical opinion and experience regarding the utilization of PROTS, which may be of value in the management of mechanical spine pain.

A 2020 report regarding US chiropractic practices reviewed six analyses conducted between 1993–2015, where 3810 US-based DCs were surveyed on whether the practitioner took radiographs in their office [34]. The report states that 47% of respondents took radiographs in their office and that 56.2% of their patients were radiographed. The 53% that did not take radiographs in their office referred 21.9% of their patients out for radiographs. Additionally, DCs that relied on radiographs were asked the frequency at which they performed or referred out for radiographs, as well as for repeat or follow-up radiographs to monitor patient progress or response to care (61.3%); to identify or rule out fracture, dislocation, and other pathology (94.1%); and to review for the possible presence of spinal displacements and (or) vertebral subluxation (66.8%). While this 2020 study had a large sample and included multiple questions regarding use of radiographs in chiropractic practice, the binary nature of the questions limited respondents' ability to convey the extent of their preferences regarding utilization of plain radiography. A 2021 survey suggests that the DCs' preference towards use of radiographs correlated with their view on DCs' role in healthcare; however, the limited response options and few questions related to PROTS are insufficient to conclude the comprehensive opinions and experience of DCs use of PROTS [35]. Another study from 2017 surveyed a select group of 190 members from the

American Chiropractic College of Radiology, known as chiropractic radiologists, and only had 73 respondents [36]. The study is limited by the small sample size of chiropractors and possible bias from members belonging to a select organization.

The current study was comprised of a combination of binary and Likert questions given to practicing DCs. The aim of the study was to examine the chiropractic profession's opinions on the utilization of PROTS, based on their experience, in an attempt to provide the most in-depth evaluation of such opinions to date. As a result, the authors coordinated with a statistician in the development of the Clinician Opinion & Experience on Chiropractic Radiography (COECR) scale. Our hypothesis for the survey, due to recent national association press releases [28], is that the survey results would be heavily weighted against the utilization of PROTS and that we would see conflicting responses.

2. Materials and Methods

In creating the survey for this study, the authors intended to be consistent with EBP and developed a series of 11 questions to adequately reflect the clinical opinion and experience of the US DCs on the utilization of PROTS in a chiropractic clinical setting. All procedures performed in this study were in accordance with the ethical standards of the 1964 Helsinki declaration and its later amendments or comparable ethical standards. The authors developed 8 revisions of the survey over a period of 6 months with the goal to design neutral survey questions that represent the clinicians' decision process and to minimize bias. The survey included a variety of both Likert and binary response options that could accurately reflect each DCs' clinical opinions and experience rather than solely binary response options. Many aspects of the clinicians' decision process were considered during the process, including why practitioners would or would not order PROTS, what value DCs attribute to PROTS, how to adequately reflect DCs' clinical opinion and experience of PROTS as it relates to patient care, and issues related to plain radiography utilization safety and research.

The first question requested the participant's name and address. Participants were notified in the introduction of the survey that their personal information would remain anonymous; identifying information was only available for the data analyst to ensure that survey responses were not duplicated since some DCs may have received multiple survey invitations. The intention to use the response for future publications was clearly indicated. If participants consented to participate, they proceeded to questions 2 through 11.

Questions 2 through 9 surveyed the participants about reasons that DCs may or may not order plain radiography and to determine the presence of radiographic equipment in the office. Additional findings from these questions include determining the level of agreement to utilization on a graded scale, questions pertaining to how, why, and when these procedures are valuable, how and if they have value as it relates to the direction and outcome of patient treatment and care, and to assess the clinical opinions and experience regarding the level of risk or safety associated with these procedures.

The 11th and last question of the survey was an open-response textbox that allowed DCs to explain the rationale that guided their respective answers to survey questions and to provide additional comments on the subject matter. A summary is provided in Appendix D, but these responses are not included in the analysis of this publication and will be reserved for future projects.

2.1. Survey Distribution

To gather a broad sample, we aimed to distribute the survey to as many US DCs as possible using three main data sources. The survey was distributed through email invitations (Appendix A) on multiple occasions during a period of 18 months between 2019 and 2021. The survey was formatted using SurveyMonkey, a cloud-based software platform developed to support online survey data collection. Although sampling weights were not developed, distribution of emails by state was provided from the database source.

The primary source of survey distribution was through an opt-in email database purchased from a leading chiropractic magazine publication resulting in email invitations on two separate occasions to the database, which included 49,747 DCs located throughout the US. Appendix B shows the distribution numbers and percentages based on the state of residence.

Next, the survey link was distributed utilizing an opt-in email source from a private company database. The survey link was distributed to approximately 20,400 US DCs on two separate occasions. Third, the survey was disseminated to the non-profit organization Chiro Congress (formerly known as the Congress of Chiropractic State Associations, COCSA) email database. Chiro Congress was selected since it is a national organization that has affiliated state chiropractic associations from nearly all US states. The state associations affiliated with the Chiro Congress network were invited to send the survey link to their members. Lastly, survey recipients were encouraged to share the survey with their colleagues: all survey email invitations stated, "Please send this survey link and encourage your colleagues to take the survey as well".

Overall, the survey was emailed to an estimated 50,000 unique email addresses of licensed DCs. Approximately 5788 DCs opened the survey (an open rate of approximately 3.99–9.20%), of which 4301 DCs completed responses. If a DC submitted a survey response more than once, only the most recent submission was used in the analysis. Although the aim of the survey was to collect responses from practicing DCs in the US (n = 3641), some responses came from Canada (n = 459) and the rest of the world (n = 201). The survey submissions were widespread across the US, as represented in Appendix C.

2.2. Statistical Analyses

2.2.1. Procedures and Sample

The analysis included all 10 quantitative survey questions (question 11 was qualitative and omitted from the analysis of the current study). Question 1 (Q1) collected demographic information; questions 2 (Q2) and 10 (Q10) had 5 response options each and allowed participants to choose multiple responses. Question 7 (Q7) offered 5 different categorical responses, limiting the participants to a single-category response. The remaining questions collected responses on a 5-point Likert-type scale.

To prepare the data for the analyses, variables were re-coded to account for item structure and to ensure that higher values corresponded to stronger clinical opinions. The dependent variable, Q7, originally contained 5 response options, but was dichotomously re-coded. Q2 and Q10 were dummy-coded, turning each response option into a stand-alone survey item. Dummy coding is a recategorization of discrete variables into a series of dichotomous items to ensure a linear relationship [37]. Additionally, by re-coding Q2 and Q10, the overlapping responses were eliminated. The remaining questions were re-coded in a way that higher values represented higher levels of the variable. Specifics about re-coding are detailed in the measures section.

2.2.2. Dependent Variable

The utilization of plain radiography in chiropractic practices was assessed by the following survey item: Please select one answer that best describes your use of general spinal radiography in your practice. (This is NOT regarding advanced imaging such as CT/MRI). Respondents were provided with 5 response options to indicate use of spinal radiography:

(1) I do NOT take radiographs in my clinic, I refer patients out to another facility (coded as 0);
(2) I DO have an X-ray machine in my practice, but I still refer patients out to another facility for the majority of my spinal radiographs (coded as 0);
(3) I have a plain film X-ray system in my practice and use it for the majority of my radiographs (coded as 1);
(4) I have a DR (digital radiography) digital X-ray system in my practice and use it for the majority of my radiographs (coded as 1);

(5) I have a CR (computed radiography) digital X-ray system in my practice and use it for the majority of my radiographs (coded as 1).

2.2.3. Predictors

Appendix D provides the full list of survey questions that were used as predictors.

2.3. Clinician Opinion & Experience on Chiropractic Radiography (COECR) Scale

Q2.1–Q2.5 and Q10.1–Q10.5 (Table 1) establish a set of items that capture the clinical opinions of practicing DCs towards using spinal radiology in chiropractic practices. In an effort to construct a new scale, this study subjected the COECR scale to psychometric evaluation by investigating internal consistency of the scale, performing confirmatory factor analysis, and specifying and testing an Item-Response Theory (IRT) model [38–40].

Table 1. List of survey questions and response options.

Q2.1: Radiographic procedures in a chiropractic office have value beyond identification of pathology.	0 = No	1 = Yes			
Q2.2: Radiographs for biomechanical analysis have significant value.	0 = No	1 = Yes			
Q2.3: I order radiographs only for red flags or pathology.	0 = No	1 = Yes			
Q2.4: Radiographic procedures are vital to the chiropractic care I provide in my clinic.	0 = No	1 = Yes			
Q2.5: I utilize radiographic procedures to aid in the measurement of clinical outcomes.	0 = No	1 = Yes			
Q3: What is your level of agreement/disagreement with the following statement: Based on the educational training and past clinical experiences, the Doctor of Chiropractic should be able to make their own clinical decision regarding the utilization of spinal radiographs on their patients?	1 = Strongly disagree	2 = Mostly disagree	3 = Neutral	4 = Mostly agree	5 = Strongly Agree
Q4: The foundation of an Evidence-Based Practice (EBP) is based on 3 integrated components: (1) Doctor's Clinical Expertise, (2) Patient Preferences/Values, and (3) Best Research Evidence. When making the clinical decision to obtain spinal radiographs of your patient, should all three EBP components be equally considered?	1 = Strongly disagree	2 = Mostly disagree	3 = Neutral	4 = Mostly agree	5 = Strongly Agree
Q5: What is your level of agreement/disagreement with the following statement: In my clinical opinion, patient outcomes would benefit from continued research regarding appropriate utilization of spinal radiographs in the practice of chiropractic?	1 = Strongly disagree	2 = Mostly disagree	3 = Neutral	4 = Mostly agree	5 = Strongly Agree
Q6: What is your level of agreement/disagreement with the following statement: In the absence of published chiropractic research evidence, the doctor's clinical experience combined with patient preferences are adequate for the appropriate recommendation of spinal radiographs in the practice of chiropractic?	1 = Strongly disagree	2 = Mostly disagree	3 = Neutral	4 = Mostly agree	5 = Strongly Agree
Q8: What level of risk do you believe is present in your chiropractic practice affecting your patients' health, as a result of X-ray radiation from your utilization of radiography?	1 = No risk	2 = Very low risk	3 = Low risk	4 = Moderate Risk	5 = High risk
Q7.1: I do not take radiographs in my clinic. I refer out to another facility.					

Table 1. Cont.

Q9: What is your level of agreement/disagreement with the following statement: In my clinical experience, sharing chiropractic clinical findings from radiographic studies with the patient is beneficial to their clinical outcome?	1 = Strongly disagree	2 = Mostly disagree	3 = Neutral	4 = Mostly agree	5 = Strongly Agree
Q10.1: To determine adjusting technique or vertebral levels to be adjusted.		0 = No		1 = Yes	
Q10.2: Mechanical analysis or obtaining measurements of spinal alignment.		0 = No		1 = Yes	
Q10.3: Future plan modification and considerations.		0 = No		1 = Yes	
Q10.4: Determine spinal complications such as degenerative changes, anomalies, or defects.		0 = No		1 = Yes	
Q10.5: Investigate red flags (fracture, neurologic deficits, suspected pathology).		0 = No		1 = Yes	

2.4. Analytic Plan

The statistical analysis began with an examination of descriptive statistics and evaluating group differences using chi-square tests and t-tests. For categorical variables, percentages were reported. For continuous variables, the averages and standard deviations were described. Subsequently, binary logistic regression with logit link [41] was estimated and tested using the survey data. Binary logistic regression is a regression model where the outcome is following a binomial distribution with predictors of any form including continuous, categorical, or both [42]. Preference was given to binary logistic regression due to the distribution of the dependent variable (Q7). The descriptive statistics, chi-square tests, and logistic regression analyses were conducted in Statistical Package for Social Sciences (SPSS) version 24.0 [43].

To further understand DCs' utilization of plain radiology, we performed Rasch analysis on the set of items that capture DCs' clinician opinion and experience on PROTS. Fitting the Rasch model [44] to the data, we were able to evaluate the difficulty of endorsing each item included in the analysis as well as to estimate the relationship of each item with the underlying latent trait [45]. In this study, the latent trait, denoted by θ, is the clinical opinion towards DCs' utilization of plain radiography in chiropractic practice.

2.5. Study 1: Predicting the Use of Plain Radiography of the Spine in Chiropractic Practice

A multiple binary logistic regression was estimated and tested to understand the relationship between DCs' utilization of plain radiography of the spine in chiropractic practice and the rest of the variables included in the survey. Logistic regression can be considered an approach similar to multiple linear regression (with Gaussian outcome) except that the dependent variable is binary [46].

2.6. Study 2: COECR Scale Development and Validation

The Cronbach's coefficient alpha [47] statistics was used to estimate the internal consistency of the COECR Scale. A one-factor CFA model was applied to responses Q2.1–Q-2.5 and Q10.1–Q10.5 in order to ensure the unidimensionality of the scale. Mplus 8.6 [48] was used to conduct the dimensionality study. To evaluate the statistical fit of the CFA models, we used likelihood ratio tests [49], chi-square tests, and model fit indices available for latent variable modeling. Following the recommendation of Hu and Bentler [50], we used the root-mean-square error of approximation [51], the comparative fit index [52], and normed fit index [53].

Rasch Model

The goal of this analysis was to evaluate the psychometric properties of the items on the COECR scale. Item Response Theory [54] was selected as the framework to test the psychometric qualities of items. Two important assumptions made for IRT models are unidimensionality [55] and local independence [56,57]. The assumption of unidimensionality was tested with CFA. To test the assumption of local independence, Q3 statistics were estimated [58]. The Q3 statistics are pairwise residual correlations after fitting the Rasch model for every item pair on a scale. Yen [59] provided the guidance for the assessment of local independence: "The expected value of Q3, when local independence holds, is approximately $-1/(n-1)$" (p. 198). The Q3 statistics for COECR ranged from -0.37 to 0.26, indicating that the assumption of local independence was not violated [59,60]. The Rasch model was estimated and graphed in R Statistical Software using irtoys and eRm [61]. The Q3 statistics were estimated using the mirt package [62].

3. Results

3.1. Initial Results

A summary of the overall 4301 survey respondents is provided (see Tables 2 and 3). Not all respondents responded to every question. While the survey was intended to focus on US licensed DCs, there were additional respondents from Canada and other countries. The collected data allowed for statistical analysis of US responses, comparative analysis between US and non-US DC responses, and comparative analysis between those respondents with radiographic facilities and those who lack them as described in the methods section.

Table 2. Summary of binary survey responses (Questions 2, 7, 10).

Predictor	%
Q2: Please select all statements that you agree with regarding spinal radiographs (multiple choices allowed). (n = 4231)	
Q2.1: Radiographic procedures in a chiropractic office have value beyond identification of pathology.	91.9
Q2.2: Radiographs for biomechanical analysis have significant value.	86.7
Q2.3: I order radiographs only for red flags or pathology.	16.5
Q2.4: Radiographic procedures are vital to the chiropractic care I provide in my clinic.	82.9
Q2.5: I utilize radiographic procedures to aid in the measurement of clinical outcomes.	67.4
Q7: Please select the one answer that best describes your use of general spinal radiography in your practice (This is not regarding advanced imaging such as CT/MRI). (n = 4138)	
Q7.1: I do not take radiographs in my clinic. I refer out to another facility.	24.7
Q7.2: I do have an X-ray machine in clinic, but I still refer patients out to another facility for the majority of my spinal radiographs.	2.1
Q7.3: I have a plain film X-ray system in my practice and us it for the majority of my radiographs.	16
Q7.4: I have a DR digital X-ray system in my practice and use it for the majority of my radiographs.	47.7
Q7.5: I have a CR digital X-ray system in my practice and use it for the majority of my radiographs. (CR digital requires the cassette to be placed into the image processor to process images)	9.5
Q10: Based on your clinical experience, which reasons are valid to obtain a spinal radiograph in the practice of chiropractic? (choose all that apply): (n = 4106)	
Q10.1: To determine adjusting technique or vertebral levels to be adjusted.	72.1
Q10.2: Mechanical analysis or obtaining measurements of spinal alignment.	84.5
Q10.3: Future plan modification and considerations.	81.9
Q10.4: Determine spinal complications such as degenerative changes, anomalies, or defects.	97.1
Q10.5: Investigate red flags (fracture, neurologic deficits, suspected pathology).	98.2

Table 3. Summary of responses to Likert-type scale items (Questions 3–6, 8, 9).

Predictor	n	Strongly Agree	Mostly Agree	Neutral	Mostly Disagree	Strongly Disagree
Q3	4223	92.9	5.3	0.7	0.6	0.5
Q4	4198	43.3	34.4	9.2	7.6	4.6
Q5	4188	60.9	21.4	11.0	4.4	2.3
Q6	4156	56.6	27.5	7.1	5.7	3.1
Q8 (No Risk-High Risk)	4138	0.2	1.1	10.1	61.2	27.4
Q9	4111	79.1	13.9	3.8	2.2	0.9

n = number of respondents per question.

3.2. Descriptive Statistics, Chi-Square, and Mean Differences

A complete case analysis (also known as listwise deletion) for missing data was performed. Listwise deletion is a method that excludes an entire record from the analysis if any single value is missing [63]. The analysis revealed 232 cases with missing responses, which were removed from the dataset. Exclusion of cases with missing data on key variables resulted in an analytic sample of n = 4069. There were no systematic differences between the original and analysis samples.

Practicing DCs who obtain spinal radiographs using radiology devices/machines within their practice (n = 2985) compared with those who do not have radiology devices/machines in their practice who subsequently refer out to other facilities for PROTS (n = 1084) were systematically dissimilar on a number of predictors. Pearson chi-square tests revealed that a country where DCs practiced is a significant predictor of utilizing plain radiography. Additionally, utilizers versus non-utilizers of spinal radiology significantly differed on all but one COECR scale item (Q10.5; Investigate red flags [fracture, neurologic deficits, suspected pathology]). The results for these comparisons are presented in Table 4.

Table 4. Percentage of respondents who do and do not obtain radiographs in their office.

		No Radiograph		Radiograph		
Predictor		%	n	%	n	χ^2
Country						106.34 **
US		24.4%	842	75.6%	2603	
Canada		30.8%	137	69.2%	308	
Outside US and Canada		58.7%	105	41.3%	74	
Q 2.1						442.97 **
	No	76.4%	246	23.6%	76	
	Yes	22.4%	838	77.6%	2909	
Q 2.2						450.15 **
	No	64.3%	343	35.4%	188	
	Yes	20.9%	741	79.1%	2797	
Q 2.3						603.52 **
	No	19.1%	649	80.9%	2751	
	Yes	65.0%	435	35.0%	234	
Q 2.4						950.1 **
	No	73.9%	510	26.1%	180	
	Yes	17.0%	574	83.0%	2805	
Q 2.5						564.44 **
	No	50.5%	663	49.5%	650	
	Yes	15.3%	421	84.7%	2335	

Table 4. Cont.

Predictor		No Radiograph %	n	Radiograph %	n	χ^2
Q 10.1						407.49 **
	No	49.1%	558	50.9%	578	
	Yes	17.9%	526	82.1%	2407	
Q 10.2						551.13 **
	No	64.5%	409	35.5%	225	
	Yes	19.7%	657	80.3%	2760	
Q 10.3						174.09 **
	No	46.0%	341	54.0%	400	
	Yes	22.3%	743	77.7%	2585	
Q 10.4						153.05 **
	No	75.0%	93	25.0%	31	
	Yes	25.1%	991	74.9%	2954	
Q 10.5						0.95
	No	31.3%	26	68.7%	57	
	Yes	26.5%	1058	73.5%	2928	

Note: ** $p < 0.001$.

The factor analytic model showed that the items considered for the COECR scale assess a single trait—clinical opinion and experience regarding the utilization of PROTS in chiropractic practice. This is a prerequisite for establishing a unidimensional scale. The only item that impacted the factor in a different (negative) direction was "*I order radiography only for pathology and red flags.*" There is an inverse relationship for doctors that only order radiography for pathology and red flags and the total score on the scale. This means that DCs scoring higher on this item will score lower on the entire scale and vice versa. The results of this survey demonstrate that DCs who only order radiography for pathology and red flags responded in opposition to the other respondents to the survey (see Table 5).

Table 5. Average responses to clinical opinion questions.

Predictor	n	Mean	SD
Q3	4069	4.9	0.44
Q4	4069	4.07	1.12
Q5	4069	4.35	0.98
Q6	4069	4.3	1.02
Q8	4069	1.85	0.65
Q9	4069	4.68	0.73

n = Number of Survey Respondents. SD = Standard Deviation.

Table 5 depicts the differences between utilizers and non-utilizers of plain radiography as a function of continuous variables included in the survey (Q3, Q4, Q5, Q6, Q8, and Q9).

Independent t-tests revealed that the DCs who were more likely to have X-ray units in their office believed that their educational and clinical experiences should allow them to decide whether to utilize plain radiology ($p < 0.01$; Q3); believed that patient outcomes would benefit from continued research regarding appropriate utilization of spinal radiology (Q5); were confident that DCs' clinical experience together with patient preferences are adequate and appropriate for recommending PROTS (Q6); and/or believed that sharing spinal radiographic findings with the patient is beneficial for patient outcomes (Q9).

DCs who believed that PROTS may be risky to a patient's health were less likely to have an X-ray unit in their chiropractic office ($p < 0.01$). Finally, DCs who believed that they should equally consider all three EBP components when making clinical decisions to obtain spinal radiographs were not statistically different from those who did not believe this in terms of having plain radiography in their office. The effect sizes for statistically significant results ranged from small to large (see Table 6).

Table 6. Binary logistic regression model predicting position on radiographing chiropractic patients.

Predictor	B	SE	Wald	OR
Country				
US	1.99	0.17	130.88	7.36 **
Canada	1.16	0.2	33.18	3.17 **
Q 2.1	0.43	0.22	3.96	1.54 *
Q 2.2	0.54	0.18	9.15	1.72 **
Q 2.3	−0.98	0.13	58.52	0.38 **
Q 2.4	1.78	0.13	178.23	5.93 **
Q 2.5	0.80	0.11	57.18	2.23 **
Q 3	−0.02	0.11	0.03	0.98
Q 4	0.01	0.04	0.09	1.01
Q 5	−0.03	0.05	0.38	0.97
Q 6	0.06	0.05	1.82	1.06
Q 8	0.02	0.07	0.07	1.02
Q 9	0.17	0.07	5.27	1.18 *
Q 10.1	0.35	0.11	9.52	1.42 **
Q 10.2	0.34	0.16	4.48	1.4 *
Q 10.3	0.45	0.13	11.45	1.57 **
Q 10.4	0.41	0.31	1.74	1.51
Q 10.5	−0.32	0.31	1.04	0.73

B = Beta. SE = Standard Error. $Wald$ = Wald test. OR = Odds Ratio. ** $p < 0.001$, * $p < 0.05$.

3.3. Study 1: Logistic Regression

Binary logistic regression was estimated and tested to determine which of the variables remain predictive of DCs' utilization of PROTS after controlling for the variability associated with all other predictors. Therefore, a binary logistic regression model with Q7 being the outcome variable and 18 categorical and continuous predictors was estimated and tested. For the country of practice, the US and Canada were included in the model while the rest of the world category (outside US and Canada) served as the reference group. For categorical variables, the lower level (coded as 0) served as a comparison level for the levels coded as 1. The continuous predictors were included in the model as continuous variables.

The overall model revealed statistical significance. The model was evaluated using Nagelkerke pseudo R^2. All predictors, taken together, accounted for 38% of the variability in utilization of spinal radiography. The classification of cases was acceptable as the model correctly classified 48.6% and 94.5%, respectively, of DCs who utilized PROTS in their chiropractic practice and those who did not. The overall classification was 82% and was calculated using the following equation:

$$P(\text{correct classification}) = P(y = 1 \text{ and } \hat{y} = 1) + P(y = 0 \text{ and } \hat{y} = 0)$$
$$= P(\hat{y} = 1|y = 1)P(y = 1) + P(\hat{y} = 0|y = 0)P(y = 0)$$

which is a weighted average of sensitivity and specificity [64].

As presented in Table 7, DCs in the US are seven times more likely to utilize plain radiography, $OR = 7.36$, $p < 0.01$, compared to the rest of the world (outside US and Canada), while DCs practicing in Canada are three times more likely to utilize PROTS, $OR = 3.17$, $p < 0.01$. The DCs who utilized PROTS believed that:

(1) radiographic procedures in a chiropractic office have value beyond the identification of pathology, $OR = 1.54$, $p < 0.05$
(2) radiographs for biomechanical procedures have significant value, $OR = 1.72$, $p < 0.01$
(3) radiographic procedures are vital to chiropractic care, $OR = 5.93$, $p < 0.01$

(4) radiographic procedures aid in the measurement of clinical outcomes, OR = 2.23, $p < 0.01$
(5) that sharing chiropractic clinical findings from radiographic studies with the patient is beneficial to their clinical outcome, OR = 1.18, $p < 0.05$
(6) biomechanical analysis or measurements of spinal alignment are valid reasons for obtaining spinal radiograph, OR = 1.4, $p < 0.05$
(7) and care plan modification consideration is a valid reason to obtain a spinal radiograph, OR = 1.57, $p < 0.01$.

Table 7. Factorial structure of unidimensional model.

Item	Loadings	Standard Error
Q 2.1	0.95 **	0.01
Q 2.2	0.95 **	0.01
Q 2.3	0.71 **	0.02
Q 2.4	0.87 **	0.01
Q 2.5	0.82 **	0.01
Q 10.1	0.88 **	0.01
Q 10.2	0.95 **	0.01
Q 10.3	0.84 **	0.01
Q 10.4	0.97 **	0.01
Q 10.5	0.87 **	0.01

Note: χ^2 (35) = 1685.68, $p < 0.001$; RMSEA = 0.05, 90% CI (0.04, 0.06); CFI = 0.97; TLI = 0.97. ** $p < 0.001$. RMSEA = Root-Mean-Square Error of Approximation; CFI = Comparative Fit Index TLI = Tucker–Lewis Index.

Respondents who believed that PROTS should be utilized only for pathology or red flags were much less likely to use PROTS for the chiropractic practice, OR = 0.38, $p < 0.01$.

3.4. Study 2: Scale Construction

CFA was conducted using CFA procedures for binary or categorical items. The one-factor model regressed categorical indicators on a single factor: clinician opinions and experience on chiropractic radiography. Despite the significant value of the chi-square statistics, the model produced a good fit to the data: RMSEA = 0.05, 90% CI = (0.04, 0.06); CFI = 0.97; TLI = 0.97. In general, the chi-square is not considered to be a practical fit index, because it is strongly affected by sample size [65,66]. The item loadings ranged from 0.71 to 0.97 and were statistically significant ($p < 0.001$). Initially, item Q2.3 revealed negative loading on the factor, which was consistent with the previous analyses. The item was reverse coded to ensure positive loading. The CFA results are presented in Table 7.

The internal consistency reliabilities were estimated using alpha coefficient [47]. The estimate with original coding of Q2.3 was $\alpha = 0.8$. There was an increase in internal consistency after recoding Q2.3: $\alpha = 0.84$. Both coefficients are high and in support of a unidimensional scale. Two Rasch models were specified and tested using R Statistical Software. The first model (M1) was estimated with Q2.3 being originally coded, while the second model (M2) was estimated with Q2.3 being reverse coded. The results for Rasch models are presented in Table 6. Two types of fit statistics—infit and outfit indices—were estimated to assess the fit of the derived scale to the data. The infit is sensitive to unexpected responses near the item, whereas the outfit is sensitive to unexpected responses far from the item [67]. In M1, Q2.3 showed a misfit with *Outfit MSQ* = 12.6. In M2, the infit/outfit mean square estimates for all COECR items were within their reasonable bounds; thus, the sequence is considered stable and scalable. Figures 1 and 2 show the item characteristic curves (ICC) for M1 and M2. The ICC is an S-shaped curve that portrays the probability of endorsing an item as a function of the latent trait. For M2, the location characteristic (item difficulty level) was higher for Q2.5 ($b = -0.84$) and Q10.1 ($b = -1.0$), while the items that were easiest to endorse were Q10.5 ($b = -3.23$) and Q10.4 ($b = -3.24$).

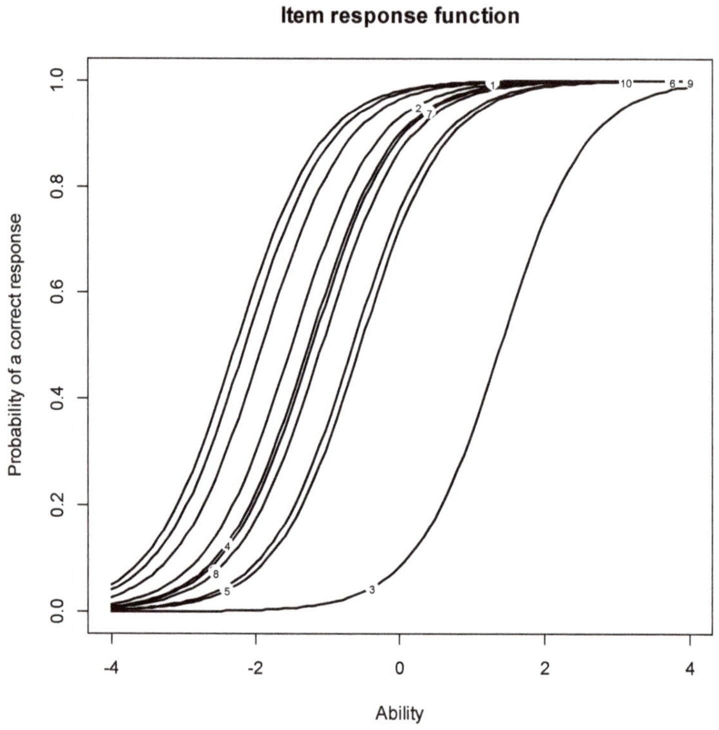

Item response function

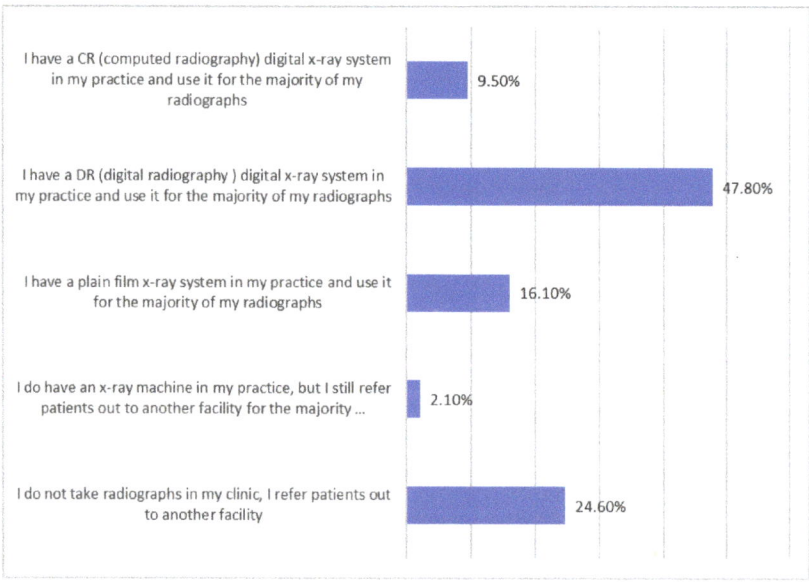

Figure 1. IRT Characteristic Curves for Survey Items.

Figure 2. Original (Before Recoding) Distribution of Item Q7.

3.5. Item Response Theory

The authors used the Rasch IRT model to rank the scale items by difficulty, a common step in scale development. Table 8 presents the results of the Rasch model fit and Figures 1 and 2 present the graphical ranking of the items before and after the "*I order radiography for pathology and red flags*" is recorded. Once again, the Rasch model showed that DCs who utilize plain radiography of the spine *only* to rule out pathology in the presence of red flags are statistical outliers and are significantly inconsistent with the clinical opinion of the chiropractic profession.

Table 8. Item-level estimates and fit statistics for the Rasch model.

Item	χ^2	df	Difficulty	Outfit MSQ	Infit MSQ
Q 2.1	1111.56	4110	−1.92	0.27	0.69
Q 2.2	1409.32	4110	−1.51	0.34	0.69
Q 2.3	51,793.5	4110	1.39	12.60	1.32
Q 2.4	2074.18	4110	−1.27	0.51	0.82
Q 2.5	2657.84	4110	−0.55	0.65	0.76
Q 10.1	2027.26	4110	−0.66	0.49	0.66
Q 10.2	1210.89	4110	−1.22	0.30	0.52
Q 10.3	1983.27	4110	−1.09	0.48	0.75
Q 10.4	773.515	4110	−2.15	0.19	0.65
Q 10.5	1707.58	4110	−2.28	0.42	0.86

χ^2 = Chi-square. *df* = degrees of freedom. *Outfit MSQ* = Outlier-sensitive Fit Mean Square. *Infit MSQ* = Inlier-sensitive Fit Mean Square.

3.6. Results Summary

There is an inverse relationship in the responses between DCs that do and do not utilize PROTS in their practice; however, the clinical opinion of US DCs who utilized PROTS in their practice assigns a high value to the utilization of PROTS (Tables 5 and 6). These doctors believe PROTS to be safe and that the DCs' clinical experience is adequate for recommending PROTS. (Q6) In summary, 77.6% of these US-based DCs indicated that PROTS has value beyond the identification of pathology, 79.1% indicate that PROTS is important regarding biomechanical analysis of the spine, 83.0% noted PROTS to be vital to chiropractic practice and 84.7% believe PROTS aids in measuring outcomes (Table 4).

4. Discussion

While there is not consensus on the use of PROTS for chiropractic patient management, we surveyed a national sample of DCs to help clarify this topic with the most extensive investigation into the clinical expertise of the chiropractic profession regarding utilization of plain radiography to date. We demonstrate that DCs embrace a spectrum of opinions, ranging from possible perspectives that, due to safety concerns, utilization of PROTS be limited to diagnosing pathology in the presence of red flags [68–71] to an absolute necessity of X-ray images to determine spine and biomechanical parameters [71–73].

EBP includes three categories: published literature, patient preference, and clinician experience. The clinical experience and expertise of the practicing DCs has been neglected in the development of guidelines using EBP guidelines despite being an essential component of the EBP. The results of this study demonstrate that DCs' clinical experience and expertise regards PROTS as vital to practice, valuable for patient diagnosis, care, management, biomechanical assessment, and overall outcomes.

Recent evidence suggests that 73.4% of practicing DCs read peer-reviewed research about patient management between several times a day to about once a month, and an additional 22.8% of DCs review published research 1–6 times per year. Further, 40.2% of practicing DCs review best practice guidelines from several times a day to about once per month, with another 37.6% reviewing EBP about 1–6 times per year [34] (pp. 106–108). Given the increasing evidence that chiropractic care has a positive impact on spinal health, the clinical experience and opinion of DCs should be considered in any practice guideline development that utilizes EBP as a foundation. Recall that EBP is the equivalent balance of three components: (1) the best research evidence, (2) clinical experience, and (3) the patient's preferences [74]. The best research evidence is clinically relevant, peer-reviewed research that has been conducted using sound methodology. Clinical experience refers to the clinician's cumulative experience, education, and clinical skills in managing patient care, and patient preference refers to the patient's unique concerns, expectations, and values. These three components should be taken into consideration in the decision-making process for patient care [75].

The results of the survey show that a majority of the respondents utilize plain radiography (73.3%) within their practice facility, with 82.9% believing that plain radiography procedures are vital for chiropractic care. Additionally, 17.1% of DCs who do not utilize PROTS in their clinics believed that plain radiography is vital for chiropractic care provided. These findings indicate that the majority of DCs consider plain radiography vital to practice (Table 4). Respondents were disaggregated into two groups, those who owned an X-ray machine in their clinic and those who did not, which served as the dependent variable. The authors of the study analyzed the responses of the two groups on every item in the survey (the analysis of dichotomous items is presented in Figure 1, and the analysis of continuous items is presented in Figure 2). The two groups were statistically dissimilar on almost every survey item, which may suggest that the decision of owning a radiograph system in a chiropractic clinic goes above and beyond affordability. Believing that utilization of PROTS is vital to the chiropractic case and these radiographic procedures aid in the measurement of clinical outcomes emerged as the strongest predictors of having a radiographic system in a chiropractic clinic. These analyses (see Table 4) confirmed and strengthened previous findings (see Tables 2 and 3). In addition to analyzing the survey data and reporting the results, the authors of the study utilized the collected survey responses to construct a scale (a measurement instrument) for future use. The authors provided a valid and reliable scale with good internal consistency to assess clinical opinions toward the use of plain radiography in chiropractic clinical management and is so named the Clinician Opinion and Experience on Chiropractic Radiography (COECR) scale.

Results from the present study unveiled intriguing differences between those who choose to perform in-office PROTS and those who do not. The binary logistic regression analysis revealed that, aside from geography, the strongest predictor of having a radiography system in a chiropractic practice was an opinion that radiographic procedures are essential to chiropractic care: DCs who endorsed this item were 6 times more likely ($OR = 5.9$) to have a radiography system in their clinics. The second strongest predictor was the utilization of PROTS to aid measurement of clinical outcomes. DCs adhering to these views were twice as likely ($OR = 2.2$) to own a radiographic system. On the other hand, DCs who took radiographs only when suspecting pathology in the presence of red flags were much less likely to own a radiographic system in their clinic ($OR = 0.4$).

The data do not support the assumption that DCs who fully adhere to EBP are less likely to utilize PROTS for chiropractic case management. The strength of adherence to EBP was assessed by asking respondents if the clinical decision to obtain spinal radiographs should be based on all three EBP components. While the majority of respondents agreed or strongly agreed that all three components should be equally considered (77.7%), there were no statistically significant differences in utilization of plain film radiography between those who agreed that all three EBP components should be equally considered and those who did not (22.3%). Moreover, this question did not emerge as a significant predictor of the utilization of plain film radiography. These findings suggest that most DCs believe that all three components of EBP should be considered together.

Regarding the overall clinical opinions and experience of practicing DCs towards PROTS, 9.5% own a CR digital X-ray system in their practice; 47.7% have a DR digital X-ray system in the practice; 16.0% own a plain film radiography system; 2.1% do have a plain radiography system in their facility, but they refer the majority of patients out for PROTS; and 24.7% do not own any plain radiographic equipment in their chiropractic practice. It is evident from the survey that DCs who undervalue the use of PROTS are less likely to own a plain radiography system, while the reverse is true for those who value PROTS as they are likely to own a radiography system.

There is evidence in the literature to support the rationale for the high clinical opinions reflected in the survey regarding value of PROTS, the relevance to biomechanical analysis and the relationship to measuring the outcome. Radiographic measurements such as frontal and sagittal spine alignment are well demonstrated to be important factors in predicting spinal health, quality of life and neurological dysfunction [76–82]. Frontal and sagittal spinal alignment are also correlated with many other radiographic parameters, including thoracic and pelvic morphology [83–86] Altered spinal balance remains associated with higher mechanical load and dysfunctional movement patterns and is a possible source of increased risk of pain and degeneration [87].

It is important to note that the literature also suggests that many of these radiographic parameters such as sagittal cervical spinal alignment and posture can be corrected with conservative care and these corrections can be corelated with improved function and health outcomes [88–102]. Other studies indicate that conservative care can result in radiographic changes to sagittal lumbar spinal alignment and posture, which is correlated with improved pain scores and health-related quality of life (HRQOL) [103–107]. Research has demonstrated that abnormal sagittal thoracic spinal alignment can be corrected, which is correlated with improvement in the risk of falls, headaches, forced expiratory volume, and HRQOL [108–115]. Additional studies have demonstrated that conservative correction of cervical lordosis and forward head posture can be associated with increased HRQOL, reduced back pain, and improved nervous system adaptability [100]. Coincidently, similar studies exist within the orthopedic research suggesting that the utilization of PROTS to measure surgical correction of biomechanical parameters such as sagittal vertical axis, lumbar lordosis, sacral slope, pelvic tilt and pelvic incidence angle have a direct impact on predictive surgical outcome, improved Oswestry Disability Index and improved patient HRQOL [116–120]. The current research suggesting the ability to correct radiographic parameters provides rationale for the clinical opinion of DCs indicated in the survey that more research should be dedicated to radiographic utilization in practice.

4.1. Other Findings

Additional findings also offer important insights. Item Q2.3 (*I only order radiographs for pathology or red flags*) showed negative factor loading when a one-factor CFA model was considered. This shows that the item measures the opposite pole of the intended construct, suggesting a negative linear correlation between the observed item and the latent construct measured [121]. The issue was echoed when the initial Rasch model was considered in the estimate of difficulty (the item was the most difficult to endorse) and the values of MSQ. After the item was reverse coded, the fit of the CFA and Rasch models was improved.

When considering the COECR scale, all items are consistent in producing a total score except Q2.3 (prior to recoding), which may suggest a different mindset for practitioners who take radiographs only when pathology is suspected. Although a minority, they strongly believe that the prudent use of plain radiography does not significantly improve long-term management of chiropractic patients and that there should be limitations on utilization due to concerns about safety, ethics, and economics. According to our findings, this is not the view of today's practicing DCs.

4.2. Strengths

Methodologically, this is the strongest study in the literature regarding clinical experience for plain radiography utilization. So far, no study reported in the last 10 years implemented this level of sophisticated statistical methods combining descriptive analyses, group differences, predictive modeling, factor analysis, and IRT. The only study that used predictive methods was that of Pearce et al. [122], but the model in the study was challenged by the limitations described in the previous sections. For the first time, researchers collected a sizable, national sample surveying clinical expertise of the chiropractic profession toward plain radiograph utilization for chiropractic case management. Although the data from previous studies show systematic dissimilarities in clinical opinions toward the use of PROTS for chiropractic management between DCs who own radiographs in their clinics and those who do not, the items were considered one by one. The predictive model developed by the researchers in this study considered all items at once. This approach allows for predictors to reveal statistical significance while controlling for all other variables in the model. Additionally, our study shows that those who agreed with the statement *"I order radiography for pathology and red flags"* are in the minority, which contradicts current trends in evidence-based practice recommendations. These guidelines tend to dictate the political stance for the rest of the profession using research that is highly susceptible to bias and that does not consider biomechanical analysis, treatment strategies, or patient outcome. This requires further research and visibility in the literature to improve the professional understanding of the value of plain radiography on patient outcome that is evident in the clinical opinion of practicing DCs.

4.3. Limitations

This study is an examination of DCs' clinical opinions and experience on using plain radiography for chiropractic case management. The findings in this study are novel and important; however, limitations should be considered. Methodologically, our study's design involved a non-experimental approach evaluating cross-sectional variables. Thus, causal relationships cannot be established between the predictors and the outcomes. As with many self-report surveys, there were limitations regarding sampling and response biases. While we informed participants that the survey was anonymous, results may have been affected by social desirability bias [123]. The authors did not seek outside expertise in the creation of the survey and did not utilize an initial pilot study; some respondents may have misinterpreted the definition of red flags which could have skewed some of the responses. Additionally, it is possible that some DCs have no interest in the topic of utilization of PROTS, which would have resulted in self-selection bias and a lack of representation from DCs who are not strongly opinionated toward PROTS. When considering the EBP definition of clinical experience [75], our survey lacked the ability to determine the level of expertise and experience as it did not consider items such as years in practice, practice setting, levels of advanced education, hours of study per week and the financial implications of owning a radiographic unit. The distribution of the survey link to licensed DCs was based on email lists that were purchased from publication distribution lists and organizations that had access to significant national distribution of professionals. Therefore, we did not assign a priori probabilities to all population units to be selected in the sample. Although we attempted to minimize subjectivity, the inference of the findings to the target population may be susceptible to bias [124].

Question-related subjectivity and bias were minimized by constructing questions that were neutral, answer options that were not leading, survey results that were anonymous, and ensuring the anonymity of the organizing group. That said, there is no single correct way to structure a question or provide response options. Different respondents may have had different perceptions of the same question, which may influence survey responses and inference of the findings to the target population [124]. Additionally, the dependent variable in the predictive analysis (Q7) did not ask DCs directly whether they do or do not support taking spinal radiographs for chiropractic case management, so measuring clinical opinion was captured indirectly. Despite the limitations, this study provides novel information about DCs' clinical opinions toward utilization of PROTS. Researching the opinions and experience of practicing DCs may clarify the utilization of plain radiography in chiropractic.

4.4. Future Research

Respondents indicated a desire for the chiropractic profession to align itself with the current trends in healthcare and refine our understanding of how to better utilize radiographic interpretation in the prediction and management of spinal health. There is a need for expanded research from the chiropractic profession to help determine the efficacy of the clinical opinions represented in this survey. Continued research may include additional surveys, qualitative studies, and observational studies. Additionally, longitudinal comparative studies are necessary to help understand the impact of spinal correction as measured with PROTS on patient QOL. Cooperation and joint research with the orthopedic profession may be beneficial, as there are already many orthopedic studies related to PROTS and the relationship between surgical biomechanical correction of the spine on QOL.

5. Conclusions

This survey provides the most extensive insight into the clinical opinion of the US chiropractic profession regarding PROTS and suggests that the majority of the DCs consider utilization of PROTS to have value beyond the identification of pathology, to be vital to chiropractic practice and essential to biomechanical analysis. The US DCs who utilized PROTS *only* to rule out pathology in the presence of red flags are, in fact, statistical outliers in this study and may represent a minority of US DCs. A majority of the DCs also consider the doctors' clinical experience and expertise, coupled with patient preferences, to be appropriate for recommending PROTS. Most DCs in this survey found that sharing spinal radiographic findings with the patient is beneficial for patient outcomes. All participants in the survey believed that patient outcomes would benefit from continued research regarding appropriate utilization of PROTS. The results of this survey clearly indicate the value of PROTS reflected by DCs and demonstrate the need for continued research to help understand how this value can affect the quality of care, conservative correction of spinal alignment and patient health.

Author Contributions: Conceptualization, P.A.A.; methodology, S.J.K.; software, S.J.K.; validation, S.J.K.; formal analysis, P.A.A., S.J.K., D.F.L.; investigation, P.A.A., S.J.K. and D.F.; data curation, P.A.A., S.J.K. and J.J.; writing—original draft preparation, P.A.A., S.J.K., J.J., D.F.L., D.F. and C.T.; writing—review and editing, D.F.L. and D.F.; visualization, S.J.K.; supervision, P.A.A.; project administration, P.A.A. All authors have read and agreed to the published version of the manuscript.

Funding: This research received no external funding.

Institutional Review Board Statement: The study was approved by the Institutional Review Board of Sherman College of Chiropractic (protocol code ECEUPR09162022).

Informed Consent Statement: Informed consent was obtained from all subjects involved in the study.

Data Availability Statement: All data is represented within the manuscript. Archived datasets analyzed during this study can be accessed publicly at the following link: https://radevidence.org/evidence-based-practice/ (accessed on 6 March 2023).

Conflicts of Interest: The authors declare no conflict of interest. Author Steven J. Kraus is an employee and stock holder in Biokinemetrics, Inc., a digital X-ray company.

Appendix A

Invitation to complete the Survey
Chiropractic Radiology Evidence-Based Practice Survey

Your identity is required to validate you are a DC and only complete the survey once.
This 10-question survey is only for licensed Doctors of Chiropractic. Please complete this independent survey to help the chiropractic profession evaluate opinions on general spinal radiography. The survey is not sponsored by any state or national association, nor any technique group, nor business. None of your contact information will be shared or published without your permission. Your survey responses, except for name and street

address and email identification data, will be tabulated and published. Your identity is needed to validate the survey was completed only once by an actual licensed DC. After completing the survey responses with integrity, you agree to these terms described.

Overall survey results will be emailed to you at the email you provide after all the survey results are closed, fully tabulated, and published. Please encourage other licensed DCs to take the survey so that the largest representative sample can be achieved.

Estimated survey completion time: 5 min. Thank you for your thoughtful participation.

Appendix B

Survey distribution numbers and percentage by state of residence.

State	N	%
AL	352	0.72%
AK	146	0.29%
AZ	1032	2.07%
AR	478	0.96%
CA	7617	15.31%
CO	1304	2.62%
CT	716	1.44%
DE	81	0.16%
DC	30	0.06%
FL	4346	8.74%
GA	1447	2.90%
HI	63	0.13%
ID	399	0.80%
IL	2656	5.34%
IN	465	0.93%
IA	718	1.44%
KS	393	0.79%
KY	722	1.45%
LA	340	0.68%
MA	667	1.34%
MD	375	0.75%
ME	134	0.27%
MI	1823	3.66%
MN	1010	2.03%
MS	264	0.53%
MO	1107	2.23%
MT	172	0.35%
NE	610	1.23%
NV	315	0.63%
NH	188	0.38%
NJ	2455	4.93%
NM	179	0.36%
NY	3462	6.96%
NC	864	1.74%
ND	133	0.27%
OH	2153	4.33%
OK	355	0.71%
OR	654	1.31%
PA	1998	4.02%
RI	80	0.16%
SC	616	1.24%
SD	158	0.32%
TN	557	1.12%
TX	2657	5.34%
UT	519	1.04%
VT	97	0.19%

State	N	%
VA	601	1.21%
WA	1200	2.41%
WV	108	0.22%
WI	869	1.75%
WY	62	0.42%
Total	49,747	100.00%

Appendix C

Completed survey responses by state and percentage.

State	n	%
AL	16	0.44%
AK	14	0.38%
AZ	51	1.40%
AR	16	0.44%
CA	423	11.62%
CO	89	2.44%
CT	27	0.74%
DE	3	0.08%
DC	5	0.14%
FL	198	5.44%
GA	199	5.47%
HI	8	0.22%
ID	59	1.62%
IL	159	4.37%
IN	89	2.44%
IA	77	2.11%
KS	31	0.85%
KY	13	0.36%
LA	84	2.30%
MA	41	1.13%
MD	47	1.29%
ME	8	0.22%
MI	259	7.11%
MN	73	2.00%
MS	5	0.14%
MO	38	1.04%
MT	25	0.69%
NE	26	0.71%
NV	43	1.18%
NH	13	0.36%
NJ	87	2.39%
NM	19	0.52%
NY	108	2.97%
NC	71	1.95%
ND	13	0.36%
OH	104	2.86%
OK	23	0.63%
OR	164	4.50%
PA	192	5.27%
RI	7	0.19%
SC	59	1.62%
SD	52	1.42%
TN	37	1.02%
TX	121	3.32%
UT	126	3.46%
VT	6	0.16%

State	N	%
VA	69	1.89%
WA	152	4.17%
WV	6	0.16%
WI	68	1.87%
WY	18	0.49%
Total	3641	100.00%

Appendix D

Out of 4301 respondents, 1292 clinicians provided additional comments ranging from one sentence to four paragraphs, which resulted in valuable insights regarding the clinician decision process for utilization of plain radiography. Some responses commented on multiple topics. A summary of these the responses could be divided as follows:

- 41% were short comments emphasizing the need for X-rays as an integral and essential tool within their chiropractic practice.
- 37% commented on the differences between utilization in a chiropractic clinical setting versus a medical setting.
- 37% described conditions that they found on numerous occasions in which the patient had no red flags or complaints yet required alteration of care.
- 5% of the comments were related to clinicians supporting the need for this type of survey.
- 4% revolved around comments related to safety.
- Less than 1% commented on question selection.

References

1. Koch, C.; Hänsel, F. Non-specific Low Back Pain and Postural Control During Quiet Standing—A Systematic Review. *Front. Psychol.* **2019**, *10*, 586. [CrossRef] [PubMed]
2. Cassidy, J.D.; Boyle, E.; Côté, P.; Hogg-Johnson, S.; Bondy, S.J.; Haldeman, S. Risk of Carotid Stroke after Chiropractic Care: A Population-Based Case-Crossover Study. *J. Stroke Cerebrovasc. Dis. Off. J. Natl. Stroke Assoc.* **2017**, *26*, 842–850. [CrossRef] [PubMed]
3. Todd, A.J.; Carroll, M.T.; Robinson, A.; Mitchell, E.K.L. Adverse Events Due to Chiropractic and Other Manual Therapies for Infants and Children: A Review of the Literature. *J. Manipulative Physiol. Ther.* **2015**, *38*, 699–712. [CrossRef]
4. Rubinstein, S.M.; de Zoete, A.; van Middelkoop, M.; Assendelft, W.J.J.; de Boer, M.R.; van Tulder, M.W. Benefits and harms of spinal manipulative therapy for the treatment of chronic low back pain: Systematic review and meta-analysis of randomised controlled trials. *BMJ* **2019**, *364*, l689. [CrossRef]
5. Ward, K.L.; Smith, M. Association Between Chiropractic Utilization and Opioid Prescriptions Among People With Back or Neck Pain: Evaluation of the Medical Expenditure Panel Survey. *J. Manipulative Physiol. Ther.* **2022**, *45*, 315–322. [CrossRef]
6. Acharya, M.; Chopra, D.; Smith, A.M.; Fritz, J.M.; Martin, B.C. Associations Between Early Chiropractic Care and Physical Therapy on Subsequent Opioid Use Among Persons With Low Back Pain in Arkansas. *J. Chiropr. Med.* **2022**, *21*, 67–76. [CrossRef]
7. Emary, P.C.; Brown, A.L.; Oremus, M.; Mbuagbaw, L.; Cameron, D.F.; DiDonato, J.; Busse, J.W. Association of Chiropractic Care With Receiving an Opioid Prescription for Noncancer Spinal Pain Within a Canadian Community Health Center: A Mixed Methods Analysis. *J. Manipulative Physiol. Ther.* **2022**, *45*, 235–247. [CrossRef]
8. Whedon, J.M.; Uptmor, S.; Toler, A.W.J.; Bezdjian, S.; MacKenzie, T.A.; Kazal, L.A. Association between chiropractic care and use of prescription opioids among older medicare beneficiaries with spinal pain: A retrospective observational study. *Chiropr. Man. Ther.* **2022**, *30*, 5. [CrossRef] [PubMed]
9. Keeney, B.J.; Fulton-Kehoe, D.; Turner, J.A.; Wickizer, T.M.; Chan, K.C.G.; Franklin, G.M. Early predictors of lumbar spine surgery after occupational back injury: Results from a prospective study of workers in Washington State. *Spine* **2013**, *38*, 953–964. [CrossRef]
10. Trager, R.J.; Daniels, C.J.; Perez, J.A.; Casselberry, R.M.; Dusek, J.A. Association between chiropractic spinal manipulation and lumbar discectomy in adults with lumbar disc herniation and radiculopathy: Retrospective cohort study using United States' data. *BMJ Open* **2022**, *12*, e068262. [CrossRef] [PubMed]
11. Goertz, C.M.; Long, C.R.; Vining, R.D.; Pohlman, K.A.; Walter, J.; Coulter, I. Effect of Usual Medical Care Plus Chiropractic Care vs Usual Medical Care Alone on Pain and Disability Among US Service Members With Low Back Pain: A Comparative Effectiveness Clinical Trial. *JAMA Netw. Open* **2018**, *1*, e180105. [CrossRef]
12. Mueller, K.; Wang, D.; Lea, R.; Murphy, D. Chiropractic Care for Workers with Low Back Pain. *Work. Compens. Res. Inst.* **2022**.
13. Cifuentes, M.; Willetts, J.; Wasiak, R. Health maintenance care in work-related low back pain and its association with disability recurrence. *J. Occup. Environ. Med.* **2011**, *53*, 396–404. [CrossRef] [PubMed]
14. Ndetan, H.; Hawk, C.; Evans, W.; Tanue, T.; Singh, K. Chiropractic Care for Spine Conditions: Analysis of National Health Interview Survey. *J. Health Care Res.* **2020**, *1*, 105–118. [CrossRef]

15. Young, K.J. Historical influence on the practice of chiropractic radiology: Part II—Thematic analysis on the opinions of diplomates of the American Chiropractic College of Radiology about the future. *Chiropr. Man. Ther.* **2017**, *25*, 15. [CrossRef]
16. Chang, M. The Chiropractic Scope of Practice in the United States: A Cross-Sectional Survey. *J. Manipulative Physiol. Ther.* **2014**, *37*, 363–376. [CrossRef]
17. Oakley, P.A.; Betz, J.W.; Harrison, D.E.; Siskin, L.A.; Hirsh, D.W.; International Chiropractors Association Rapid Response Research Review Subcommittee. Radiophobia Overreaction: College of Chiropractors of British Columbia Revoke Full X-Ray Rights Based on Flawed Study and Radiation Fear-Mongering. *Dose-Response Publ. Int. Hormesis Soc.* **2021**, *19*, 15593258211033142. [CrossRef]
18. Lumbreras, B.; Donat, L.; Hernández-Aguado, I. Incidental findings in imaging diagnostic tests: A systematic review. *Br. J. Radiol.* **2010**, *83*, 276–289. [CrossRef]
19. Ammendolia, C.; Côté, P.; Hogg-Johnson, S.; Bombardier, C. Do Chiropractors Adhere to Guidelines for Back Radiographs?: A Study of Chiropractic Teaching Clinics in Canada. *Spine* **2007**, *32*, 2509–2514. [CrossRef]
20. Ferrari, R. Imaging studies in patients with spinal pain: Practice audit evaluation of Choosing Wisely Canada recommendations. *Can. Fam. Physician* **2016**, *62*, e129–e137. [PubMed]
21. Hoffman, J.R.; Zucker, M.I. Validity of a Set of Clinical Criteria to Rule Out Injury to the Cervical Spine in Patients with Blunt Trauma. *N. Engl. J. Med.* **2000**, *6*, 94. [CrossRef]
22. Cardarelli, J.J.; Ulsh, B.A. It Is Time to Move Beyond the Linear No-Threshold Theory for Low-Dose Radiation Protection. *Dose-Response* **2018**, *16*, 155932581877965. [CrossRef]
23. Pollycove, M.; Feinendegen, L.E. Molecular biology, epidemiology, and the demise of the linear no-threshold (LNT) hypothesis. *Comptes Rendus Académie Sci. Ser. III Sci. Vie* **1999**, *322*, 197–204. [CrossRef] [PubMed]
24. Siegel, J.A.; Pennington, C.W.; Sacks, B. Subjecting Radiologic Imaging to the Linear No-Threshold Hypothesis: A Non Sequitur of Non-Trivial Proportion. *J. Nucl. Med.* **2017**, *58*, 1–6. [CrossRef] [PubMed]
25. Tubiana, M.; Feinendegen, L.E.; Yang, C.; Kaminski, J.M. The Linear No-Threshold Relationship Is Inconsistent with Radiation Biologic and Experimental Data. *Radiology* **2009**, *251*, 13–22. [CrossRef] [PubMed]
26. Siegel, J.A.; Welsh, J.S. Does Imaging Technology Cause Cancer? Debunking the Linear No-Threshold Model of Radiation Carcinogenesis. *Technol. Cancer Res. Treat.* **2016**, *15*, 249–256. [CrossRef] [PubMed]
27. Orton, C.G.; Williamson, J.F. *Controversies in Medical Physics: A Compendium of Point/Counterpoint Debates Volume 3*; American Association of Physicists in Medicine: Alexandria, VA, USA, 2017; 349p.
28. Available online: https://www.choosingwisely.org/wp-content/uploads/2017/08/ACA-Choosing-Wisely-List.pdf (accessed on 18 November 2022).
29. II) Chiropractic Guideline for Spine Radiography for the Assessment of Spinal Subluxation in Children and Adults. *Pract. Chiropr. Comm. Radiol. Protoc.* **2006**. Available online: http://www.pccrp.org/docs/PCCRP%20Section%20II.pdf (accessed on 14 September 2022).
30. Guyatt, G.H. Evidence-based medicine. *ACP J. Club* **1991**, *114*, A-16. [CrossRef]
31. Ulrich, R.S.; Zimring, C.; Zhu, X.; DuBose, J.; Seo, H.-B.; Choi, Y.-S.; Quan, X.; Joseph, A. A Review of the Research Literature on Evidence-Based Healthcare Design. *HERD Health Environ. Res. Des. J.* **2008**, *1*, 61–125. [CrossRef]
32. Bhargava, K.; Bhargava, D. Evidence Based Health Care: A scientific approach to health care. *Sultan Qaboos Univ. Med. J.* **2007**, *7*, 105–107.
33. Haynes, R.B.; Devereaux, P.J.; Guyatt, G.H. Physicians' and patients' choices in evidence based practice. *BMJ* **2002**, *324*, 1350. [CrossRef]
34. Practice Analysis of Chiropractic 2020—NBCE Survey Analysis. Available online: https://www.nbce.org/practice-analysis-of-chiropractic-2020/ (accessed on 14 September 2022).
35. Gliedt, J.A.; Perle, S.M.; Puhl, A.A.; Daehler, S.; Schneider, M.J.; Stevans, J. Evaluation of United States chiropractic professional subgroups: A survey of randomly sampled chiropractors. *BMC Health Serv. Res.* **2021**, *21*, 1049. [CrossRef] [PubMed]
36. Young, K.J. Historical influence on the practice of chiropractic radiology: Part I—A survey of Diplomates of the American Chiropractic College of Radiology. *Chiropr. Man. Ther.* **2017**, *25*, 14. [CrossRef]
37. Tabachnick, B.G.; Fidell, L.S.; Ullman, J.B. *Using Multivariate Statistics*, 7th ed.; Pearson: New York, NY, USA, 2019; ISBN 978-0-13-479054-1.
38. van der Linden, W.J.; Hambleton, R.K. (Eds.) *Handbook of Modern Item Response Theory*; Springer: New York, NY, USA, 1997; ISBN 978-1-4419-2849-8.
39. Reise, S.P.; Widaman, K.F.; Pugh, R.H. Confirmatory factor analysis and item response theory: Two approaches for exploring measurement invariance. *Psychol. Bull.* **1993**, *114*, 552–566. [CrossRef] [PubMed]
40. Reise, S.P.; Revicki, D.A. (Eds.) *Handbook of Item Response Theory Modeling: Applications to Typical Performance Assessment*; Multivariate Applications Series; Routledge, Taylor & Francis Group: New York, NY, USA, 2015; ISBN 978-1-84872-972-8.
41. Faraway, J.J. Generalized linear models. In *International Encyclopedia of Education*; Peterson, P., Baker, E., McGaw, B., Eds.; Elsevier: Amsterdam, The Netherlands, 2010; pp. 178–183. ISBN 978-0-08-044894-7.
42. Midi, H.; Sarkar, S.K.; Rana, S. Collinearity diagnostics of binary logistic regression model. *J. Interdiscip. Math.* **2010**, *13*, 253–267. [CrossRef]
43. *IBM SPSS Statistics for Windows*; IBM Corp: Armonk, NY, USA, 2017.

44. Rasch, G. An Item Analysis Which Takes Individual Differences into Account. *Br. J. Math. Stat. Psychol.* **1966**, *19*, 49–57. [CrossRef]
45. Toit, M.D. *IRT from SSI: BILOG-MG, MULTILOG, PARSCALE, TESTFACT*; Scientific Software International: Skokie, IL, USA, 2003; ISBN 978-0-89498-053-4.
46. Tranmer, M.; Murphy, J.; Elliot, M.; Pampaka, M. *Multiple Linear Regression*, 2nd ed.; Cathie Marsh Institute: Manchester, UK, 2020; 59p.
47. Cronbach, L.J. Coefficient alpha and the internal structure of tests. *Psychometrika* **1951**, *16*, 297–334. [CrossRef]
48. Muthén, B.; Muthén, L. *Mplus User's Guide*, 6th ed.; Muthén & Muthén: Los Angeles, CA, USA, 1998.
49. Lawley, D.N. VI.—The Estimation of Factor Loadings by the Method of Maximum Likelihood. *Proc. R. Soc. Edinb.* **1940**, *60*, 64–82. [CrossRef]
50. Hu, L.; Bentler, P.M. Cutoff criteria for fit indexes in covariance structure analysis: Conventional criteria versus new alternatives. *Struct. Equ. Model. Multidiscip. J.* **1999**, *6*, 1–55. [CrossRef]
51. MacCallum, R.C.; Browne, M.W.; Sugawara, H.M. Power analysis and determination of sample size for covariance structure modeling. *Psychol. Methods* **1996**, *1*, 130–149. [CrossRef]
52. Bentler, P.M. Comparative fit indexes in structural models. *Psychol. Bull.* **1990**, *107*, 238–246. [CrossRef] [PubMed]
53. Tucker, L.R.; Lewis, C. A reliability coefficient for maximum likelihood factor analysis. *Psychometrika* **1973**, *38*, 1–10. [CrossRef]
54. Lord, F.M.; Novick, M.R.; Birnbaum, A. *Statistical Theories of Mental Test Scores*; Addison-Wesley: Oxford, UK, 1968.
55. Hambleton, R.K.; Swaminathan, H. *Item Response Theory: Principles and Applications*; Springer Science & Business Media: Berlin/Heidelberg, Germany, 2013.
56. Lazarsfeld, P.F. *Latent Structure Analysis [by] Paul F. Lazarsfeld [and] Neil W. Henry*; Houghton, Mifflin: Boston, MA, USA, 1968.
57. Rosenbaum, P.R. Testing the Local Independence Assumption in Item Response Theory. *ETS Res. Rep. Ser.* **1984**, *1984*, i-26. [CrossRef]
58. Yen, W.M. Effects of local item dependence on the fit and equating performance of the three-parameter logistic model. *Appl. Psychol. Meas.* **1984**, *8*, 125–145. [CrossRef]
59. Yen, W.M. Scaling Performance Assessments: Strategies for Managing Local Item Dependence. *J. Educ. Meas.* **1993**, *30*, 187–213. [CrossRef]
60. Christensen, K.B.; Makransky, G.; Horton, M. Critical Values for Yen's Q3: Identification of Local Dependence in the Rasch Model Using Residual Correlations. *Appl. Psychol. Meas.* **2017**, *41*, 178–194. [CrossRef]
61. Mair, P.; Hatzinger, R. CML based estimation of extended Rasch models with the eRm package in R. *Psychol. Sci.* **2007**, *49*, 26.
62. Chalmers, R.P. mirt: A multidimensional item response theory package for the R environment. *J. Stat. Softw.* **2012**, *48*, 1–29. [CrossRef]
63. Allison, P.D. *Missing Data*; SAGE Publications: Southend Oaks, CA, USA, 2001; ISBN 978-1-4522-0790-2.
64. Agresti, A. *Introduction to Categorical Data Analysis*; John and Wiley and Sons: Hoboken, NJ, USA, 2007; 394p.
65. Jöreskog, K.G.; Sörbom, D. *LISREL 8: Structural Equation Modeling with the SIMPLIS Command Language*; Scientific Software International: Skokie, IL, USA, 1993; ISBN 978-0-89498-033-6.
66. Bentler, P.M.; Bonett, D.G. Significance tests and goodness of fit in the analysis of covariance structures. *Psychol. Bull.* **1980**, *88*, 588. [CrossRef]
67. Masters, G.N.; Wright, B.D. *A Model for Partial Credit Scoring*; Statistical Laboratory, Department of Education, University of Chicago: Chicago, IL, USA, 1981.
68. Jenkins, H.J.; Downie, A.S.; Moore, C.S.; French, S.D. Current evidence for spinal X-ray use in the chiropractic profession: A narrative review. *Chiropr. Man. Ther.* **2018**, *26*, 48. [CrossRef]
69. Corso, M.; Cancelliere, C.; Mior, S.; Kumar, V.; Smith, A.; Côté, P. The clinical utility of routine spinal radiographs by chiropractors: A rapid review of the literature. *Chiropr. Man. Ther.* **2020**, *28*, 1–15. [CrossRef]
70. Anderson, B. Critical analysis of "X-ray imaging is essential for contemporary chiropractic and manual therapy spinal rehabilitation: Radiography increases benefits and reduces risks" by Oakley et al. *Dose-Response* **2018**, *16*, 1559325818813509. [CrossRef]
71. Kawchuk, G.; Goertz, C.; Axén, I.; Descarreaux, M.; French, S.; Haas, M.; Hartvigsen, J.; Kolberg, C.; Jenkins, H.; Peterson, C.; et al. Letter to the Editor Re: Oakley PA, Cuttler JM, Harrison DE. X-Ray Imaging Is Essential for Contemporary Chiropractic and Manual Therapy Spinal Rehabilitation: Radiography Increases Benefits and Reduces Risks. *Dose-Response* **2018**, *16*, 1559325818811521. [CrossRef]
72. Oakley, P.A.; Harrison, D.E. Radiophobic Fear-Mongering, Misappropriation of Medical References and Dismissing Relevant Data Forms the False Stance for Advocating Against the Use of Routine and Repeat Radiography in Chiropractic and Manual Therapy. *Dose-Response Publ. Int. Hormesis Soc.* **2021**, *19*, 1559325820984626. [CrossRef]
73. Oakley, P.A.; Harrison, D.E. Death of the ALARA Radiation Protection Principle as Used in the Medical Sector. *Dose-Response* **2020**, *18*, 1559325820921641. [CrossRef]
74. Pape, T.M. Evidence-Based Nursing Practice: To Infinity and Beyond. *J. Contin. Educ. Nurs.* **2003**, *34*, 154–161. [CrossRef]
75. Sackett, D.L. Evidence-based medicine and treatment choices. *The Lancet* **1997**, *349*, 570. [CrossRef]
76. Miyakoshi, N.; Itoi, E.; Kobayashi, M.; Kodama, H. Impact of postural deformities and spinal mobility on quality of life in postmenopausal osteoporosis. *Osteoporos. Int.* **2003**, *14*, 1007–1012. [CrossRef]

77. Diebo, B.G.; Oren, J.H.; Challier, V.; Lafage, R.; Ferrero, E.; Liu, S.; Vira, S.; Spiegel, M.A.; Harris, B.Y.; Liabaud, B.; et al. Global sagittal axis: A step toward full-body assessment of sagittal plane deformity in the human body. *J. Neurosurg. Spine* **2016**, *25*, 494–499. [CrossRef]
78. Hasegawa, K.; Okamoto, M.; Hatsushikano, S.; Shimoda, H.; Ono, M.; Watanabe, K. Normative values of spino-pelvic sagittal alignment, balance, age, and health-related quality of life in a cohort of healthy adult subjects. *Eur. Spine J. Off. Publ. Eur. Spine Soc. Eur. Spinal Deform. Soc. Eur. Sect. Cerv. Spine Res. Soc.* **2016**, *25*, 3675–3686. [CrossRef]
79. Mac-Thiong, J.-M.; Transfeldt, E.E.; Mehbod, A.A.; Perra, J.H.; Denis, F.; Garvey, T.A.; Lonstein, J.E.; Wu, C.; Dorman, C.W.; Winter, R.B. Can c7 plumbline and gravity line predict health related quality of life in adult scoliosis? *Spine* **2009**, *34*, E519–E527. [CrossRef]
80. Harrison, D.E.; Cailliet, R.; Harrison, D.D.; Troyanovich, S.J.; Harrison, S.O. A review of biomechanics of the central nervous system–Part I: Spinal canal deformations resulting from changes in posture. *J. Manip. Physiol. Ther.* **1999**, *22*, 227–234. [CrossRef]
81. Mohanty, C.; Massicotte, E.M.; Fehlings, M.G.; Shamji, M.F. Association of preoperative cervical spine alignment with spinal cord magnetic resonance imaging hyperintensity and myelopathy severity: Analysis of a series of 124 cases. *Spine* **2015**, *40*, 11–16. [CrossRef]
82. Sun, J.; Zhao, H.-W.; Wang, J.-J.; Xun, L.; Fu, N.-X.; Huang, H. Diagnostic Value of T1 Slope in Degenerative Cervical Spondylotic Myelopathy. *Med. Sci. Monit. Int. Med. J. Exp. Clin. Res.* **2018**, *24*, 791–796. [CrossRef]
83. Lee, S.-H.; Son, E.-S.; Seo, E.-M.; Suk, K.-S.; Kim, K.-T. Factors determining cervical spine sagittal balance in asymptomatic adults: Correlation with spinopelvic balance and thoracic inlet alignment. *Spine J. Off. J. North Am. Spine Soc.* **2015**, *15*, 705–712. [CrossRef]
84. Lee, D.-H.; Ha, J.-K.; Chung, J.-H.; Hwang, C.J.; Lee, C.S.; Cho, J.H. A retrospective study to reveal the effect of surgical correction of cervical kyphosis on thoraco-lumbo-pelvic sagittal alignment. *Eur. Spine J. Off. Publ. Eur. Spine Soc. Eur. Spinal Deform. Soc. Eur. Sect. Cerv. Spine Res. Soc.* **2016**, *25*, 2286–2293. [CrossRef]
85. Weng, C.; Wang, J.; Tuchman, A.; Wang, J.; Fu, C.; Hsieh, P.C.; Buser, Z.; Wang, J.C. Influence of T1 Slope on the Cervical Sagittal Balance in Degenerative Cervical Spine: An Analysis Using Kinematic MRI. *Spine* **2016**, *41*, 185–190. [CrossRef]
86. Jun, H.S.; Kim, J.H.; Ahn, J.H.; Chang, I.B.; Song, J.H.; Kim, T.H.; Park, M.S.; Kim, Y.C.; Kim, S.W.; Oh, J.K. T1 slope and degenerative cervical spondylolisthesis. *Spine* **2015**, *40*, E220–E226. [CrossRef]
87. Keorochana, G.; Taghavi, C.E.; Lee, K.-B.; Yoo, J.H.; Liao, J.-C.; Fei, Z.; Wang, J.C. Effect of sagittal alignment on kinematic changes and degree of disc degeneration in the lumbar spine: An analysis using positional MRI. *Spine* **2011**, *36*, 893–898. [CrossRef]
88. Fortner, M.O.; Oakley, P.A.; Harrison, D.E. Alleviation of chronic spine pain and headaches by reducing forward head posture and thoracic hyperkyphosis: A CBP® case report. *J. Phys. Ther. Sci.* **2018**, *30*, 1117–1123. [CrossRef]
89. Moustafa, I.M.; Diab, A.A.M.; Hegazy, F.A.; Harrison, D.E. Does rehabilitation of cervical lordosis influence sagittal cervical spine flexion extension kinematics in cervical spondylotic radiculopathy subjects? *J. Back Musculoskelet. Rehabil.* **2017**, *30*, 937–941. [CrossRef]
90. Silber, J.S.; Lipetz, J.S.; Hayes, V.M.; Lonner, B.S. Measurement variability in the assessment of sagittal alignment of the cervical spine: A comparison of the gore and cobb methods. *J. Spinal Disord. Tech.* **2004**, *17*, 301–305. [CrossRef]
91. Bsdc, C.C.; Robinson, D.H. Improvement of Cervical Lordosis and Reduction of Forward Head Posture with Anterior Head Weighting and Proprioceptive Balancing Protocols. *J. Vertebral Subluxation Res.* Available online: https://vertebralsubluxationresearch.com/2017/09/06/improvement-of-cervical-lordosis-and-reduction-of-forward-head-posture-with-anterior-head-weighting-and-proprioceptive-balancing-protocols/ (accessed on 15 September 2022).
92. Morningstar, M. Cervical curve restoration and forward head posture reduction for the treatment of mechanical thoracic pain using the pettibon corrective and rehabilitative procedures. *J. Chiropr. Med.* **2002**, *1*, 113–115. [CrossRef]
93. Ferrantelli, J.R.; Harrison, D.E.; Harrison, D.D.; Stewart, D. Conservative treatment of a patient with previously unresponsive whiplash-associated disorders using clinical biomechanics of posture rehabilitation methods. *J. Manip. Physiol. Ther.* **2005**, *28*, e1–e8. [CrossRef]
94. Harrison, D.E.; Cailliet, R.; Harrison, D.D.; Janik, T.J.; Holland, B. A new 3-point bending traction method for restoring cervical lordosis and cervical manipulation: A nonrandomized clinical controlled trial. *Arch. Phys. Med. Rehabil.* **2002**, *83*, 447–453. [CrossRef] [PubMed]
95. Harrison, D.E.; Harrison, D.D.; Betz, J.J.; Janik, T.J.; Holland, B.; Colloca, C.J.; Haas, J.W. Increasing the cervical lordosis with chiropractic biophysics seated combined extension-compression and transverse load cervical traction with cervical manipulation: Nonrandomized clinical control trial. *J. Manipulative Physiol. Ther.* **2003**, *26*, 139–151. [CrossRef] [PubMed]
96. Moustafa, I.M.; Diab, A.A.; Taha, S.; Harrison, D.E. Addition of a Sagittal Cervical Posture Corrective Orthotic Device to a Multimodal Rehabilitation Program Improves Short- and Long-Term Outcomes in Patients With Discogenic Cervical Radiculopathy. *Arch. Phys. Med. Rehabil.* **2016**, *97*, 2034–2044. [CrossRef]
97. Fortner, M.O.; Oakley, P.A.; Harrison, D.E. Non-surgical improvement of cervical lordosis is possible in advanced spinal osteoarthritis: A CBP® case report. *J. Phys. Ther. Sci.* **2018**, *30*, 108–112. [CrossRef] [PubMed]
98. Moustafa, I.M.; Diab, A.A.; Hegazy, F.; Harrison, D.E. Does improvement towards a normal cervical sagittal configuration aid in the management of cervical myofascial pain syndrome: A 1- year randomized controlled trial. *BMC Musculoskelet. Disord.* **2018**, *19*, 396. [CrossRef]

99. Moustafa, I.M.; Diab, A.A.; Harrison, D.E. The effect of normalizing the sagittal cervical configuration on dizziness, neck pain, and cervicocephalic kinesthetic sensibility: A 1-year randomized controlled study. *Eur. J. Phys. Rehabil. Med.* **2017**, *53*, 57–71. [CrossRef]
100. Fedorchuk, C.; Lightstone, D.F.; McCoy, M.; Harrison, D.E. Increased Telomere Length and Improvements in Dysautonomia, Quality of Life, and Neck and Back Pain Following Correction of Sagittal Cervical Alignment Using Chiropractic BioPhysics® Technique: A Case Study. *J. Mol. Genet. Med.* **2017**, *11*, 1. [CrossRef]
101. Fortner, M.O.; Oakley, P.A.; Harrison, D.E. Alleviation of posttraumatic dizziness by restoration of the cervical lordosis: A CBP® case study with a one year follow-up. *J. Phys. Ther. Sci.* **2018**, *30*, 730–733. [CrossRef]
102. Wickstrom, B.M.; Oakley, P.A.; Harrison, D.E. Non-surgical relief of cervical radiculopathy through reduction of forward head posture and restoration of cervical lordosis: A case report. *J. Phys. Ther. Sci.* **2017**, *29*, 1472–1474. [CrossRef]
103. Fedorchuk, C.; Lightstone, D.F.; McRae, C.; Kaczor, D. Correction of Grade 2 Spondylolisthesis Following a Non-Surgical Structural Spinal Rehabilitation Protocol Using Lumbar Traction: A Case Study and Selective Review of Literature. *J. Radiol. Case Rep.* **2017**, *11*, 13–26. [CrossRef]
104. Harrison, D.E.; Cailliet, R.; Harrison, D.D.; Janik, T.J.; Holland, B. Changes in sagittal lumbar configuration with a new method of extension traction: Nonrandomized clinical controlled trial. *Arch. Phys. Med. Rehabil.* **2002**, *83*, 1585–1591. [CrossRef]
105. Diab, A.A.; Moustafa, I.M. Lumbar lordosis rehabilitation for pain and lumbar segmental motion in chronic mechanical low back pain: A randomized trial. *J. Manip. Physiol. Ther.* **2012**, *35*, 246–253. [CrossRef]
106. Moustafa, I.M.; Diab, A.A. Extension traction treatment for patients with discogenic lumbosacral radiculopathy: A randomized controlled trial. *Clin. Rehabil.* **2013**, *27*, 51–62. [CrossRef]
107. Harrison, D.E.; Oakley, P.A. Non-operative correction of flat back syndrome using lumbar extension traction: A CBP® case series of two. *J. Phys. Ther. Sci.* **2018**, *30*, 1131–1137. [CrossRef]
108. Mendoza-Lattes, S.; Ries, Z.; Gao, Y.; Weinstein, S.L. Natural history of spinopelvic alignment differs from symptomatic deformity of the spine. *Spine* **2010**, *35*, E792–E798. [CrossRef]
109. Yu, M.; Zhao, W.-K.; Li, M.; Wang, S.-B.; Sun, Y.; Jiang, L.; Wei, F.; Liu, X.-G.; Zeng, L.; Liu, Z.-J. Analysis of cervical and global spine alignment under Roussouly sagittal classification in Chinese cervical spondylotic patients and asymptomatic subjects. *Eur. Spine J. Off. Publ. Eur. Spine Soc. Eur. Spinal Deform. Soc. Eur. Sect. Cerv. Spine Res. Soc.* **2015**, *24*, 1265–1273. [CrossRef]
110. Oakley, P.A.; Jaeger, J.O.; Brown, J.E.; Polatis, T.A.; Clarke, J.G.; Whittler, C.D.; Harrison, D.E. The CBP® mirror image® approach to reducing thoracic hyperkyphosis: A retrospective case series of 10 patients. *J. Phys. Ther. Sci.* **2018**, *30*, 1039–1045. [CrossRef]
111. Fortner, M.O.; Oakley, P.A.; Harrison, D.E. Treating "slouchy" (hyperkyphosis) posture with chiropractic biophysics®: A case report utilizing a multimodal mirror image® rehabilitation program. *J. Phys. Ther. Sci.* **2017**, *29*, 1475–1480. [CrossRef]
112. Miller, J.E.; Oakley, P.A.; Levin, S.B.; Harrison, D.E. Reversing thoracic hyperkyphosis: A case report featuring mirror image® thoracic extension rehabilitation. *J. Phys. Ther. Sci.* **2017**, *29*, 1264–1267. [CrossRef]
113. Betz, J.W.; Oakley, P.A.; Harrison, D.E. Relief of exertional dyspnea and spinal pains by increasing the thoracic kyphosis in straight back syndrome (thoracic hypo-kyphosis) using CBP® methods: A case report with long-term follow-up. *J. Phys. Ther. Sci.* **2018**, *30*, 185–189. [CrossRef]
114. Mitchell, J.R.; Oakley, P.A.; Harrison, D.E. Nonsurgical correction of straight back syndrome (thoracic hypokyphosis), increased lung capacity and resolution of exertional dyspnea by thoracic hyperkyphosis mirror image® traction: A CBP® case report. *J. Phys. Ther. Sci.* **2017**, *29*, 2058–2061. [CrossRef]
115. Oakley, P.A.; Harrison, D.E. Reducing thoracic hyperkyphosis subluxation deformity: A systematic review of Chiropractic Biophysics® methods employed in its structural improvement. *J. Contemp. Chiropr.* **2018**, *1*, 59–66.
116. Ochtman, A.E.A.; Kruyt, M.C.; Jacobs, W.C.H.; Kersten, R.F.M.R.; le Huec, J.C.; Öner, F.C.; van Gaalen, S.M. Surgical Restoration of Sagittal Alignment of the Spine: Correlation with Improved Patient-Reported Outcomes: A Systematic Review and Meta-Analysis. *JBJS Rev.* **2020**, *8*, e1900100. [CrossRef]
117. Rhee, C.; Visintini, S.; Dunning, C.E.; Oxner, W.M.; Glennie, R.A. Does restoration of focal lumbar lordosis for single level degenerative spondylolisthesis result in better patient-reported clinical outcomes? A systematic literature review. *J. Clin. Neurosci.* **2017**, *44*, 95–100. [CrossRef]
118. Kim, C.-W.; Hyun, S.-J.; Kim, K.-J. Surgical Impact on Global Sagittal Alignment and Health-Related Quality of Life Following Cervical Kyphosis Correction Surgery: Systematic Review. *Neurospine* **2020**, *17*, 497–504. [CrossRef]
119. Zhang, Y.; Shao, Y.; Liu, H.; Zhang, J.; He, F.; Chen, A.; Yang, H.; Pi, B. Association between sagittal balance and adjacent segment degeneration in anterior cervical surgery: A systematic review and meta-analysis. *BMC Musculoskelet. Disord.* **2019**, *20*, 430. [CrossRef] [PubMed]
120. Mehta, V.A.; Amin, A.; Omeis, I.; Gokaslan, Z.L.; Gottfried, O.N. Implications of spinopelvic alignment for the spine surgeon. *Neurosurgery* **2015**, *76* (Suppl. S1), S42–S56; discussion S56. [CrossRef] [PubMed]
121. Kline, R.B. *Principles and Practice of Structural Equation Modeling*; Guilford Publications: New York, NY, USA, 2015.
122. Pearce, M.S.; Salotti, J.A.; Little, M.P.; McHugh, K.; Lee, C.; Kim, K.P.; Howe, N.L.; Ronckers, C.M.; Rajaraman, P.; Craft, A.W.; et al. Radiation exposure from CT scans in childhood and subsequent risk of leukaemia and brain tumours: A retrospective cohort study. *The Lancet* **2012**, *380*, 499–505. [CrossRef] [PubMed]

123. Crano, W.D.; Brewer, M.B.; Lac, A. *Principles and Methods of Social Research*, 3rd ed.; Routledge: New York, NY, USA, 2014; ISBN 978-1-315-76831-1.
124. Groves, R.M.; Fowler, J.F., Jr.; Couper, M.P.; Lepkowski, J.M.; Singer, E.; Tourangeau, R. *Survey Methodology*; John Wiley & Sons: Hoboken, NJ, USA, 2011; ISBN 978-1-118-21134-2.

Disclaimer/Publisher's Note: The statements, opinions and data contained in all publications are solely those of the individual author(s) and contributor(s) and not of MDPI and/or the editor(s). MDPI and/or the editor(s) disclaim responsibility for any injury to people or property resulting from any ideas, methods, instructions or products referred to in the content.

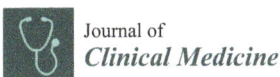

Systematic Review

Current Knowledge on the Different Characteristics of Back Pain in Adults with and without Scoliosis: A Systematic Review

Fabio Zaina [1,*], Rosemary Marchese [2], Sabrina Donzelli [1], Claudio Cordani [3,4], Carmelo Pulici [1], Jeb McAviney [2] and Stefano Negrini [3,4]

1. ISICO (Italian Scientific Spine Institute), 20141 Milan, Italy; sabrina.donzelli@isico.it (S.D.); carmelo.pulici@isico.it (C.P.)
2. ScoliCare, Sydney 2217, Australia; rosemary.marchese@scolicare.com (R.M.); jeb@scolicare.com (J.M.)
3. Department of Biomedical, Surgical and Dental Sciences, University "La Statale", 20122 Milan, Italy; claudio.cordani@unimi.it (C.C.); stefano.negrini@unimi.it (S.N.)
4. IRCCS Istituto Ortopedico Galeazzi, 20157 Milan, Italy
* Correspondence: fabio.zaina@isico.it

Abstract: Patients with scoliosis have a high prevalence of back pain (BP). It is possible that scoliosis patients present with specific features when experiencing back or leg pain pathology. The aim of this systematic review is to report the signs, symptoms and associated features of BP in patients with scoliosis compared to adults without scoliosis during adulthood. From inception to 15 May 2023, we searched the following databases: PubMed, EMBASE, the Cumulative Index to Nursing and Allied Health Literature (CINAHL), and Scopus. We found 10,452 titles, selected 25 papers for full-text evaluation and included 8 in the study. We found that scoliosis presents with asymmetrical pain, most often at the curve's apex, eventually radiating to one leg. Radiating symptoms are usually localised on the front side of the thigh (cruralgia) in scoliosis, while sciatica is more frequent in non-scoliosis subjects. These radiating symptoms relate to rotational olisthesis. The type and localization of the curve have an impact, with lumbar and thoracolumbar curves being more painful than thoracic. Pain in adults with scoliosis presents specific features: asymmetrical localization and cruralgia. These were the most specific features. It remains unclear whether pain intensity and duration can differentiate scoliosis and non-scoliosis-related pain in adults.

Keywords: scoliosis; low back pain; back pain; disability; lumbar spine

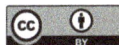

1. Introduction

Idiopathic scoliosis is a three-dimensional spine and trunk deformity of unknown origin [1]. There are several classifications based on the location and size of the curves and according to the age of diagnosis [1]. Usually, idiopathic scoliosis becomes evident during adolescence (AIS), which is the riskiest period for worsening due to rapid growth. Infantile and juvenile scoliosis are less common but, in many cases, show a more unfavourable prognosis [2]. Occasionally, idiopathic scoliosis is diagnosed later, during adulthood, while primary (de novo) degenerative scoliosis refers to a structural curve that develops after skeletal maturity in a previously normal spine [3]. It is also a fairly frequent condition, especially in females, with a prevalence of up to 37.6% in people older than 60 years [4].

Despite etiological differences, the clinical impact on Quality of Life (QoL) of idiopathic and degenerative scoliosis during adulthood can be similar. Studies have shown that patients with scoliosis have a higher prevalence of back pain (BP) and experience a more severe and longer duration of pain than controls without scoliosis [5]. Pain can eventually radiate distally to one or both legs. Features that distinguish BP related to scoliosis, as opposed to other potential causes of BP, have yet to be identified. Pain in scoliosis patients seems to have specific features, including increasing with prolonged standing while reducing when lying down [5]. Also, the localization of pain seems different in patients with scoliosis, with the pain being more asymmetric and principally at the apex of the curve, on either the side of the prominence or the concavity and frequently radiating to one of the inferior limbs [6]. Most of the time, the pain is localised in the lumbar spine, which is subjected to faster degeneration effects; however, in some cases, pain is localised in the thoracolumbar or in the thoracic spine in the prominent area where the biomechanics play a major role [7]. This is why authors sometimes refer to BP and other times to low back pain (LBP).

According to current knowledge, AIS should reach the threshold of 30° to be significant in adulthood [8,9], while degenerative scoliosis can be painful even at lower degrees [4]. Unfortunately, in everyday clinical practice, it is not always possible to differentiate between the two forms. We can diagnose scoliosis as indeed being degenerative only if it is lumbar/thoracolumbar and we have a previous radiograph showing a straight spine. However, degenerative phenomena may also affect idiopathic scoliosis during adulthood.

According to some estimates, we can expect that by 2050, the proportion of the world's population aged greater than 60 years will nearly double [10]. This event will increase the number of patients with scoliosis presenting to doctors with BP [11]. Therefore, there is a need to better identify the clinical and associated features of BP in adult patients living with scoliosis to distinguish whether scoliosis is the underlying cause of BP. Understanding the features of BP in this group of patients would have clinically relevant outcomes related to the treatment and prevention of pain.

The primary aim of this systematic review is to report and characterise the signs, symptoms and associated features of pain (e.g., localization, intensity, duration, modifying factors) in patients with idiopathic or degenerative scoliosis during adulthood compared to adults without scoliosis. The hypothesis is that scoliosis patients present specific features when experiencing back or leg pain connected to the peculiarities of the structural changes of their spine.

The secondary aim is to differentiate LBP and leg pain features between idiopathic and degenerative scoliosis.

2. Materials and Methods

2.1. Design

We developed this systematic review based on the MOOSE Reporting Guidelines for Meta-analyses of Observational Studies [12]. We registered the protocol on PROSPERO (CRD42023364455).

2.2. Selection Criteria

2.2.1. Type of Study

We included original peer-reviewed primary research articles that were considered a control group. We considered studies in any language, and we obtained translations where needed. We excluded secondary research (review articles), case reports and studies that did not meet the inclusion criteria.

2.2.2. Population

We included adults with scoliosis and BP or LBP. The definition of scoliosis in adults included adults diagnosed with idiopathic scoliosis as an infant, juvenile or adolescent or those diagnosed with scoliosis during adulthood (idiopathic or degenerative). We included these different types of scoliosis because, in clinical practice, it can sometimes be difficult to be certain whether they are degenerative, idiopathic or even both. Moreover, most of the published studies presented a mixed population. Finally, despite some differences, we can expect similar complaints. We excluded studies if the scoliosis was not idiopathic or degenerative, such as neuromuscular, congenital and other secondary scoliosis. We also excluded studies if the patients underwent surgical management for their scoliosis. We included studies of patients treated during adulthood, provided they did not receive any treatments in the last six months, and considered only the baseline information (i.e., before any treatment is applied).

2.2.3. Search Strategy

From inception to 15 May 2023, we conducted a literature search in the following databases: PubMed (via https://pubmed.ncbi.nlm.nih.gov/ accessed on 15 May 2023), CINHAL (via EBSCOhost), EMBASE (via Embase.com) and Scopus. In addition, we searched the reference lists of the included studies for other possible studies. We contacted the authors for studies in which the full text was unavailable. We first developed the search strategy for PubMed and adapted it to the other databases.

Search strings were composed of search terms defining the "scoliosis" OR "spinal deformities" AND "low back pain", "spinal pain" OR "pain".

The complete search strategies for each database are available in Appendix A. We imported the search results into the bibliographic management online software Rayyan (https://www.rayyan.ai accessed on 15 May 2023) after we discarded duplicates on EndNote X9. We reported the results of the search as per the MOOSE flow diagram (Figure 1).

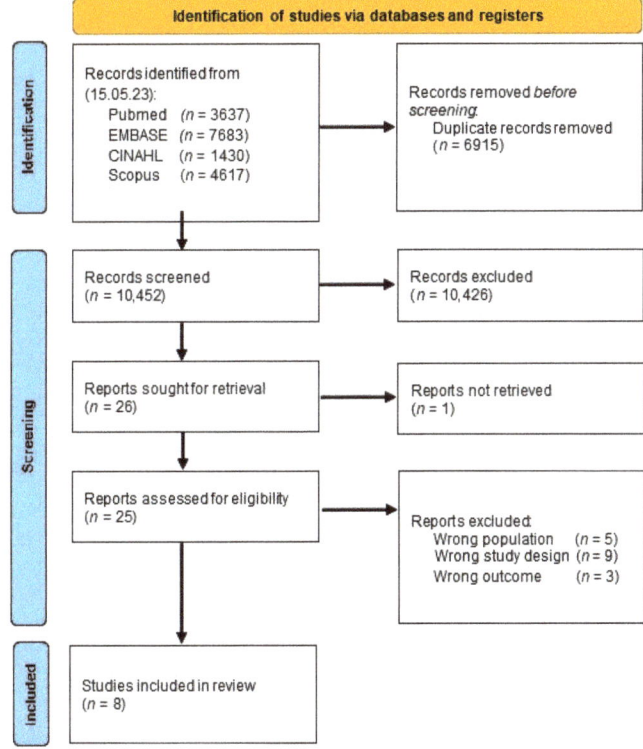

Figure 1. Study flow chart.

2.2.4. Outcome Measures

The outcomes of interest are the signs, symptoms and associated features of BP and LBP in adults with and without scoliosis. Pain-related outcomes may include but are not limited to intensity, duration, type, location (back or distal), onset and triggering factors/positions, relieving factors/positions, and time-related behaviour. Associated features may include but are not limited to patient demographics (gender, age, occupation), number of pregnancies, family history of scoliosis and pain, Cobb angle, number of curves, types of curve and X-ray features, e.g., osteoporosis, rotational olisthesis.

2.2.5. Study Screening

Two reviewers (CP, FZ) independently screened the titles and abstracts retrieved by the search strategy and assessed the full-text articles for their potential inclusion. Disagreements were resolved through discussion with another author (RM) to reach a consensus. We managed these phases by using the Rayyan software.

2.2.6. Data Extraction

Two reviewers (CP, FZ) independently extracted the general characteristics (first author, publication year, study design, study setting, sample size, participant characteristics) and outcome data into an Excel form. We solved any differences in opinion about the study characteristics with a third review author (RM).

2.3. Quality Assessment

Two reviewers (CC, SD) independently assessed the studies' quality. We solved any differences in opinion about the methodological quality with a third review author (SN). We used the JBI checklist, as appropriate.

2.4. Evidence Synthesis and Statistical Analysis

We tabulated the characteristics of the included studies for comparison. We intended to assess for heterogeneity (e.g., visually, using I^2 or the χ^2 test) and, if possible, include a prevalence meta-analysis with weighted proportions. However, due to the small number and some limitations of the included studies, we performed a narrative synthesis with frequencies because the meta-analysis was not applicable.

3. Results

3.1. Study Selection

After removing the duplicates from the different databases, we found 10,452 titles (Figure 1). After the title screening, we selected 25 papers for a full-text evaluation and included 8 in the study. (Figure 1, Table 1).

Table 1. Characteristics of the included studies.

Authors	Design	Setting	Country	Evaluated Pain	Participants	Sample N° scoliosis; Female (F) %;	Sample N° non-scoliosis; Female (F)	Age Scoliosis Mean (SD), Range in years (as reported by study)	Age Non-Scoliosis Mean (SD), Range in years (as reported by study)	Type of Scoliosis (AAIS or De Novo)	Lumbar Curve Severity in Degrees (Before Treatment)	Presence of More than One Curve
		Recruitment from hospital/outpatient/general population		Low back pain (LBP); Back pain (BP)						As reported by study	As reported by study	As reported by study
Perennou 1994 [13]	prospective controlled	Spine Rehabilitation Unit	France	LBP	671	50 (7.5%); F 36 (72%)	621 (92.5%); F 298 (48%)	62.1 ± 12.4 (5 pz < 45 y)	49.6 ± 15.5	14% AIS, 86% discovered during examination	21.2 ± 11.4° (56% <20°, 28% 20–29; 10% 30–39; 6% ≥40°	only lumbar curves
Gremeaux 2008 [6]	prospective controlled	Spine Rehabilitation Unit	France	LBP	100	50 (50%) F 68%	50 (50%); F 66%	62 ± 13.1	62 ± 13.7	idiopathic and degenerative scoliosis	23.1 ± 13.1° (10–75°)	only lumbar curves
Yuan 2019 [14]	cross-sectional	Department of Physical Therapy and Rehabilitation	China	LBP	90	41 (45.5%) F 100%	49 (54.5%); F 100%	24.95 ± 2.90	24.73 ± 2.83	100% AIS	26°	only lumbar curves
Jackson 1983 [7]	retrospective controlled	Department of Orthopaedics	Canada	BP	377–245 report pain	197 pts (52%)–101 pts (51%) report pain;	180 pts (48%)–144 pts (80%) report pain	31	36	idiopathic scoliosis	16 pts lumbar 38°	45 pts thoracic curve 60°; 26 pts thoracolumbar 50°; 14 pts double curve 55°;
Mayo 1994 [5]	retrospective cohort study	Departments of Medicine and Department of Occupational Health, and Epidemiology and Biostatistics	Canada/USA	BP	3231 (724 report pain)	1476 (45.6%)–295 pts report pain;	1755 (55.4%)–429 report pain			100% AIS		

Table 1. Cont.

Authors	Design	Setting	Evaluated Pain	Participants	Sample	Age	Type of Scoliosis (AAIS or De Novo)	Lumbar Curve Severity in Degrees (Before Treatment)	Presence of More than One Curve
Hoevenars 2022 [15]	retrospective controlled	Outpatient	Netherlands	LBP	320	80 (25%); F 79%	240 (75%); F 79%	50.9 (SD 14.1, min-max 21–76)	50.1 (±12.0, 21–74)	24 adult idiopathic scoliosis, 56 de novo degenerative lumbar scoliosis;	21.4 (9.4, 11–72)	only lumbar curves
Bissolotti 2013 [16]	cross-sectional	Outpatient	Italy	LBP	80	40 (50%); F 75%	40 (50%); F 77.5%	61.8 ± 11.5	58.2 ± 10.9	Adult scoliosis	27.1 ± 11.5° primary curve (range, 15–63°); thoracic curve 25.5 ± 22.3° (range, 8–58°)	
Weinstein 2003 [17]	prospective controlled	Department of Orthopaedic Surgery	USA	BP	179 (88 report pain)	117 (65.3)–71 (60%) pts report pain; F 89%	62 (34.6%)–17 (10.4%) pts report pain; F 79.4%	66 (range, 54–80 y)	<65 y: 23/62 (37); >65 y 39/62 (63)	Late-onset idiopathic scoliosis	49.41 (SD 26.38 (range 15–90) lumbar, 89.54 (32.69) (range 50–155) Thoracolumbar, 84.50 (30.17) (range 23–156) thoracic	48 (41%) thoracic curve, 14 (12%) thoracolumbar, 32 (27%) lumbar, 23 (20%) double major

The reasons for exclusion were no study design of interest (nine papers), no population of interest (five papers) and no outcome of interest (three papers).

Three studies were prospective controlled [6,13,17], three were retrospective [5,7,15], and two were cross-sectional [14,16]. One of the cross-sectional studies was a congress abstract [16]. Two studies were from France, two were from Canada, and the others were from the USA, The Netherlands, China and Italy.

The total number of scoliosis patients was 727, and the controls were 1590.

Three studies included a larger number of adults with scoliosis and healthy controls but were included because they presented data for the subgroup of patients with BP [5,7,17].

Five studies focused on LBP [6,13–16], while the other three reported on BP, including both thoracic and lumbar or without giving details on the location [5,7,17].

3.2. Critical Appraisal

Following the JBI checklist, in the cross-sectional studies [14,16], the major limitations were the absence of strategies to identify and manage confounding factors. Moreover, in one study [16], the selection criteria and statistical analysis were not completely clear. Regarding the longitudinal studies [5–7,13,15,17], the main methodological limitations were associated with the absence of the confounding factors' identification and the strategies for managing them, as well as the application of strategies to address incomplete follow-up visits. Table 2 provides the results of the critical appraisal performed on the studies included in the present review.

Table 2. Critical appraisal of the included studies.

Cross-Sectional	1	2	3	4	5	6	7				
Bissolotti 2013 [16] *	Unclear	No	Yes	No	No	Yes	Unclear				
Yuan 2019 [14]	Yes	Yes	Yes	No	No	Yes	Yes				
Longitudinal	1	2	3	4	5	6	7	8	9	10	11
Gremeaux 2008 [6]	No	Yes	Yes	No	No	No	Yes	Yes	No	No	Yes
Hoevenars 2022 [15]	Yes	Yes	Yes	No	No	No	Yes	Yes	No	No	Yes
Jackson 1983 [7]	Yes	Yes	Yes	No	No	No	Yes	Unclear	Yes	Unclear	Unclear
Mayo 1994 [5]	No	Yes	Yes	Yes	Yes	No	Yes	Yes	No	No	Yes
Perennou 1994 [13]	No	Yes	Yes	No	No	No	Yes	Unclear	Unclear	Unclear	Yes
Weinstein 2003 [17]	No	Yes	Yes	No	No	No	Yes	Yes	No	No	Yes

Cross-sectional studies items: (1) Were the criteria for inclusion in the sample clearly defined? (2) Were the study subjects and setting described in detail? (3) Were objective, standard criteria used for the measurement of the condition? (4) Were confounding factors identified? (5) Were strategies to deal with confounding factors stated? (6) Were the outcomes measured in a valid and reliable way? (7) Was appropriate statistical analysis used? **Longitudinal studies items**: (1) Were the two groups similar and recruited from the same population? (2) Were the exposures measured similarly to assign people to both exposed and unexposed groups? (3) Was the exposure measured in a valid and reliable way? (4) Were the confounding factors identified? (5) Were strategies to deal with the confounding factors stated? 6) Were the groups/participants free of the outcome at the start of the study (or at the moment of exposure)? (7) Were the outcomes measured in a valid and reliable way? (8) Was the follow-up time reported and was it sufficient to be long enough for outcomes to occur? (9) Was a follow-up complete, and if not, were the reasons for the lack of a follow-up described and explored? (10) Were strategies to address incomplete follow-up utilised? (11) Were the strategies to address the incomplete follow-up utilised? * Conference abstract.

3.3. Main Findings

The description of symptoms (localization, intensity, disability and functional status) varied among the different papers. Five studies reported pain localization, five studies reported pain severity and/or disability in adults with scoliosis compared to non-scoliosis subjects and two papers reported on the factors influencing pain (Table 3).

Table 3. Symptom characteristics provided by the included studies.

Authors	Severity/Intensity of Pain		Location of BP		Referred/Lower Extremity Symptoms		Functional Status	
	Scoliosis	Non-Scoliosis	Scoliosis	Non-Scoliosis	Scoliosis	Non-Scoliosis	Scoliosis	Non-Scoliosis
Perennou 1994 [13]	–	–	–	–	40% radicular pain: 26% Sciatica, 14% cruralgia	44.3% radicular pain: 38% Sciatica, 6.3% cruralgia	–	–
Gremeaux 2008 [6]	60% little or usual; 40% considerable or severe	68% little or usual, 32% considerable or severe	–	–	56% (sciatica 26%; cruralgia 26%, neurological claudication 10%, buttock pain 30%); Inguinal dysesthesia 30%, 10% costo-iliac syndrome; Buttock Pain (20% little or usual; 45% considerable or severe) Inguinal pain (16.6%; 70%) Obturator neuralgia (3.3%; 30%)	44% (sciatica 32%; cruralgia 12%, neurological claudication 8%; buttock pain 34%) Inguinal dysesthesia 6%; 0% costo-iliac syndrome	–	–
Yuan 2019 [14]	3.5 NRS	5.5 NPRS	32 (78%) left-sided lumbar pain, 9 (21%) right-sided lumbar pain; 78% pain on the convex side	83.7% midline or symmetrical pain	–	–	–	–
Jackson 1983 [7]	3.3 (scale from 0 to 5)	–	44% pain at lower junctional segment /compensatory curves below the major deformity; DM: 35% mainly junctional area, 44% localised pain in lower junctional levels and in lesser curves below. TL and L mainly junctional and fractional curve segments below MC in 46% and 44%; lumbosacral half-curve segment was most painful.	–	65% of patients complained of limb distress, including buttock and thigh pain, before treatment.	–	–	–

Table 3. Cont.

Authors	Severity/Intensity of Pain		Location of BP		Referred/Lower Extremity Symptoms		Functional Status	
	Scoliosis	Non-Scoliosis	Scoliosis	Non-Scoliosis	Scoliosis	Non-Scoliosis	Scoliosis	Non-Scoliosis
Mayo 1994 [5]	–	–	Spreading pain (curves > 40°), generalised back pain (curves > 20°)	–	–	–	Limitations in lifting, walking, standing, travel, sitting. Need to change position and lie down/rest.	–
Hoevenaars 2022 [15]	58.4 (19.1) NRS	60.4 (19.1)	–	–	–	–	39.5 (±12) ODI	40.2 (±12.1) ODI
Bissolotti 2013 [16]	NRS 5.9 ± 1.8 (range 2–10)	5.1 ± 2.2	–	–	27% sciatic pain	47% (sciatic pain)	33.9 ± 17% ODI	32.6 ± 18.8% ODI
Weinstein 2003 [17]	Little/moderate score 1–2: 48/71 (68%); quite bad/unbearable score 3–5: 23/71 (32%)	Little/moderate score 1–2: 12/17 (71%); quite bad/unbearable score 3–5: 5/17 (29%)	–	–	–	–	37 pts (39%) felt they had a disability	16 pts (30%) felt they had a disability

Abbreviations: pts: patients; BP: back pain; DM: double major; TL: thoracolumbar; L: lumbar; MC: major curve.

3.4. Pain Localization

Five papers reported pain localization [6,7,13,14,16]. Two papers reported on a similar population of older people, and therefore we pooled their data [6,13]. One was about younger subjects [14]. One congress abstract reported sciatica prevalence [16].

In two studies, adults with scoliosis and LBP experienced more frequent radiating pain and cruralgia (defined as compressive nerve root irritation of L3–L4 [18]) than the control group of LBP patients without scoliosis (48 vs. 37.5% and 20% vs. 6.7%, respectively), and sciatica was more frequent in patients without scoliosis (26% vs. 44%) [6,13]. A congress abstract reported similar significant findings (27 vs. 47%) [16]. Cruralgia was associated with rotatory dislocation (olisthesis) [6,13].

In one paper reporting on the younger adult population, all the scoliosis patients experienced unilateral lumbar pain (78% of the time on the convex side), while 83.7% of patients without scoliosis experienced midline or symmetrical lumbar pain [14].

Considering the back area, the most common localization of pain was over the major deformity in scoliosis. In a double major curve, the pain was frequently at the distal curve, while in thoracic curves, the pain was at the distal junctional level [7].

3.5. Pain Intensity and Disability

Five studies described pain intensity and disability [5,12,14,16,18]. One study reported pain intensity and frequency at 50 years of follow-up [17]. The authors reported that pain intensity and duration were similar between scoliosis and non-scoliosis adult patients with BP [17]. They also created a more complete pain composite, summing the pain intensity and duration. Also, this parameter showed similar trends in both groups [17].

One congress abstract reported similar findings for pain and disability in scoliosis and non-scoliosis adults with LBP [16]. The numerical rating scale (NRS) values were 5.9 ± 1.8 for scoliosis patients versus 5.1 ± 1.2 for the controls, while the Oswestry Disability Index (ODI) values were $33.9 \pm 17.6\%$ versus $32.6 \pm 18.8\%$ [16].

A retrospective study included subjects with chronic BP who failed a primary care conservative treatment approach and were referred to a combined physical and psychological program. The authors found no differences at the baseline for pain intensity (58.4 ± 19.1 vs. 60.4 ± 19.1 for NRS), functional status (39.5 ± 12.0 vs. 40.2 ± 12.1 for ODI), or pain duration (15.5 vs. 13.6 years) [15].

On the contrary, two retrospective studies reported more frequent pain in scoliosis patients [5,7]. One study found that current BP and prevalence of BP over the last year were higher for scoliosis than non-scoliosis adults, without any impact of curve entity [5]. In scoliosis patients, the pain was more continuous and chronic [5]. The other study found that adults with scoliosis had more severe, constant or frequent pain, while non-scoliosis patients referred more occasional or recurrent pain [7].

3.6. Factors Influencing Pain

Two papers reported data on the factors influencing pain [5,7]. One paper reported details from the Roland Morris Scale (RM), the ODI and McGill Pain Questionnaire [5]. Compared to non-scoliosis BP patients, adults with scoliosis and BP showed a more frequent need to change position, with limitations in standing and sitting for a long time [4]. Patients with curves larger than 40° also showed limitations in walking, and those with curves between 20° and 40° had limitations in lifting and travelling [5]. Issues related to social activity, personal care and the need for pain control were similar among the two groups [4]. One retrospective study reported that major lumbar, thoracolumbar and lumbosacral curves were the most painful, while major thoracic was the least painful [7].

4. Discussion

There is evidence that adults with scoliosis frequently report pain issues. In clinical practice, it is sometimes difficult to understand whether the pain relates to the spinal deformity or is nonspecific [19]. BP is so common that there are cases in which it affects someone with scoliosis just by chance. To help clinicians, we designed this systematic review to report the available information on the topic. Only a few studies compared BP in scoliosis and non-scoliosis subjects. According to the data reported in our review, scoliosis presents with asymmetrical pain, which is, for most of the time, lumbar and at the curve's apex, eventually radiating to one leg. Radiating symptoms are usually localised on the front side of the thigh (cruralgia), while sciatica is more frequent in non-scoliosis subjects. These radiating symptoms relate to rotational olisthesis [6,13], consistently with other reports [20,21]. Also, the type and localization of the curve have an impact, with lumbar and thoracolumbar ones being more painful than thoracic [7]. In thoracic curves, the painful area is usually distal to the curve [7].

Other features of pain in scoliosis are related to difficulty standing and eventually sitting for a prolonged time, where lying down seems to relieve symptoms [5]. Travelling and lifting seem challenging for patients with curves between 20° and 40°, while for those with larger curves, walking seems problematic [5]. We can hypothesise that these symptoms are associated with spine stiffness, which typically characterises scoliosis, and the altered biomechanics of the spine due to frontal and/or sagittal imbalance. We can also speculate that upper spine pain and fatigue are symptoms that start earlier, before degeneration, and could be more related to the altered biomechanics of the spine, whereas radiating LBP is a typical complaint of patients with degeneration in the lumbar spine; however, more clinically descriptive studies are needed to investigate these speculations.

Data from the papers included in this review are inconsistent regarding pain intensity and the duration of symptoms. Some studies reported more intensity and duration of symptoms in adults with scoliosis and BP [5,7]. In contrast, others found no difference compared to the control groups of non-scoliosis subjects [16,17].

Reporting about disability is challenging, too. Data collected from the ODI show no differences between scoliosis and non-scoliosis subjects [16]; however, some differences appear with the Roland Morris Scale and the McGill Questionnaire [5]. The ODI may not be suitable for capturing the disability of scoliosis patients. Recently, a study about bracing in adults with scoliosis and BP reported good results on pain and the Core Outcome Measurement Index (COMI), but no changes were recorded for the ODI [22,23]. Therefore, the application of the ODI in this specific group of patients seems questionable, and more specific tools are under investigation and applied in routine clinical practice [24,25].

Scoliosis is a three-dimensional trunk deformity that leads to global imbalance. In adult scoliosis, trunk imbalance has been suggested as one of the most crucial elements in pain generation; however, the studies that suggest this fell outside of the inclusion criteria of our study, mostly because they lacked control groups. The Schwab classification tried to help understand the pattern and risk factors of pain [9]; however, some papers questioned the role of such parameters in lumbar degenerative scoliosis [26]. As the evidence grows, we hope that the quality of evidence is such that we can compare the role of trunk imbalance in scoliosis and non-scoliosis populations and the relationship to LBP. As we already stated, it is possible that a patient with scoliosis experienced nonspecific LBP, and the findings of this review will help clinicians in everyday practice. It is important to recognise specific features of pain to correctly classify patients with scoliosis and BP to provide appropriate specific treatment. We need to bear in mind that LBP is very frequent in the adult population, and the disadvantaged biomechanics of the spine with scoliosis can represent a risk factor for these patients. If the features of pain are well-known, specific treatment can be applied when appropriate, with exercise [27] and bracing showing different degrees of effectiveness [28].

Due to the increasing prevalence of spinal deformities in adulthood, linked to the progressive ageing of the population, and the need for clinicians to identify a clear clinical picture for appropriate treatments, it is of major importance to identify what is known (signposting the relevant papers to clinicians) and what is unknown (driving future research efforts). A systematic review is an appropriate methodology to answer these needs. Due to the expected scarcity of papers, we considered a wide approach to collect all possible information. What we found clearly shows the need for much more and higher quality research in the field. Clinicians need to know if their patient's BP is due to a spinal deformity or if it is a common BP similar to patients without deformities. The next research step can be gathering consensus among experts to determine the current clinical understanding and develop research hypotheses for future studies.

Study Limitations

One limitation was the different outcome measures used in the different studies. A standard method for measuring pain was missing. Some papers applied ordinal scales, and others the NRS. For pain frequency and duration, some reported the year, and others used descriptive scales. All these elements, together with the small number of retrieved studies, prevented performing a meta-analysis. Some adults with scoliosis seek a clinical visit to check the evolution of their curves, while other times, for disability or pain. They may be used to experiencing some pain and fatigue in their everyday life, and therefore it is possible that they are frequently not concerned about their symptoms but may be worried about progression. This behaviour may justify the confusion regarding the pain's features and characterization. This highlights the need for further studies describing the pain features in scoliosis adults compared to adults with BP without scoliosis.

No study reported a direct comparison of pain in degenerative and idiopathic scoliosis, making it impossible to determine any difference between the two populations. Degenerative de novo scoliosis is not easy to diagnose, and it is possible that clinicians are not sure if it is a de novo scoliosis rather than idiopathic with a delayed diagnosis.

Unfortunately, the quality of the included studies is low. Moreover, just a few of them focused on the clinical features of LBP in adults with scoliosis. More research is needed in the field; therefore, we suggest starting with a consensus among experts to better define the most relevant features to investigate according to the available data and clinical experience and then designing appropriate clinical studies.

5. Conclusions

Pain in adults with scoliosis and BP seems to present specific features. Its localization, usually asymmetrical and associated with cruralgia, was the most specific feature. It remains unclear whether pain intensity and duration can differentiate scoliosis and non-scoliosis adults with BP. Further studies are needed to better understand BP in adults with scoliosis and provide specific treatment recommendations.

Author Contributions: Conceptualization, F.Z. and R.M.; methodology, C.C., C.P. and S.D.; data extraction F.Z., C.P. and R.M.; formal analysis, J.M. and S.N.; writing—original draft preparation, F.Z. and R.M.; writing—review and editing, all authors; supervision, S.N. and J.M. All authors have read and agreed to the published version of the manuscript.

Funding: This research received no external funding.

Institutional Review Board Statement: Not applicable.

Informed Consent Statement: Not applicable.

Data Availability Statement: Not applicable.

Acknowledgments: This study was supported and funded by the Italian Ministry of Health—Ricerca Corrente (2023). The authors wish to thank Federico Zaina for the original drawings of the graphical abstract.

Conflicts of Interest: S.N. owns ISICO stock. J.M. owns Scolicare stock. All other authors have no conflict of interest to declare.

Appendix A

Inception to May 2023

Databases: PubMed (via pubmed-ncbi.nlm.nih.gov/ accessed on 15 May 2023), CINHAL (via EBSCOhost), EMBASE (via Embase.com) and Scopus, from inception to May 2023.

PubMed (via pubmed-ncbi.nlm.nih.gov/ accessed on 15 May 2023)

1. ("spinal curvatures"[MeSH Terms]) OR (scoliosis[MeSH Terms]);
2. ((("spinal curvatures*"[Title/Abstract]) OR (scoliosis*[Title/Abstract]) OR ("spinal deformit*"[Title/Abstract]);
3. #1 OR #2;
4. (back pain[MeSH Terms] OR sciatica[MeSH Terms] OR radiculopathy[MeSH Terms]);
5. ((low back pain*[Title/Abstract]) OR (back pain*[Title/Abstract]) OR (spinal pain[Title/Abstract]) OR (backache*[Title/Abstract]) OR (back ache*[Title/Abstract]) OR (aching[Title/Abstract]) OR (lumbar pain[Title/Abstract]) OR (lumbo*[Title/Abstract]) OR (back disorder*[Title/Abstract]) OR sciatic*[Title/Abstract] OR radiculopat*[Title/Abstract]);
6. #4 OR #5;
7. #3 AND #6.

EMBASE (via Embase.com)

8. ('scoliosis'/exp OR 'spinal pain'/exp OR 'spine malformation'/exp);
9. ('spine diseas*':ab,ti,kw OR 'spinal curvature*':ti,ab,kw OR 'idiopathic* scoliosis':ti,ab,kw OR 'degenerative* scoliosis':ti,ab,kw OR 'de novo* scoliosis':ti,ab,kw OR 'spine malformat*':ti,ab,kw OR 'spinal deformit*':ti,ab,kw OR 'scoliosis*':ti,ab,kw);
10. #1 OR #2;
11. 'backache'/exp OR 'sciatica'/exp;
12. ('backache*':ti,ab,kw OR 'back pain*':ti,ab,kw OR 'low back pain*':ti,ab,kw OR 'scoliosis*':ti,ab,kw OR 'spinal pain*':ti,ab,kw OR 'back ache*':ti,ab,kw OR 'lumbar pain*':ti,ab,kw OR 'lumbo*':ti,ab,kw OR 'aching':ti,ab,kw OR 'back disorder*':ti,ab,kw OR 'sciatic*':ti,ab,kw OR 'radiculopat*':ti,ab,kw);
13. #4 OR #5;
14. #3 AND #6.

Scopus

15. TITLE-ABS-KEY("spinal curvature*" OR "scoliosis*" OR (("idiopathic*" OR "degenerativ*" OR "de novo*") W/1 ("scoliosis")));
16. TITLE-ABS-KEY("back pain*" OR "low back pain*" OR (("spinal" OR "lumbar") W/1 ("pain*")) OR "backache*" OR "back ache*" OR "aching" OR "lumbo*" OR "back disorder*" OR "sciatic*" OR "radiculopat*")));
17. #1 AND #2.

CINAHL (via EBSCOhost)

18. (MH "Spinal Curvatures+") OR (MH "Scoliosis+");
19. TI ((spinal W1 curvatures*) OR "scoliosis*" OR ((idiopathic* OR degenerativ* OR de novo*) N1 (scoliosis))) OR AB ((spinal W1 curvatures*) OR "scoliosis*" OR ((idiopathic* OR degenerativ* OR de novo*) N1 (scoliosis))) OR SU ((spinal W1 curvatures*) OR "scoliosis*" OR ((idiopathic* OR degenerativ* OR de novo*) N1 (scoliosis)));
20. #1 OR #2;
21. (MH "Back Pain+") OR (MH "Sciatica") OR (MH "Radiculopathy");
22. TI (((back OR spinal OR lumbar) N1 (pain*)) OR backache OR sciatic* OR radiculopat*OR (back W1 ache*) OR aching OR lumbo* OR (back W1 disorder*)) OR AB (((back OR spinal OR lumbar) N1 (pain*)) OR backache OR sciatic* OR radiculopat*OR (back W1 ache*) OR aching OR lumbo* OR (back W1 disorder*)) OR SU (((back OR spinal OR lumbar) N1 (pain*)) OR backache OR sciatic* OR radiculopat*OR (back W1 ache*) OR aching OR lumbo* OR (back W1 disorder*));

23. #4 OR #5;
24. #3 AND #6.

References

1. Negrini, S.; Donzelli, S.; Aulisa, A.G.; Czaprowski, D.; Schreiber, S.; de Mauroy, J.C.; Diers, H.; Grivas, T.B.; Knott, P.; Kotwicki, T.; et al. 2016 SOSORT Guidelines: Orthopaedic and Rehabilitation Treatment of Idiopathic Scoliosis during Growth. *Scoliosis Spinal Disord.* **2018**, *13*, 3. [CrossRef] [PubMed]
2. Hresko, M.T. Clinical Practice. Idiopathic Scoliosis in Adolescents. *N. Engl. J. Med.* **2013**, *368*, 834–841. [CrossRef] [PubMed]
3. Aebi, M. The Adult Scoliosis. *Eur. Spine J.* **2005**, *14*, 925–948. [CrossRef] [PubMed]
4. McAviney, J.; Roberts, C.; Sullivan, B.; Alevras, A.J.; Graham, P.L.; Brown, B.T. The Prevalence of Adult de Novo Scoliosis: A Systematic Review and Meta-Analysis. *Eur. Spine J.* **2020**, *29*, 2960–2969. [CrossRef] [PubMed]
5. Mayo, N.E.; Goldberg, M.S.; Poitras, B.; Scott, S.; Hanley, J. The Ste-Justine Adolescent Idiopathic Scoliosis Cohort Study. Part III: Back Pain. *Spine* **1994**, *19*, 1573–1581. [CrossRef]
6. Gremeaux, V.; Casillas, J.-M.; Fabbro-Peray, P.; Pelissier, J.; Herisson, C.; Perennou, D. Analysis of Low Back Pain in Adults with Scoliosis. *Spine* **2008**, *33*, 402–405. [CrossRef]
7. Jackson, R.P.; Simmons, E.H.; Stripinis, D. Incidence and Severity of Back Pain in Adult Idiopathic Scoliosis. *Spine* **1983**, *8*, 749–756. [CrossRef]
8. Weinstein, S.L. Natural History. *Spine* **1999**, *24*, 2592–2600. [CrossRef]
9. Schwab, F.; Farcy, J.-P.; Bridwell, K.; Berven, S.; Glassman, S.; Harrast, J.; Horton, W. A Clinical Impact Classification of Scoliosis in the Adult. *Spine* **2006**, *31*, 2109–2114. [CrossRef] [PubMed]
10. Nations, U. World Population Projected to Reach 9.8 Billion in 2050, and 11.2 Billion in 2100. Available online: https://www.un.org/en/desa/world-population-projected-reach-98-billion-2050-and-112-billion-2100 (accessed on 14 February 2023).
11. Diebo, B.G.; Shah, N.V.; Boachie-Adjei, O.; Zhu, F.; Rothenfluh, D.A.; Paulino, C.B.; Schwab, F.J.; Lafage, V. Adult Spinal Deformity. *Lancet* **2019**, *394*, 160–172. [CrossRef] [PubMed]
12. Stroup, D.F.; Berlin, J.A.; Morton, S.C.; Olkin, I.; Williamson, G.D.; Rennie, D.; Moher, D.; Becker, B.J.; Sipe, T.A.; Thacker, S.B. Meta-Analysis of Observational Studies in Epidemiology: A Proposal for Reporting. Meta-Analysis Of Observational Studies in Epidemiology (MOOSE) Group. *JAMA* **2000**, *283*, 2008–2012. [CrossRef]
13. Pérennou, D.; Marcelli, C.; Hérisson, C.; Simon, L. Adult Lumbar Scoliosis. Epidemiologic Aspects in a Low-Back Pain Population. *Spine* **1994**, *19*, 123–128. [CrossRef] [PubMed]
14. Yuan, W.; Shen, J.; Chen, L.; Wang, H.; Yu, K.; Cong, H.; Zhou, J.; Lin, Y. Differences in Nonspecific Low Back Pain between Young Adult Females with and without Lumbar Scoliosis. *Pain Res. Manag.* **2019**, *2019*, 9758273. [CrossRef] [PubMed]
15. Hoevenaars, E.H.W.; Beekhuizen, M.; O'Dowd, J.; Spruit, M.; van Hooff, M.L. Non-Surgical Treatment for Adult Spinal Deformity: Results of an Intensive Combined Physical and Psychological Programme for Patients with Adult Spinal Deformity and Chronic Low Back Pain-a Treatment-Based Cohort Study. *Eur. Spine J.* **2022**, *31*, 1189–1196. [CrossRef]
16. Bissolotti, L.; Sani, V.; Gobbo, M.; Orizio, C. Analysis of Differences in Pain and Disability in People with Adult Scoliosis and Nonspecific Low Back Pain. *Scoliosis* **2013**, *8*, O11. [CrossRef]
17. Weinstein, S.L.; Dolan, L.A.; Spratt, K.F.; Peterson, K.K.; Spoonamore, M.J.; Ponseti, I.V. Health and Function of Patients with Untreated Idiopathic Scoliosis: A 50-Year Natural History Study. *JAMA* **2003**, *289*, 559–567. [CrossRef] [PubMed]
18. Mostofi, K.; Gharaie Moghaddam, B.; Karimi Khouzan, R.; Daryabin, M. The Reliability of LERI's Sign in L4 and L3 Radiculalgia. *J. Clin. Neurosci.* **2018**, *50*, 102–104. [CrossRef] [PubMed]
19. Rigo, M. Differential Diagnosis of Back Pain in Adult Scoliosis (Non Operated Patients). *Scoliosis* **2010**, *5*, O44. [CrossRef]
20. Kleimeyer, J.P.; Liu, N.; Hu, S.S.; Cheng, I.; Alamin, T.; Grottkau, B.E.; Kukreja, S.; Wood, K.B. The Relationship Between Lumbar Lateral Listhesis and Radiculopathy in Adult Scoliosis. *Spine* **2019**, *44*, 1003–1009. [CrossRef] [PubMed]
21. Daniels, A.H.; Durand, W.M.; Lafage, R.; Zhang, A.S.; Hamilton, D.K.; Passias, P.G.; Kim, H.J.; Protopsaltis, T.; Lafage, V.; Smith, J.S.; et al. Lateral Thoracolumbar Listhesis as an Independent Predictor of Disability in Adult Scoliosis Patients: Multivariable Assessment Before and After Surgical Realignment. *Neurosurgery* **2021**, *89*, 1080–1086. [CrossRef] [PubMed]
22. Zaina, F.; Poggio, M.; Donzelli, S.; Negrini, S. Can Bracing Help Adults with Chronic Back Pain and Scoliosis? Short-Term Results from a Pilot Study. *Prosthet. Orthot. Int.* **2018**, *42*, 410–414. [CrossRef]
23. Zaina, F.; Poggio, M.; Di Felice, F.; Donzelli, S.; Negrini, S. Bracing Adults with Chronic Low Back Pain Secondary to Severe Scoliosis: Six Months Results of a Prospective Pilot Study. *Eur. Spine J.* **2021**, *30*, 2962–2966. [CrossRef] [PubMed]
24. Zaina, F.; Ferrario, I.; Caronni, A.; Scarano, S.; Donzelli, S.; Negrini, S. Measuring Quality of Life in Adults with Scoliosis: A Cross-Sectional Study Comparing SRS-22 and ISYQOL Questionnaires. *J. Clin. Med.* **2023**, *12*, 5071. [CrossRef]
25. Mannion, A.F.; Elfering, A.; Bago, J.; Pellise, F.; Vila-Casademunt, A.; Richner-Wunderlin, S.; Domingo-Sàbat, M.; Obeid, I.; Acaroglu, E.; Alanay, A.; et al. Factor Analysis of the SRS-22 Outcome Assessment Instrument in Patients with Adult Spinal Deformity. *Eur. Spine J.* **2017**, *27*, 685–699. [CrossRef]
26. Ha, K.-Y.; Jang, W.-H.; Kim, Y.-H.; Park, D.-C. Clinical Relevance of the SRS-Schwab Classification for Degenerative Lumbar Scoliosis. *Spine* **2016**, *41*, E282–E288. [CrossRef]

27. Monticone, M.; Ambrosini, E.; Cazzaniga, D.; Rocca, B.; Motta, L.; Cerri, C.; Brayda-Bruno, M.; Lovi, A. Adults with Idiopathic Scoliosis Improve Disability after Motor and Cognitive Rehabilitation: Results of a Randomised Controlled Trial. *Eur. Spine J.* **2016**, *25*, 3120–3129. [CrossRef] [PubMed]
28. McAviney, J.; Mee, J.; Fazalbhoy, A.; Du Plessis, J.; Brown, B.T. A Systematic Literature Review of Spinal Brace/Orthosis Treatment for Adults with Scoliosis between 1967 and 2018: Clinical Outcomes and Harms Data. *BMC Musculoskelet. Disord.* **2020**, *21*, 87. [CrossRef]

Disclaimer/Publisher's Note: The statements, opinions and data contained in all publications are solely those of the individual author(s) and contributor(s) and not of MDPI and/or the editor(s). MDPI and/or the editor(s) disclaim responsibility for any injury to people or property resulting from any ideas, methods, instructions or products referred to in the content.

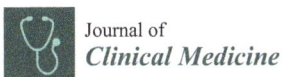

Article

Measuring Quality of Life in Adults with Scoliosis: A Cross-Sectional Study Comparing SRS-22 and ISYQOL Questionnaires

Fabio Zaina [1], Irene Ferrario [1], Antonio Caronni [2,3,*], Stefano Scarano [2,3], Sabrina Donzelli [1] and Stefano Negrini [4,5]

1. ISICO (Italian Scientific Spine Institute), Via Roberto Bellarmino 13/1, 20141 Milan, Italy
2. IRCCS, Istituto Auxologico Italiano, Department of Neurorehabilitation Sciences, Ospedale San Luca, 20149 Milan, Italy
3. Department of Biomedical Sciences for Health, Università degli Studi di Milano, 20133 Milan, Italy
4. Department of Biomedical, Surgical and Dental Sciences, University "La Statale", 20122 Milan, Italy
5. IRCCS Istituto Ortopedico Galeazzi, 20157 Milan, Italy
* Correspondence: a.caronni@auxologico.it

Abstract: Idiopathic scoliosis is common in adulthood and can impact patients' physical and psychological health. The Scoliosis Research Society-22 Questionnaire (SRS-22) has been designed to assess health-related quality of life (HRQOL) in idiopathic scoliosis, and it is the most used disease-specific outcome tool from adolescence to adulthood. More recently, the Italian Spine Youth Quality of Life (ISYQOL) international questionnaire was developed, which performs better than SRS-22 in adolescent spinal deformities. However, the ISYQOL questionnaire has never been tested in adults. This study compares the construct validity of ISYQOL and SRS-22 with the Rasch analysis (partial credit model). We recruited 150 adults and 50 adolescents with scoliosis (≥30° Cobb). SRS-22, but not ISQYOL, showed disordered categories and one item not fitting the Rasch model. A 21-item SRS-22 version with revised categories was arranged and further compared to ISYQOL. Both questionnaires showed multidimensionality, and some items (SRS-22 in a greater number) functioned differently in persons of different ages. However, the artefacts caused by multidimensionality and differential functioning had a low impact on the questionnaires' measures. The construct validity of ISYQOL International and the revised SRS-22 are comparable. Both questionnaires (but not the original SRS-22) can return measures of disease burden in adults with scoliosis.

Keywords: quality of life; adult scoliosis; rasch analysis; psychometrics

Citation: Zaina, F.; Ferrario, I.; Caronni, A.; Scarano, S.; Donzelli, S.; Negrini, S. Measuring Quality of Life in Adults with Scoliosis: A Cross-Sectional Study Comparing SRS-22 and ISYQOL Questionnaires. *J. Clin. Med.* **2023**, *12*, 5071. https://doi.org/10.3390/jcm12155071

Academic Editors: Deed Harrison, Ibrahim Moustafa and Paul Oakley

Received: 28 June 2023
Revised: 20 July 2023
Accepted: 29 July 2023
Published: 1 August 2023

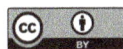

Copyright: © 2023 by the authors. Licensee MDPI, Basel, Switzerland. This article is an open access article distributed under the terms and conditions of the Creative Commons Attribution (CC BY) license (https://creativecommons.org/licenses/by/4.0/).

1. Introduction

Spinal deformities, such as scoliosis, may significantly impact patients' physical and psychological health [1]. Adolescents with idiopathic scoliosis can show psychological and emotional distress, with anxiety as the most common symptom [2]. They may exhibit poorer psychosocial functioning and body image than their healthy peers, while adults with scoliosis show concerns about the risk of disability, body image, and physical health problems [3]. During adulthood, this pathology can cause lower back pain, bent posture, shortness of breath, and reduced autonomy in everyday activities [4]. Disease-specific outcome tools can assess the extent of this impact, e.g., the Scoliosis Research Society-22 Questionnaire (SRS-22), the most used instrument to assess health-related quality of life (HRQOL) in patients with idiopathic scoliosis [5]. Initially developed [5,6] in a young population, many studies have examined its application for adult spinal deformities, demonstrating its usefulness in this population [7–9]. Nevertheless, other papers showed drawbacks and limitations [10].

When used as an HRQOL measure, the SRS-22, developed in the classical test theory framework (CTT), the oldest set of psychometrics techniques for developing scales and questionnaires, has a significant flaw: its total ordinal score is not a measure but a measure approximation at best [11]. Equal changes in ordinal scores do not necessarily reflect identical changes in the quantity of the variable of interest. This fact has practical consequences: customary statistics such as effect size can be misleading when calculated on ordinal scores.

Like CTT, the Rasch analysis is a statistical method designed to build and assess questionnaires. If a questionnaire's score empirically demonstrates compliance with the assumptions of the Rasch analysis, it is possible to turn these total scores into actual interval measures [11].

Rasch's analysis revealed that the SRS-22 has poor metric properties, failing to assess HRQOL properly in non-surgical adolescents and children [12]. Therefore, we developed the Italian Spine Youth Quality of Life (ISYQOL), using Rasch analysis, as a new patient-reported outcome measure to assess HRQOL in adolescents with spinal deformities [13]. ISYQOL had satisfactory construct validity and, compared to SRS-22, better known-groups validity, detecting the impact of disease severity on HRQOL [14]. More recently, a different version called "ISYQOL International" has been validated in a multicentre international study, the cross-culturally equivalent version of the questionnaire [15].

To our knowledge, no other Rasch-consistent questionnaire measuring HRQOL in adults with spinal deformities is available, and the data on ISYQOL's and ISYQOL International's validity come solely from the adolescent population. Therefore, the present study aims to verify the construct validity of ISYQOL International and to compare its properties to the SRS-22 in adults with scoliosis. We hypothesize that the ISYQOL can perform at least as well as the SRS-22 in adults with scoliosis. Moreover, we expect ISYQOL to perform similarly in adults and adolescents with scoliosis.

2. Materials and Methods

2.1. Study Characteristics

We conducted a cross-sectional study based on data from an ongoing prospective database collecting records from patients attending a tertiary outpatient clinic specializing in the conservative treatment of spinal deformities in Italy.

2.2. Data Collection

As standard practice, all patients attending our rehabilitation centre complete the self-administered SRS-22 and ISYQOL questionnaires before every medical consultation.

2.3. Participants

On 8 October 2022, we extracted all consecutive patients respecting the following criteria: (1) age ≥ 18 years, (2) diagnosis of idiopathic scoliosis with a curve of 30° Cobb or more, and (3) availability of both the ISYQOL and SRS-22 questionnaires. Exclusion criteria were the following: (1) history of spine surgery, (2) history of relevant diseases, surgery, or trauma, and (3) a positive neurologic examination. Only questionnaires not exceeding two missing answers were included in the analysis. From this group, we randomly extracted 150 patients. Since we expected that age could impact the results of the questionnaires, we made a cluster sampling based on age and sex. We had six groups based on age: 20–29, 30–39, 40–49, 50–59, 60–69, and 70–79 years. For each group, we extracted 20 females and five males as per the different sex prevalence of spinal deformities. This is based on the published literature and our data. A systematic review has reported a prevalence of degenerative scoliosis of 41.2% for females versus 27.5% for males [16]. Considering idiopathic scoliosis, the ratio is 7/1 in favour of females [1]. In our database, which includes a mixed population, the ratio is about 4–5/1 for all kinds of scoliosis during adulthood.

Moreover, we randomly extracted a sample of 50 individuals aged between 14 and 18 years from the dataset we analysed in our previous study for the ISYQOL validation study [14]. We included ten participants for each of the five years of age (eight females and two males), all affected by idiopathic scoliosis and all not wearing a brace.

2.4. Sample Size Calculation

In the Rasch analysis framework, about 200 questionnaires are usually enough to produce stable estimates [17]. In addition, we arranged age subgroups of equal size to comply with some recent guidelines and recommendations for the differential item functioning (DIF) analysis (see below) [18,19].

2.5. Health-Related Quality-of-Life Questionnaires: SRS-22 and ISYQOL

The SRS-22 questionnaire [5] consists of 22 items scored on five ordinal categories (1–5), with higher scores corresponding to a lower disease burden and, thus, better quality of life. It measures specific aspects of HRQOL, covering five domains: self-image, mental health, pain, function, and treatment satisfaction [20,21].

ISYQOL International derives from ISYQOL. We translated ISYQOL into different languages and assessed its cross-cultural validity. We removed four items from the original questionnaire [15]. The ISYQOL International consists of 16 items scored on three categories (0–2); the higher the category numeral, the more the disease burden. The ordinal ISYQOL total score is converted into an interval measure with logit as the measurement unit (the higher the logit measure, the higher the disease burden). The ISYQOL ordinal score can also be expressed on an interval scale ranging from 0 to 100%, with 100% indicating an excellent quality of life. It consists of two subscales, one (9 items) regarding spine health and the other (7 items) regarding brace wearing. Only the ISYQOL International spine domain was collected here since no participant wore a brace at the point of inclusion in the study.

2.6. Statistical Analysis

We ran the Rasch analysis in the following steps [12,13,15] (Appendices A and B).

2.6.1. Categories' Functioning

The categories' functioning was evaluated by assessing their average order, as per Linacre [22], and the order of the modal thresholds, as per Andrich [23].

2.6.2. Fit the Model

We can extract measures from the questionnaire's scores if categories are ordered and data fit one of the Rasch family models (here, Masters' partial credit model [24]).

We used the mean square (MnSq) and the z-standardised (Z-Std) statistics ("infit" and "outfit" variants) to quantify the departure of the observed data from the model's prediction and the probability that this departure was due to chance, respectively.

Here, an item was considered to "misfit", i.e., not fit the model adequately, if:
outfit MnSq > 2.0 and absolute outfit Z-Std > 1.96, or
infit MnSq > 1.5 and absolute infit Z-Std > 1.96.

2.6.3. Dimensionality

Measures are unidimensional, meaning they reflect a single variable's amount. In the Rasch framework, principal components with an eigenvalue >2 from a principal component analysis (PCA) calculated on the model's residuals indicate multidimensionality.

In the case that multidimensionality is found, whether this multidimensionality harms measurements can be tested by assessing if cluster 1 items (items with a large and positive loading on the principal component) and cluster 3 items (items with a large and negative loading) return a different participants measure from cluster 2 items (those items loading low on the principal component, thus reflecting only the variable grasped by the model of Rasch).

Suppose persons' measures from cluster 1 and cluster 3 are comparable. In that case, the artefact caused by the hidden variable highlighted from the principal component is not strong enough to cause a severe measurement artefact [25]. For this comparison, we used ANOVA.

2.6.4. Differential Item Functioning

Differential item functioning (DIF) indicates that an item does not work the same in different groups of respondents. Given the study's aim, the current analysis focused on the DIF for age. We reorganized the participants' sample into the following age classes: adolescents (from 14 to 18 years), young adults (from 20 to 39 years), middle-aged adults (from 40 to 59 years) and older adults (from 60 to 79 years). As a complementary analysis, we evaluated DIF for gender (males vs. females). We tested the DIF of SRS-22 and ISYQOL International items following Linacre [25].

Suppose the calibration of an item is different in a subgroup of participants and in the primary analysis. If this difference is <0.5 logit with $p > 0.01$, the DIF can be considered too small to matter.

In the case of a large (>0.5 logit) and significant ($p < 0.01$) DIF being found for an item, the observed scores of the participants' subset on this item and their expected scores are compared to provide an easy understanding of the artefact caused by the DIF in terms of the questionnaire's total score.

2.6.5. Questionnaire Reliability and Targeting

We reported the ISYQOL International and the SRS-22 reliability as "Rasch persons' reliability", similar to Cronbach's alpha. From this reliability index, we calculated the number of strata, the number of significantly different levels of the disease burden a person can progress through (Supplementary Materials 1 in [26]).

Floor and ceiling effects were calculated as the percentage of respondents obtaining the minimum and maximum total questionnaire scores, respectively. The size of the difference between the persons and the items measures complements this information. A questionnaire with no floor effect, no ceiling effect, and 0 logit difference between participants and items mean measure targets appropriately the recruited sample participants. The item and person maps graphically show the targeting of persons compared to the measurement instrument.

Finally, we provide the score-to-measure tables to allow future users to turn the questionnaires' total scores into interval measures.

We used FACETS 3.84.0 and WINSTEPS 5.4.3.0 for the Rasch analysis (partial credit model). We performed the statistics using the R (R version 4.2.3 "Shortstop Beagle") software. Type 1 error probability was set to 0.05 as customary in all analyses, but we lowered this threshold for DIF to 0.01 because of multiple statistical testing [15,27].

2.7. Ethical Approval

The local ethics committee approved the study (Comitato Etico Milano Area 2, 215_2022bis), and we registered the protocol on clinicaltrials.gov (NCT05333757). This study did not receive dedicated funding support. All participants gave written informed consent.

3. Results

At the time of data extraction, our database included 3254 adult patients with scoliosis or other spinal deformities (2540 females, 714 males), fulfilling the inclusion criteria. From these, we randomly selected 150 subjects (120 females, 30 males). For each group, we had 20 females and five males diagnosed with scoliosis based on clinical and radiological assessment.

Table 1 reports the clinical features of the participants included in the current analysis.

Table 1. Participants' clinical data.

	Adults	Adolescents
Males vs. females, N	30 vs. 120	10 vs. 40
Mean age (SD), years	49 (17.8)	16 (1.4)
Mean disease severity (SD), °Cobb	46.2 (16.6)	24.7 (9)
Median TRACE score (IQR)	7 (4)	5 (3)

N: number of participants; SD: standard deviation; °Cobb: angle of scoliosis curvature measured according to Cobb; IQR: interquartile range; TRACE: trunk aesthetic clinical evaluation (ordinal score of back aesthetics ranging from 1 to 12, with a high score marking a poor trunk aesthetic appearance).

3.1. Rasch Analysis of ISYQOL International

All nine items of ISYQOL International had ordered categories and thresholds (Table A1 in Appendix B).

Regarding the fit to the model, infit and outfit MnSq were suitable for all the questionnaire's items (Table 2).

Table 2. Calibration of items of ISYQOL International and their fit to the model.

Items	Calibration	SE	Infit		Outfit	
			MnSq	Z-Std	MnSq	Z-Std
1 (1), get worse	−1.95	0.17	0.97	−0.30	0.99	0.00
2 (2), worried back pain	−0.95	0.15	1.12	1.17	1.54	3.11
3 (3), big deal	1.76	0.16	1.00	0.00	0.95	−0.23
4 (4), worried not get better	−0.13	0.14	1.01	0.10	1.08	0.61
5 (7), suffering	0.85	0.15	0.93	−0.64	0.84	−1.22
6 (8), appearance	1.10	0.15	0.82	−1.92	0.75	−1.81
7 (9), worried back problem	−1.95	0.18	0.83	−1.68	0.75	−1.72
8 (11), bother to show	0.59	0.14	1.25	2.31	1.24	1.53
9 (12), worried visible	0.69	0.15	1.07	0.69	1.02	0.23

Items: the item number and a keyword summarising the item content; the item number of ISYQOL original is also reported in brackets. Calibration: item calibration (i.e., item measure) expressed in logit. SE: standard error in the item calibration (logit). Infit: inlier sensitive fit indices; outfit: outlier sensitive fit indices. MnSq: mean square statistic; Z-std: z-standardised statistic.

The PCA of the model's residuals highlighted that another dimension, in addition to the one taken into account by the Rasch model, affects the questionnaire scores. The eigenvalue of the first principal component was 2.55, a value which indicates that the hidden dimension affects the score of three items at most.

Cluster 1, i.e., the cluster of items with a positive loading on the first principal component, included items 6, 8, and 9 (8, 11, and 12 of ISYQOL original; Figure 1). Notably, all these three items had a large (>0.60) loading. Cluster 3 (i.e., the items with negative loading) included items 1, 2, and 7 (1, 2, and 9 of ISYQOL original).

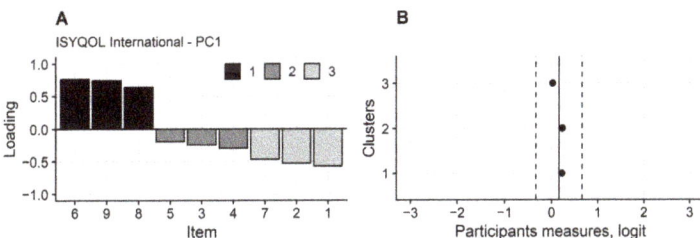

Figure 1. ISYQOL International dimensionality. The principal component analysis (PCA) calculated on the model's residuals is provided for the ISYQOL International questionnaire. Panel (**A**): loadings of the ISYQOL International items on the first principal component from the PCA. The items are grouped into three clusters (cluster 1, 2, and 3). Cluster 2 (dark grey) items load low in absolute value on the principal component. Their score is scarcely affected by the hidden variable flagged by this component but mainly reflects the variable, i.e., disease burden, grasped by the Rasch model. On the contrary, the score of cluster 1 items (black) is inflated by an additional hidden variable, while that of cluster 3 items (light grey) is reduced. Panel (**B**): participants are measured with cluster 1, 2, and 3 items, and their mean measure is compared (black dots). Vertical continuous line: participants' mean measures from the total ISYQOL International. Vertical dashed lines: participants' mean measures from the total ISYQOL International ± 0.5 logit. On average, the participants' measures from the three clusters of items are only slightly different from each other and minimally different from the participants' measures from the full ISYQOL International. In particular, the mean difference between the clusters and the total questionnaire measures is well below 0.5 logits. Even if an additional unwanted variable contaminates the scores of cluster 1 and 3 items, this variable causes a negligible

measurement artefact. Extreme persons, i.e., those obtaining the maximum or minimum questionnaire total score, whose real measure is unknown, have not been considered in this analysis.

ANOVA comparing the persons' measures from cluster 1, 2, and 3 items was not significant ($F_{2,368} = 1.09$; $p = 0.337$), indicating that on average, clusters 1 and 3, i.e., the clusters of items more severely affected by the first principal component hidden variable, measure the same as cluster 2 items, i.e., the items prominently reflecting the variable grasped by the model of Rasch.

Table 3 reports the results of the DIF analysis.

Table 3. Age-related differential item functioning of the ISYQOL International and SRS-22 questionnaires.

Item	Group	Obs − Exp	Bias	SE	*p* Value
ISYQOL International					
8 (11), bother to show	Adolescents	0.19	0.83	0.28	0.006
SRS-22					
3, nervous person	Older	0.31	0.61	0.20	0.003
4, back shape	Adolescents	−0.46	0.68	0.17	0.000
8, back pain at rest	Older	0.36	0.51	0.17	0.004
12, around the house	Adolescents	0.39	1.19	0.35	0.002

Item: item number and its keyword; the item number of ISYQOL original is also provided in brackets. Group: participants group for which the item's calibration differs from the primary analysis (e.g., the calibration of ISYQOL International item 8 is different in adolescents than in the primary analysis). Obs-Exp: artefact in the item score caused by differential item functioning (DIF) and expressed as the difference between the observed (Obs) and expected (Exp) score. The expected score is calculated given the item's calibration from the primary analysis. For example, DIF for age inflates by 0.19 the score of adolescents on ISYQOL International item 8 (i.e., their score on this item is 0.19 points higher than it should be). Bias: absolute value difference, expressed in logits, between the item's calibration from the primary analysis and the participants' group. SE: standard error (logit) of the bias. *p* value: type 1 error probability of the t-test with the null hypothesis: "item's calibrations in group and primary analysis are not different from each other". For both the ISYQOL International (upper row) and the revised SRS-22 (lower rows), only the items with DIF > 0.5 logit with $p < 0.01$ are reported. No DIF was found for gender.

One item only (item 8, corresponding to item 11 in the ISYQOL original) was affected by DIF for age.

In detail, item 8's calibration was lower in adolescents than in the primary analysis, including participants of all ages (calibration difference = 0.83 logits, $p = 0.006$).

The age-related DIF for item 8 indicates that adolescents are more likely to be bothered than young, middle-aged, and older people by showing their physical appearance despite the same overall burden of disease level.

Even if large at the item level and statistically significant, the age-related DIF of item 8 caused a minor artefact on the ISYQOL total score (and hence on the ISYQOL measures). On average, adolescents scored more than expected on item 8. However, the difference between the observed score on item 8 (biased since inflated by DIF) and the expected score given the primary analysis was 0.19 (i.e., less than one-fifth of a point of the ISYQOL International total score).

We found no DIF for gender.

The ISYQOL International's reliability (model, sample reliability, extremes included) was 0.88, which allows for distinguishing 3.91 strata. The questionnaire targeting was satisfactory, as indicated by a participant's mean measure of 0.27 logits (SD = 2.52 logits).

Regarding the ceiling and floor effect, ten participants (out of 200, i.e., 5%) obtained the maximum score and five (i.e., 2.5%) the minimum.

Figure 2 shows the item and person maps of ISYQOL International. Table 4 provides the ISYQOL International score-to-measure conversion table.

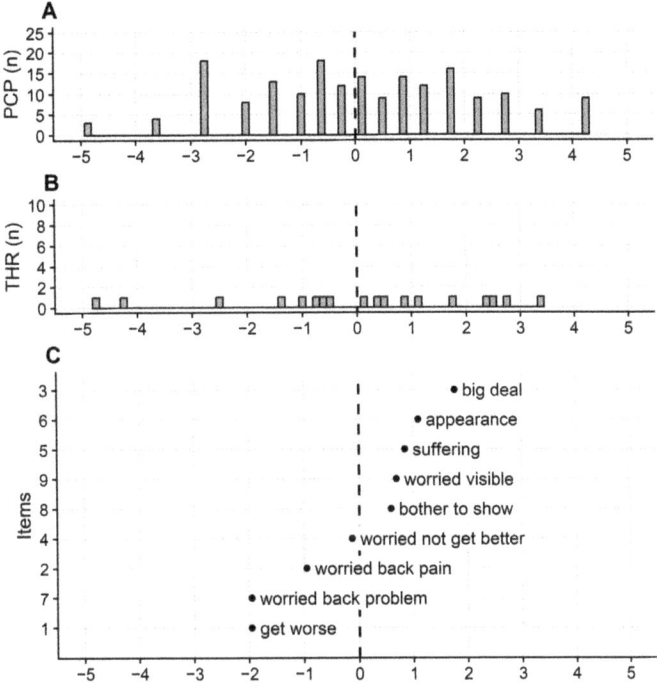

Figure 2. ISYQOL International maps. Maps of persons (**A**), thresholds (**B**), and items (**C**) of the ISYQOL International questionnaire (spine domain). PCP: participants; n: number of; THR: Andrich's thresholds. X-axis: line of the construct (i.e., the disease burden continuum) measured in logits. The disease burden increases from left to right. ISYQOL logit measures are measures of disease burden: the higher the logit measure, the more the disease burden. Rightmost persons on the disease burden line (**A**) suffer a high disease burden. The rightmost items (**C**) flag a high disease burden: only persons suffering a high disease burden will affirm the content of these items. In (**C**), the Y-axis reports the ISYQOL International item number. Labels in plot (**C**) are keywords recollecting the item content. The dot position on the X-axis returns the item measures, called here "item calibration". Vertical dashed segment: items mean calibration, set to 0 logits, as customary.

Table 4. Score-to-measure conversion table of ISYQOL International.

Score	Burden of Disease		HRQOL	
	Measure, Logit	SE, Logit	Measure, %	SE, %
0	−6.44	1.95	100.0	16.2
1	−4.89	1.24	87.1	10.3
2	−3.64	1.03	76.7	8.6
3	−2.73	0.89	69.1	7.4
4	−2.04	0.78	63.3	6.5
5	−1.49	0.71	58.8	5.9
6	−1.03	0.66	54.9	5.5
7	−0.61	0.63	51.4	5.3
8	−0.22	0.62	48.1	5.2
9	0.16	0.61	45.0	5.1

Table 4. Cont.

Score	Burden of Disease		HRQOL	
	Measure, Logit	SE, Logit	Measure, %	SE, %
10	0.54	0.61	41.9	5.1
11	0.92	0.62	38.7	5.2
12	1.32	0.64	35.4	5.3
13	1.73	0.66	31.9	5.5
14	2.19	0.69	28.1	5.8
15	2.70	0.74	23.9	6.2
16	3.32	0.84	18.7	7.0
17	4.22	1.10	11.2	9.1
18	5.56	1.88	0.0	15.7

Score: ISYQOL International (spine health domain) total ordinal score. Measure, logit: interval measures of disease burden expressed in logits, i.e., the measurement unit of the Rasch analysis. Measure, %: interval measures reported on a user-friendly scale ranging from 0 to 100%, with 100% indicating full health-related quality of life (i.e., no disease burden). SE: standard error. Note that the higher the ISYQOL International total score, the higher the problems caused by the back condition to the patient (i.e., the higher the disease burden). The relationship between logit measures and ordinal scores is monotonic. Therefore, the higher the logit measure, the more the disease burden. Originally, ISYQOL was conceptualized as an HRQOL measure rather than a disease burden measure. For this reason, measure %, which is reversed compared to the total score and the logit measure, is also reported.

3.2. Rasch Analysis of SRS-22

On the first analysis run, 11 items had disordered categories. One possible reason was that the respondents seldom selected the lower categories. As a result, the accuracy of estimating the categories' parameters was poor.

We rearranged items 7, 8, 9, 13, 17, and 20 by collapsing the original categories 1 and 2 into the new category 1. For items 5, 11, 15, 18, and 22, it was necessary to collapse categories 1, 2, and 3. Note that after this procedure, SRS-22 consisted of a mixture of items scored on five (11 items), four (6 items), and three (5 items) categories.

The collapsing procedure efficiently ordered all the items' categories (Table A2 in Appendix B)

However, modal thresholds were disordered in seven items (7, 9, 12, 15, 16, 17, and 19).

On a subsequent analysis run, item 15 did not fit the model because of a large and significant outfit (MnSq = 2.97; Z-Std = 3.30). On a new run in which item 15 was dropped from the questionnaire, all 21 items properly fit the model (Table 5). The analysis continues assessing the measurement properties of this revised version of the SRS-22.

Table 5. Calibration of items of the revised SRS-22 and their fit to the model.

Items	Calibration	SE	Infit		Outfit	
			MnSq	Z-Std	MnSq	Z-Std
1, pain six months	−0.28	0.09	0.69	−3.72	0.66	−3.67
2, pain last month	−0.15	0.09	0.75	−2.83	0.71	−3.06
3, nervous person	0.40	0.10	1.14	1.41	1.21	2.02
4, back shape	0.70	0.09	1.09	0.96	1.10	1.00
5, activity level	−0.24	0.12	0.87	−1.46	0.85	−1.13
6, look in clothes	0.32	0.10	1.04	0.41	1.04	0.45
7, down in the dumps	−0.71	0.10	0.97	−0.27	1.13	0.68
8, back pain at rest	0.30	0.09	1.42	4.07	1.52	3.90
9, work/school	−0.41	0.09	1.09	0.79	1.08	0.44
10, trunk appearance	1.19	0.10	1.00	0.03	1.01	0.10
11, pain medications	−2.13	0.18	0.96	−0.24	1.00	0.06
12, around the house	−0.19	0.08	0.74	−2.73	0.81	−1.30
13, calm and peaceful	0.72	0.11	1.17	1.73	1.18	1.72
14, personal relationships	−0.72	0.09	0.80	−1.82	0.72	−1.63

Table 5. *Cont.*

Items	Calibration	SE	Infit		Outfit	
			MnSq	Z-Std	MnSq	Z-Std
16, downhearted and blue	−0.52	0.09	1.09	0.83	1.08	0.64
17, days off	−0.99	0.12	1.35	1.67	1.80	1.21
18, going out	−0.61	0.13	0.89	−1.10	0.98	−0.07
19, feel attractive	1.29	0.09	0.97	−0.22	0.91	−0.84
20, happy person	0.67	0.11	1.03	0.37	1.05	0.48
21, satisfied with results	0.52	0.09	0.95	−0.52	0.93	−0.65
22, same management again	0.84	0.11	1.20	2.26	1.24	2.01

Same abbreviations as Table 2. SRS-22 item 15 is not reported because of outfit values beyond the tolerance limits. The item numbering of the original SRS-22 was kept. Remember that the categories of the original SRS-22 items have been extensively rearranged.

The PCA of the residuals highlighted two hidden dimensions, as indicated by the eigenvalue of the first principal component (3.45) and that of the second (2.72).

Items 1, 2, and 12 were the three items with the largest loading of cluster 1 (Figure 3). Items 4, 10, and 19 were the three with the largest negative loading (i.e., cluster 3 items with the largest loading). Regarding the second principal component, the three cluster 1 items were items 7, 13, and 16. The three most significant cluster 3 items were items 10, 19, and 21.

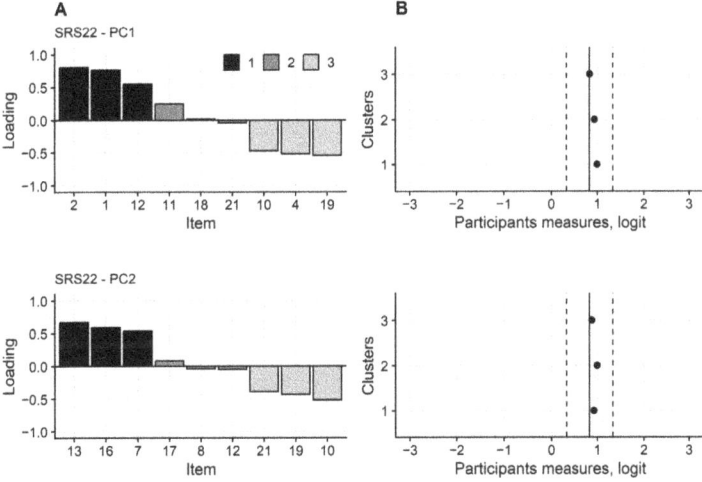

Figure 3. SRS-22 dimensionality. The principal component analysis (PCA) of the SRS-22 questionnaire (revised version) highlighted two principal components, indicating that the score of some SRS-22 items were affected by two hidden variables in addition to the Rasch dimension. Same symbols and abbreviations as Figure 1. Upper graphs in panels (**A**,**B**) report the analysis for the first principal component. The lower graphs report the clusters on the second principal component. The revised SRS-22 consists of 21 items. Here, are only the three cluster 1 items with the largest positive loadings, the three cluster 3 items with the largest negative loadings, and the three cluster 2 items with the most negligible loading.

Despite the presence of two additional dimensions, person measures from the three items clusters were not significantly different from each other (contrasts on the first principal component: $F_{2,396} = 1.57$; $p = 0.209$; contrasts on the second principal component: $F_{2,396} = 0.60$; $p = 0.549$).

Four items (i.e., items 3, 4, 8, and 12) were affected by DIF for age (Table 3).

Item 3's calibration was significantly lower when calculated in the older adults group than when we inputted the total participants' sample into the analysis. (i.e., item 3's calibration was lower in older persons than in middle-aged, young adults, and adolescents).

We found the same pattern for item 8. Item 4's calibration was higher, and item 12's was lower in adolescents.

Due to these differences in the items' calibrations, the older adults observed scores on items 3 and 8 was larger than expected. Adolescents' scores on item 4 were lower than predicted, while on item 12 were higher.

However, when we consider the artefact they cause in the SRS-22 total score, the biases of items 4 and 12 have opposite signs (the first decreases and the second increases the item's score), thus compensating each other. The bias of items 3 and 8 inflates the SRS-22 total score by 0.31 and 0.36 points (i.e., 0.67 points when considered together) in older persons. Similarly to ISYQOL International, DIF is present, but its consequences on the measures derived from the total questionnaire score seem modest.

We found no DIF for gender.

The reliability of the modified version of the SRS-22 questionnaire was 0.91, and the number of strata was 4.59.

Only one respondent obtained the SRS-22 maximum score. However, the participants' mean measure was 0.86 logits (SD = 1.18 logits), flagging poor targeting of the SRS-22 questionnaire in this sample (Figure 4).

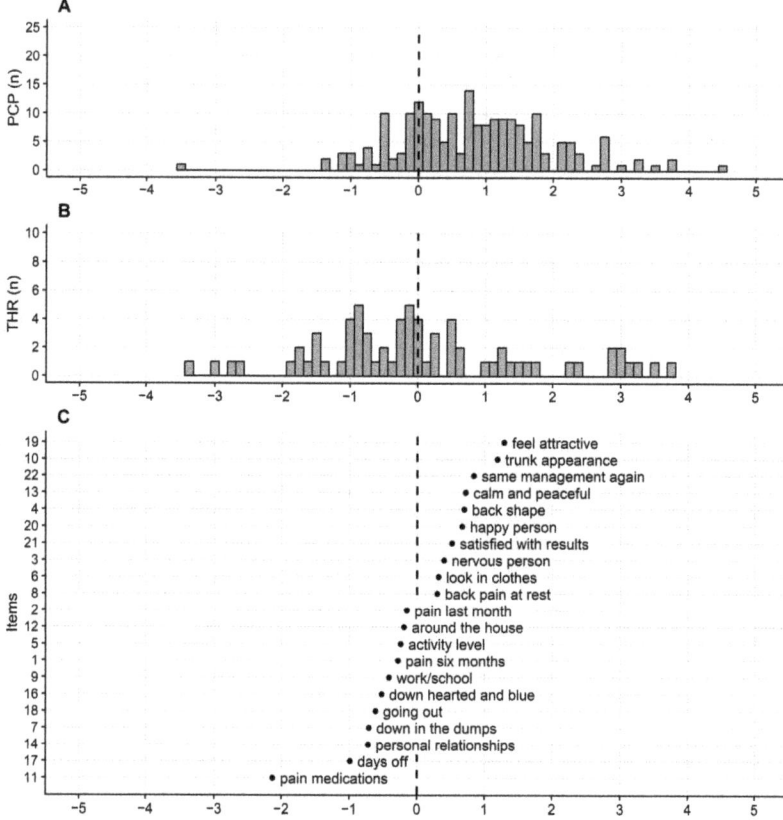

Figure 4. Revised SRS-22 maps. Same abbreviations as Figure 1. SRS-22 logit measures are measures of quality of life. So, the higher the logit measure, the higher the quality of life. People experiencing a full quality of life are on the right of the continuum, and quality of life decreases from right to left. Note that the persons map (**A**) histogram is displaced to the right (e.g., the distribution mode is about 0.75 logits). This indicates that persons score high on the questionnaire and that the SRS-22 items are

too easy to endorse for the participants' sample recruited here. The thresholds histogram (**B**) shows several thresholds with overlapping calibrations between −1 and 0 logits. While many thresholds (or items) within the same construct range increase the measurement precision, it also points out some redundancy in the questionnaire. (**C**) items map.

We provide the score-to-measure table of the revised SRS-22 version in Table 6.

Table 6. Score-to-measure conversion table of the revised SRS-22.

Score	HRQOL		HRQOL	
	Measure, Logit	SE, Logit	Measure, %	SE, %
21	−5.99	1.85	0.0	14.7
22	−4.73	1.04	10.1	8.3
23	−3.96	0.75	16.2	6.0
24	−3.49	0.63	19.9	5.0
25	−3.15	0.55	22.7	4.4
26	−2.88	0.50	24.8	4.0
27	−2.65	0.46	26.6	3.6
28	−2.46	0.42	28.2	3.4
29	−2.29	0.40	29.5	3.2
30	−2.14	0.37	30.7	3.0
31	−2.01	0.36	31.7	2.8
32	−1.89	0.34	32.7	2.7
33	−1.78	0.33	33.6	2.6
34	−1.67	0.32	34.4	2.5
35	−1.58	0.31	35.2	2.4
36	−1.49	0.30	35.9	2.4
37	−1.40	0.29	36.6	2.3
38	−1.32	0.28	37.2	2.3
39	−1.24	0.28	37.8	2.2
40	−1.17	0.27	38.4	2.2
41	−1.10	0.27	39.0	2.1
42	−1.03	0.26	39.6	2.1
43	−0.96	0.26	40.1	2.1
44	−0.89	0.26	40.7	2.1
45	−0.82	0.26	41.2	2.1
46	−0.76	0.26	41.7	2.0
47	−0.69	0.25	42.2	2.0
48	−0.63	0.25	42.7	2.0
49	−0.56	0.25	43.3	2.0
50	−0.50	0.25	43.8	2.0
51	−0.44	0.25	44.3	2.0
52	−0.37	0.25	44.8	2.0
53	−0.31	0.26	45.3	2.0
54	−0.24	0.26	45.8	2.0

Table 6. *Cont.*

Score	HRQOL Measure, Logit	SE, Logit	HRQOL Measure, %	SE, %
55	−0.18	0.26	46.4	2.1
56	−0.11	0.26	46.9	2.1
57	−0.04	0.26	47.4	2.1
58	0.03	0.26	48.0	2.1
59	0.10	0.26	48.5	2.1
60	0.17	0.27	49.1	2.1
61	0.24	0.27	49.7	2.2
62	0.31	0.27	50.2	2.2
63	0.39	0.28	50.8	2.2
64	0.47	0.28	51.5	2.2
65	0.54	0.28	52.1	2.3
66	0.63	0.29	52.7	2.3
67	0.71	0.29	53.4	2.3
68	0.80	0.30	54.1	2.4
69	0.89	0.30	54.8	2.4
70	0.98	0.31	55.6	2.5
71	1.08	0.32	56.4	2.5
72	1.18	0.32	57.2	2.6
73	1.29	0.33	58.0	2.6
74	1.40	0.34	58.9	2.7
75	1.52	0.35	59.9	2.8
76	1.65	0.36	60.9	2.9
77	1.78	0.37	61.9	2.9
78	1.92	0.38	63.0	3.0
79	2.07	0.39	64.2	3.1
80	2.22	0.40	65.5	3.2
81	2.39	0.41	66.8	3.3
82	2.57	0.43	68.2	3.4
83	2.76	0.44	69.7	3.5
84	2.96	0.46	71.4	3.7
85	3.19	0.49	73.2	3.9
86	3.44	0.52	75.2	4.1
87	3.73	0.56	77.5	4.5
88	4.09	0.63	80.3	5.0
89	4.56	0.75	84.1	6.0
90	5.31	1.03	90.1	8.2
91	6.56	1.84	100.0	14.7

Same abbreviations as Table 4. SRS-22 logit and percentage measures are quality-of-life measures: the higher the measure, the better the patient. After collection, SRS-22 item scores are rearranged so that the higher the score for each item, the better the quality of life.

4. Discussion

Spinal deformities can negatively impact a patient's quality of life during adulthood. To monitor the changes over time, clinicians need specific tools to picture the patient's pain, activity limitations, and participation restrictions. Many validated and reliable tools are available for patients with chronic LBP [28]. They can also help in the case of spinal deformities but could lack some specificity. From a psychometrics perspective, their content validity is poor. For example, some items included in the Oswestry Disability Index (ODI), such as rest quality and travelling, are not specific for spinal deformities. In a recent study about bracing, despite the significant improvements in pain, the ODI failed to show clinically significant improvements [29]. In a sample of surgically treated patients, the SRS self-image domain demonstrated higher responsiveness to change, followed by SRS total, then SRS pain, and then ODI [7]. Unfortunately, it is unclear whether it was a limit of the ODI, or an issue related to the too-small clinical changes of patients. These findings and limits suggest the need for developing specific tools. The SRS-22 was explicitly designed for adolescent scoliosis patients managed in a surgical setting. For those treated conservatively, they showed some limits and mainly a ceiling effect [12]. Many authors and clinicians use the SRS-22 also in adults even though young patients were its original target, and some limits have already been reported [10]. The SRS-22 remains the most widely used questionnaire in adults with spinal deformities. Nevertheless, the challenges with the currently accepted standard questionnaire (SRS-22) for HRQOL assessments in scoliosis are detailed in the literature and application of the SRS-22 in the adult population with scoliotic deformities has been debated [30]. Currently, there is no gold standard that is reliable and valid for the complexity of the 'patient's perception' on how their deformity impacts their life. Recently, we developed a new tool, the ISYQOL, to measure conservatively managed patients during growth appropriately, but no data are available for adults. The current one was the first study to compare the properties of the ISYQOL to the SRS-22 in adults attending a rehabilitation centre specialized in the conservative treatment of spinal deformities.

Regarding the Rasch analysis, the original SRS-22 questionnaire, but not ISYQOL International, failed to meet the two basic assumptions of the analysis: the assumption of ordered categories and data-model fit.

Several SRS-22 items had disordered categories and thresholds, and disordered thresholds remain even after rearranging the categories so that their average measure is ordered. In addition, item 15 of SRS-22 does not fit the model. Therefore, in the fundamental measurement framework [11,31], the SRS-22 should not be used in its original form to measure the disease burden in adults with spinal deformities.

Despite rearranging the SRS-22 to comply with the ordered categories and data-model fit assumptions, multidimensionality still affects it, and DIF corrupts several items for age and gender. ISYQOL International suffers similar issues in this respect. However, regarding multidimensionality, SRS-22's measures of HRQOL are disturbed by two additional unknown variables, while those from ISYQOL International are disturbed by one. The SRS-22 is tridimensional, while ISYQOL International is bidimensional: considering that accurate measures are unidimensional [11], we can assume the latter to be better than the former.

Regarding DIF, DIF for age afflicts more SRS-22 than ISYQOL items.

From a measurement theory perspective, multidimensionality and DIF are serious flaws. However, the total questionnaire score and the measures extracted with the Rasch analysis from these scores are robust to some DIF and multidimensionality [32]. If a questionnaire demonstrates this measure's robustness, we can safely use it despite these flaws. Based on our findings, the ISYQOL International and the modified SRS-22 version can measure the disease burden despite the DIF and multidimensionality, since we experimentally found these flaws are negligible. However, the artefacts caused by DIF and multidimensionality would likely be non-negligible if single or groups of items were selected from the questionnaire and used for measuring, a frequently used practice for SRS-22 [7].

ISYQOL International has two additional strengths: it is shorter and more straightforward than the SRS-22 and better targeted than SRS-22. About this last point, the average

SRS-22 measure is larger than 0 logits, indicating that several SRS-22 items investigate a (low) range of HRQOL, which the patients included here do not experience. SRS-22 is not perfectly tuned to measure patients like those recruited here.

On the contrary, SRS-22's reliability is better than that of ISYQOL International, a finding which results from its large number of categories times items. However, the modest improvement in the reliability of SRS-22 comes at the expense of a more marked increase in the number of categories and items (91 for SRS-22 and 27 for the ISQYOL International—spine domain).

We already assessed the measurement properties of the SRS-22 with the Rasch analysis [12], and our previous study also pointed out different problems. However, in the current work, a more liberal analysis has been conducted, so the SRS-22 flaws seem less severe. Nevertheless, even if adherence to the analysis requirements is relaxed as much as possible, some significant drawbacks remain, such as disordered categories and a misfitting item.

Another reason for the different results of the current and our former work is that the participants recruited here were mostly adults. At the same time, previously, we studied SRS-22 functioning in children and adolescents. The DIF analysis highlights that, in most cases, adolescents usually understand several SRS-22 items differently from adults. Hence, SRS-22 could function differently in young people than adults, but further research is needed.

Study Limitations and Further Developments

The SRS-22 and ISYQOL International questionnaires demonstrated multidimensionality, suggesting they measure multiple HRQOL aspects. It has been empirically shown here that this multidimensionality is unlikely to harm. However, multidimensionality is always a measurement threat strictly, making the questionnaires' interpretation more challenging. In this regard, the additional hidden variable in ISYQOL International's scores and the two hidden variables in the SRS-22 remain to be discovered.

The same reasoning applies to the results of the DIF analysis (to note, DIF is simply another form of multidimensionality). The study found that some questionnaire items functioned differently in individuals of different ages. Furthermore, in this case it is shown that the measurement artefact caused by DIF is negligible. However, in strict metrological terms, this response bias indicates that the questionnaires do not perform consistently across different age groups.

ISYQOL is a relatively new instrument, and studies are needed to assess it further. Recently, ISYQOL has been translated into different languages and tested in different cultures in young persons with scoliosis [15]. There is a need to compare ISYQOL International and SRS-22 in adult patients from different countries and cultures as well. We could also test ISYQOL's properties in patients who underwent spine surgery and compare it to other quality-of-life measures in addition to SRS-22. Finally, ISYQOL International has no items assessing pain, which can be a significant complaint adults make [3]. If this is an issue regarding ISQOL International's face validity when used to evaluate the scoliosis burden of disease in adults, it remains to be investigated.

5. Conclusions

Scoliosis treatment cannot be restricted solely to correcting the curvature, but it should also assess and monitor patients' satisfaction, psychological issues, and HRQOL over time. There is a need for a proper tool that allows clinicians to evaluate the impact of spinal deformities in adulthood. The results of the present work indicate that the ISYQOL spine health subscale can be administered in a clinical setting to evaluate HRQOL in adults with scoliosis. SRS-22, in its original form, showed poor construct validity in the Rasch analysis measurement framework. While the revised SRS-22 has improved metrological features, ISYQOL International is better regarding dimensionality and differential item functioning. In addition, ISYQOL International is also considerably shorter, more straightforward, and better targeted to measure the disease burden in adults with non-surgical scoliosis.

Author Contributions: Conceptualization, F.Z.; methodology, A.C. and S.S.; formal analysis, A.C. and S.S.; interpretation of results: F.Z., S.N. and S.D.; writing—original draft preparation, I.F.; writing—review and editing, all authors. All authors have read and agreed to the published version of the manuscript.

Funding: This research received no external funding.

Institutional Review Board Statement: The study was conducted in accordance with the Declaration of Helsinki, and approved by the Ethics Committee Comitato Etico Milano Area 2 (parere 215_2022bis, approved 29 March 2022).

Informed Consent Statement: Informed consent was obtained from all subjects involved in the study.

Data Availability Statement: The data presented in this study will be available on Zenodo upon acceptance of the paper.

Acknowledgments: This study was supported and funded by the Italian Ministry of Health-Ricerca Corrente (2022).

Conflicts of Interest: S.N owns stock in ISICO. I.F. is related to S.N. All other authors have no conflict to declare.

Appendix A. Methods: The Rasch Analysis of the SRS-22 and ISYQOL International Questionnaires

The Rasch analysis run in the current study has been briefly mentioned in the main text and is detailed in the present appendix. The following steps have been followed to assess the construct validity of the SRS-22 and ISYQOL International questionnaires.

1. *Categories' functioning*

First, the categories' functioning has been evaluated by assessing their order and the order of the modal thresholds.

The Rasch analysis assumes that the greater the measured variable, the higher the item numeral chosen by the respondent.

In the current study, regarding ISYQOL International, assessing the category order means verifying that the average burden of disease measure of the participants scoring 2 on an item is higher than that of those scoring 1 on the same item. In turn, those scoring 1 measure higher than those scoring 0. If this monotonic relationship between the items' numerals and the average sample measures holds for all the questionnaire's items, the questionnaire's category structure can be considered to work as intended. Regarding SRS-22, categories are ordered if those participants choosing category 5 on an item enjoy, on average, a lower burden of disease than those scoring 4 (and so on).

In addition to the category order, the order of the modal thresholds is also assessed as a complementary analysis. According to some scholars [23], ordered categories and thresholds are more robust evidence that the items category structure works appropriately.

When applied to ISYQOL International, "ordered thresholds" means that there exists a range of disease burden values for which category 0 is most likely chosen from respondents. Adjoining this range is the range of values for which the modal category is category 1 and, finally, the range of disease burden for which category 2 is the modal one. The same reasoning applies to SRS-22.

2. *Fit to the model*

Measures can be extracted from the questionnaire's scores if categories are ordered, and data fit the model of Rasch. To date, the original model of Rasch for the analysis of dichotomous items is complemented by additional models, such as the partial credit model, the one used for the current research, allowing the analysis of polytomous items.

The mean square (MnSq) and the z-standardised (Z-Std) statistics quantify the departure of the observed data from the model's prediction and the probability that this departure is due to chance, respectively.

Two versions of the MnSq and Z-Std statistics are usually considered: the "outfit", sensitive to outliers (which is obtained from the chi-squared statistics), and the "infit",

A large and significant infit MnSq indicates that items whose difficulty is well targeted on the respondents' ability do not work according to the model prescription. A large infit suggests a more severe item malfunctioning.

Here, an item is considered to "misfit", i.e., not fitting the model adequately, if

outfit MnSq > 2.0 and absolute outfit Z-Std > 1.96, or

infit MnSq > 1.5 and absolute infit Z-Std > 1.96.

Misfitting items are often dropped from the questionnaire.

As mentioned above, once the data are demonstrated to fit the model, questionnaire scores can be turned into measures on an interval scale. The logit is the measurement unit of these measures.

3. *Dimensionality*

Measures are unidimensional, i.e., reflect the amount of a single variable. However, in practice, any measurement is affected by some multidimensionality. Therefore, in addition to assessing if a measure is multidimensional, it is crucial to determine the amount of dimensionality and if multidimensionality is so extensive as to distort measures.

In the Rasch framework, multidimensionality is indicated by principal components with an eigenvalue >2 based on a principal component analysis (PCA) calculated on the model's residuals.

The idea behind this approach is straightforward: if questionnaires' scores are unidimensional, once the Rasch dimension is "peeled off" from the data, randomness remains in the residuals (i.e., the residuals are entirely uncorrelated). On the contrary, correlation among residuals indicates that a hidden, additional variable drives together the items' scores.

The PCA is simply a statistical technique that efficiently highlights the correlation pattern among residuals.

In the case of multidimensionality being found, the following approach is used here to evaluate if this multidimensionality harms the measurements.

Items are split into three clusters according to their loading on the principal component with eigenvalue >2: items belonging to cluster 1 have a large positive loading, and those belonging to cluster 3 have a large and negative loading. Finally, cluster 2 items have a low load on the principal component.

Therefore, the score of cluster 1 and 3 items depends on the quantity of the variable grasped by the Rasch model and the quantity of the variable highlighted by the principal component. The score of cluster 2 depends instead on the Rasch variable only.

Moreover, the score of cluster 1 items is inflated by the principal component variable while that of cluster 3 items is decreased, where "increased" and "decreased" are compared to what is predicted by the Rasch model.

Persons are measured with the three clusters, and the three sets of measures are compared with ANOVA (here calculated on linear mixed-effects models).

If persons' measures from cluster 1 and cluster 3 are comparable to, i.e., not significantly different from those from cluster 2 (i.e., those measures reflecting only the variable grasped by the model of Rasch), then the inflation/deflation of the items' scores caused by the hidden variable highlighted from the principal component is not strong enough to cause a severe measurement artefact. In a few words, despite multidimensionality, the Rasch variable still mainly drives the items' scores (despite multidimensionality, the measures from multidimensional items are still comparable to those from unidimensional ones).

Only non-extreme person measures are used for this analysis to improve the accuracy of the analysis (measures are approximated for persons totalling the questionnaire maximum or minimum total score).

4. *Differential Item Functioning*

Differential item functioning (DIF), also called item bias, indicates that an item does not work the same in different groups of respondents.

A prominent feature of measures is that they depend only on the measured quantity and are not affected by other features of the measured object. An example from the physical world will clarify this aspect.

Say we have 1 kg of carrots and 1 kg of potatoes. We expect that if a scales is used to measure the mass of carrots and potatoes, the scales reading will be the same (1 kg) when both vegetables are tested.

Say instead that the scales returns 1.3 kg for the (1 kg) of carrots and 0.8 kg for the (1 kg) of potatoes. We would conclude that there is something wrong with the scales. Is the scales measuring the mass and something else (maybe the volume of the vegetable)? Is the scales broken?

The DIF assessment evaluates if an item (which corresponds to the scales of the previous example) returns the same measures of persons (vegetables, in the example) belonging to different groups (e.g., carrots and potatoes). Here, testing DIF is testing if measures from an item of individuals with the same burden of disease level but belonging to different groups (e.g., adolescents vs. old persons) are the same.

Since the study aims to assess if SRS-22 and ISYQOL are suitable to quantify the burden of disease in adults and older people, the current analysis focussed on the DIF for age. The participants' sample was split into: adolescents (from 14 to 18 years), young adults (from 20 to 39 years), middle-aged adults (from 40 to 59 years), and older adults (from 60 to 79 years). As a complementary analysis, DIF for gender (males vs. females) was also evaluated.

The DIF of SRS-22 and ISYQOL International items is tested here following Linacre [25].

The observed scores for an item in a group of respondents (say older adults) are compared to their expected scores for that item given the items' calibration from the primary analysis, the analysis including the whole participants' sample (i.e., adolescents, young, middle-aged, and older people).

Now, imagine that older adults scored more than expected on item i. Item i is thus easier to endorse in older adults than in the complete participants' sample and easier to endorse than in the participants of the remaining subsets. In other words, the item's calibration is lower for older adults than for the participants of the other classes.

Item i is considered corrupted by DIF if the difference between the two calibrations is large (i.e., >0.5 logits) and significant (i.e., $p < 0.01$, see below).

Say DIF is found for some items and grouping variables (i.e., age or gender here). Similar to multidimensionality, what is essential is to assess if DIF causes such a large measurement distortion to produce an artefact in the persons' measures from the questionnaire total score.

The consequences of DIF (i.e., the malfunctioning of some items) on the measures from the questionnaire's total score can be just assessed by comparing the observed and expected scores.

Imagine a questionnaire, with each item scored in four categories. Now, consider two different scenarios in which DIF corrupts item k. In the first scenario, the average observed score by a class of respondents is 2.1 points higher than expected. In the second, the difference between the observed and the expected score is 0.14. In the first case, DIF causes a two-point artefact in the total questionnaire score (and thus on the respondents' measures). In the second, the impact of DIF on the total score are much more negligible (the total score is inflated by just 0.14).

By comparing the observed and expected scores, it is thus easy to understand the artefact caused by DIF at the questionnaire's total score level.

This way of analysing DIF clearly makes the questionnaire's total score (and thus the questionnaire measures) central. The idea behind this is all about answering the question: are item calibrations from the main analysis (biased if there is DIF) a good proxy of the exact calibration which would be obtained in the specific group of participants?

Because of multiple statistical testing, the type 1 error probability was lowered to 0.01 for the DIF significance analysis [27].

5. *Targeting and reliability*

High-quality measures have high reliability, meaning the measurement error is low compared to the measures' total variance. High reliability implies that several levels of the measured variable can be distinguished at a single subject level.

In the current work, ISYQOL International's and SRS-22's reliability is reported as "Rasch persons' reliability", a reliability index similar to Cronbach's alpha from the CTT. From this reliability index, the number of strata is calculated, i.e., the number of significantly different levels of the burden of disease a person can progress through.

For example, with a questionnaire or a scale with four strata, it is possible to follow a patient's modification of their clinical condition from severe to moderate, mild, and eventually minimal. When the patient changes stratum, their clinical condition is different in a statistically significant way (see Supplementary Materials 1 in [26]).

Finally, floor and ceiling effects are also calculated as the percentage of respondents obtaining the minimum and maximum total questionnaire scores, respectively. The size of the difference between the persons and the items measures complements this information. A questionnaire with no floor effect, no ceiling effect, and 0 logit difference between participants and items mean measure is appropriately targeted to the recruited sample participants. To take an analogy from the physical world, a questionnaire with these features is like a ruler of the proper length for measuring the object of interest (e.g., the height of a chair vs. the length of a car).

Appendix B. Supplementary Results

Table A1. Category and threshold orders of the ISYQOL International (spine domain).

Item	Score	Count Used	Average Measure	Andrich Threshold Calibration	SE
1, get worse	0	9	−1.36	-	-
	1	88	1.13	−2.27	0.39
	2	88	3.45	2.27	0.19
2, worried back pain	0	28	−0.91	-	-
	1	77	0.30	−1.49	0.26
	2	80	2.60	1.49	0.20
3, big deal	0	89	−3.03	-	-
	1	77	−0.50	−1.64	0.20
	2	19	0.71	1.64	0.29
4, worried not get better	0	47	−1.82	-	-
	1	76	0.21	−1.30	0.22
	2	62	2.01	1.30	0.21
5, suffering	0	65	−2.54	-	-
	1	86	−0.17	−1.61	0.20
	2	34	1.57	1.61	0.24
6, appearance	0	71	−2.66	-	-
	1	85	−0.41	−1.64	0.20
	2	29	1.76	1.64	0.25
7, worried back problem	0	6	−0.65	-	-
	1	106	1.08	−2.84	0.46
	2	73	3.85	2.84	0.20
8, bother to show	0	67	−1.94	-	-
	1	72	−0.29	−1.20	0.21
	2	46	1.55	1.20	0.22
9, worried visible	0	58	−2.35	-	-
	1	92	−0.18	−1.74	0.21
	2	35	1.60	1.74	0.24

Item: item number and a keyword briefly describing the item content. Score: item's categories. Counts: number of observations per category participating in the estimation (extreme scores are excluded). Average measure: the mean measure of the participants scoring a specific category to an item, calculated from the item's calibration. For example, item 3 calibration is 1.76 logits. The mean measure of the participants scoring 1 on item 3 is 1.76 − 0.50 = 1.26 logits. Andrich thresholds calibration: calibration (i.e., measure) of the Andrich (modal) thresholds. SE: standard error. All nine ISYQOL International items had ordered categories and thresholds.

Table A2. SRS-22 category and threshold orders.

Item	Score	Count Used	Average Measure	Andrich Threshold Calibration	SE
1, pain six months	1	3	−1.69	-	-
	2	37	0.08	−2.74	0.63
	3	50	0.53	0.13	0.21
	4	56	1.44	0.88	0.18
	5	53	2.21	1.73	0.19
2, pain last month	1	6	−0.91	-	-
	2	26	−0.10	−1.78	0.46
	3	51	0.37	−0.42	0.22
	4	60	1.15	0.65	0.18
	5	56	2.06	1.56	0.19
3, nervous person	1	4	−1.96	-	-
	2	46	−0.21	−3.19	0.55
	3	88	0.34	−0.67	0.19
	4	45	1.09	1.34	0.18
	5	16	1.47	2.51	0.30
4, back shape	1	18	−1.15	-	-
	2	36	−0.55	−1.54	0.28
	3	77	0.07	−1.04	0.19
	4	44	0.63	0.90	0.18
	5	24	1.39	1.67	0.26
5, activity level	1	26	0.10	-	-
	2	63	0.40	−0.54	0.23
	3	110	1.68	0.54	0.16
6, look in clothes	1	5	−0.89	-	-
	2	19	−0.67	−2.12	0.50
	3	94	0.28	−1.69	0.24
	4	65	1.02	0.97	0.17
	5	16	1.73	2.85	0.29
7, down in the dumps	1	8	0.20	-	-
	2	30	0.54	−1.00	0.40
	3	35	1.04	0.73	0.21
	4	126	2.01	0.27 (*)	0.17
8, back pain at rest	1	28	−0.30	-	-
	2	49	0.02	−0.86	0.23
	3	53	0.70	0.19	0.18
	4	69	1.09	0.68	0.18
9, work/school	1	15	−0.07	-	-
	2	26	0.47	−0.43	0.31
	3	37	0.77	0.30	0.21
	4	120	1.73	0.12 (*)	0.17
10, trunk appearance	1	13	−1.89	-	-
	2	56	−0.88	−2.73	0.31
	3	100	−0.20	−1.17	0.17
	4	23	0.54	1.64	0.23
	5	7	1.39	2.26	0.44
11, pain medications	1	2	1.97	-	-
	2	38	2.01	−1.25	0.77
	3	159	3.20	1.25	0.19
12, around the house	1	11	−0.84	-	-
	2	20	−0.05	−0.82	0.35
	3	42	0.41	−0.50	0.23
	4	38	1.04	0.82	0.19
	5	88	1.78	0.50 (*)	0.18
13, calm and peaceful	1	21	−0.89	-	-
	2	57	−0.32	−1.70	0.26
	3	98	0.36	−0.56	0.17
	4	23	1.04	2.26	0.25

Table A2. Cont.

Item	Score	Count Used	Average Measure	Andrich Threshold Calibration	SE
14, personal relationships	1	5	−0.38	-	-
	2	11	0.05	−0.78	0.52
	3	26	0.67	−0.34	0.31
	4	42	1.15	0.51	0.21
	5	115	2.12	0.62	0.17
16, down hearted and blue	1	6	−0.43	-	-
	2	8	−0.05	−0.41	0.48
	3	38	0.79	−1.16 (*)	0.32
	4	55	1.15	0.53	0.19
	5	92	1.95	1.05	0.17
17, days off	1	10	0.31	-	-
	2	6	0.83	0.92	0.39
	3	7	1.52	0.75 (*)	0.32
	4	176	1.95	−1.67 (*)	0.26
18, going out	1	18	0.27	-	-
	2	52	0.80	−0.45	0.27
	3	129	1.87	0.45	0.17
19, feel attractive	1	26	−1.70	-	-
	2	25	−1.22	−1.31	0.24
	3	104	−0.33	−2.18 (*)	0.19
	4	37	0.14	0.99	0.20
	5	7	1.81	2.51	0.43
20, happy person	1	15	−0.84	-	-
	2	65	−0.38	−2.16	0.29
	3	100	0.40	−0.40	0.17
	4	19	1.52	2.56	0.27
21, satisfied with results	1	11	−1.09	-	-
	2	26	−0.62	−1.68	0.35
	3	76	−0.01	−1.32	0.21
	4	63	0.83	0.57	0.17
	5	18	1.68	2.43	0.28
22, same management again	1	67	−0.71	-	-
	2	64	0.10	−0.37	0.18
	3	62	0.55	0.37	0.18

Same abbreviations as Table A1. Note that item 15 was removed because it did not fit the model. Note also that the original item structure on five categories has been rearranged for ten items because of disordered categories. Finally, despite ordered categories, six items have disordered Andrich thresholds (*).

References

1. Negrini, S.; Donzelli, S.; Aulisa, A.G.; Czaprowski, D.; Schreiber, S.; de Mauroy, J.C.; Diers, H.; Grivas, T.B.; Knott, P.; Kotwicki, T.; et al. 2016 SOSORT Guidelines: Orthopaedic and Rehabilitation Treatment of Idiopathic Scoliosis during Growth. *Scoliosis Spinal Disord.* **2018**, *13*, 3. [CrossRef]
2. Sanders, A.E.; Andras, L.M.; Iantorno, S.E.; Hamilton, A.; Choi, P.D.; Skaggs, D.L. Clinically Significant Psychological and Emotional Distress in 32% of Adolescent Idiopathic Scoliosis Patients. *Spine Deform.* **2018**, *6*, 435–440. [CrossRef] [PubMed]
3. Tones, M.; Moss, N.; Polly, D.W. A Review of Quality of Life and Psychosocial Issues in Scoliosis. *Spine* **2006**, *31*, 3027–3038. [CrossRef] [PubMed]
4. Weinstein, S.L.; Dolan, L.A.; Spratt, K.F.; Peterson, K.K.; Spoonamore, M.J.; Ponseti, I.V. Health and Function of Patients with Untreated Idiopathic Scoliosis: A 50-Year Natural History Study. *JAMA* **2003**, *289*, 559–567. [CrossRef]
5. Asher, M.; Min Lai, S.; Burton, D.; Manna, B. Discrimination Validity of the Scoliosis Research Society-22 Patient Questionnaire: Relationship to Idiopathic Scoliosis Curve Pattern and Curve Size. *Spine* **2003**, *28*, 74–78. [CrossRef]
6. Asher, M.; Min Lai, S.; Burton, D.; Manna, B. Scoliosis Research Society-22 Patient Questionnaire: Responsiveness to Change Associated with Surgical Treatment. *Spine* **2003**, *28*, 70–73. [CrossRef]
7. Bridwell, K.H.; Berven, S.; Glassman, S.; Hamill, C.; Horton, W.C.; Lenke, L.G.; Schwab, F.; Baldus, C.; Shainline, M. Is the SRS-22 Instrument Responsive to Change in Adult Scoliosis Patients Having Primary Spinal Deformity Surgery? *Spine* **2007**, *32*, 2220–2225. [CrossRef]
8. Bridwell, K.H.; Cats-Baril, W.; Harrast, J.; Berven, S.; Glassman, S.; Farcy, J.-P.; Horton, W.C.; Lenke, L.G.; Baldus, C.; Radake, T. The Validity of the SRS-22 Instrument in an Adult Spinal Deformity Population Compared with the Oswestry and SF-12: A Study of Response Distribution, Concurrent Validity, Internal Consistency, and Reliability. *Spine* **2005**, *30*, 455–461. [CrossRef]

9. Berven, S.; Deviren, V.; Demir-Deviren, S.; Hu, S.S.; Bradford, D.S. Studies in the Modified Scoliosis Research Society Outcomes Instrument in Adults: Validation, Reliability, and Discriminating Capacity. *Spine* **2003**, *28*, 2164–2169, discussion 2169. [CrossRef]
10. Mannion, A.F.; Elfering, A.; Bago, J.; Pellise, F.; Vila-Casademunt, A.; Richner-Wunderlin, S.; Domingo-Sàbat, M.; Obeid, I.; Acaroglu, E.; Alanay, A.; et al. Factor Analysis of the SRS-22 Outcome Assessment Instrument in Patients with Adult Spinal Deformity. *Eur. Spine J.* **2017**, *27*, 685–699. [CrossRef]
11. Tesio, L.; Scarano, S.; Hassan, S.; Kumbhare, D.; Caronni, A. Why Questionnaire Scores Are Not Measures: A Question-Raising Article. *Am. J. Phys. Med. Rehabil.* **2023**, *102*, 75–82. [CrossRef]
12. Caronni, A.; Zaina, F.; Negrini, S. Improving the Measurement of Health-Related Quality of Life in Adolescent with Idiopathic Scoliosis: The SRS-7, a Rasch-Developed Short Form of the SRS-22 Questionnaire. *Res. Dev. Disabil.* **2014**, *35*, 784–799. [CrossRef]
13. Caronni, A.; Sciumè, L.; Donzelli, S.; Zaina, F.; Negrini, S. ISYQOL: A Rasch-Consistent Questionnaire for Measuring Health-Related Quality of Life in Adolescents with Spinal Deformities. *Spine J.* **2017**, *17*, 1364–1372. [CrossRef]
14. Caronni, A.; Donzelli, S.; Zaina, F.; Negrini, S. The Italian Spine Youth Quality of Life Questionnaire Measures Health-Related Quality of Life of Adolescents with Spinal Deformities Better than the Reference Standard, the Scoliosis Research Society 22 Questionnaire. *Clin. Rehabil.* **2019**, *33*, 1404–1415. [CrossRef]
15. Negrini, S.; Zaina, F.; Buyukaslan, A.; Fortin, C.; Karavidas, N.; Kotwicki, T.; Korbel, K.; Parent, E.; Sanchez-Raya, J.; Shearer, K.; et al. Cross-Cultural Validation of the Italian Spine Youth Quality of Life Questionnaire: The ISYQOL International. *Eur. J. Phys. Rehabil. Med.* **2023**, *59*, 364. [CrossRef]
16. McAviney, J.; Roberts, C.; Sullivan, B.; Alevras, A.J.; Graham, P.L.; Brown, B.T. The Prevalence of Adult de Novo Scoliosis: A Systematic Review and Meta-Analysis. *Eur. Spine J.* **2020**, *29*, 2960–2969. [CrossRef]
17. Linacre, J.M. Sample Size and Item Calibration (or Person Measure) Stability. *Rasch Meas. Trans.* **1994**, *7*, 328.
18. Mallinson, T.; Kozlowski, A.J.; Johnston, M.V.; Weaver, J.; Terhorst, L.; Grampurohit, N.; Juengst, S.; Ehrlich-Jones, L.; Heinemann, A.W.; Melvin, J.; et al. Rasch Reporting Guideline for Rehabilitation Research (RULER): The RULER Statement. *Arch. Phys. Med. Rehabil.* **2022**, *103*, 1477–1486. [CrossRef]
19. Van de Winckel, A.; Kozlowski, A.J.; Johnston, M.V.; Weaver, J.; Grampurohit, N.; Terhorst, L.; Juengst, S.; Ehrlich-Jones, L.; Heinemann, A.W.; Melvin, J.; et al. Reporting Guideline for RULER: Rasch Reporting Guideline for Rehabilitation Research: Explanation and Elaboration. *Arch. Phys. Med. Rehabil.* **2022**, *103*, 1487–1498. [CrossRef]
20. Monticone, M.; Nava, C.; Leggero, V.; Rocca, B.; Salvaderi, S.; Ferrante, S.; Ambrosini, E. Measurement Properties of Translated Versions of the Scoliosis Research Society-22 Patient Questionnaire, SRS-22: A Systematic Review. *Qual. Life Res.* **2015**, *24*, 1981–1998. [CrossRef]
21. Aulisa, A.G.; Guzzanti, V.; Perisano, C.; Marzetti, E.; Specchia, A.; Galli, M.; Giordano, M.; Aulisa, L. Determination of Quality of Life in Adolescents with Idiopathic Scoliosis Subjected to Conservative Treatment. *Scoliosis* **2010**, *5*, 21. [CrossRef] [PubMed]
22. Linacre, J. Category Disordering (Disordered Categories) vs. Threshold Disordering (Disordered Thresholds). *Rasch Meas. Trans.* **1999**, *13*, 675.
23. Andrich, D. An Expanded Derivation of the Threshold Structure of the Polytomous Rasch Model That Dispels Any "Threshold Disorder Controversy". *Educ. Psychol. Meas.* **2013**, *73*, 78–124. [CrossRef]
24. Masters, G.N. A Rasch Model for Partial Credit Scoring. *Psychometrika* **1982**, *47*, 149–174. [CrossRef]
25. Linacre, J.M. Facets Computer Program for Many-Facet Rasch Measurement. 2022. Available online: https://www.winsteps.com/facets.htm (accessed on 29 June 2023).
26. Caronni, A.; Picardi, M.; Redaelli, V.; Antoniotti, P.; Pintavalle, G.; Aristidou, E.; Gilardone, G.; Carpinella, I.; Lencioni, T.; Arcuri, P.; et al. The Falls Efficacy Scale International Is a Valid Measure to Assess the Concern about Falling and Its Changes Induced by Treatments. *Clin. Rehabil.* **2021**, *36*, 558–570. [CrossRef]
27. Lange, R.; Irwin, H.J.; Houran, J. Top-down Purification of Tobacyk's Revised Paranormal Belief Scale. *Personal. Individ. Differ.* **2000**, *29*, 131–156. [CrossRef]
28. Fairbank, J.C.; Pynsent, P.B. The Oswestry Disability Index. *Spine* **2000**, *25*, 2940–2953. [CrossRef]
29. Zaina, F.; Poggio, M.; Di Felice, F.; Donzelli, S.; Negrini, S. Bracing Adults with Chronic Low Back Pain Secondary to Severe Scoliosis: Six Months Results of a Prospective Pilot Study. *Eur. Spine J.* **2021**, *30*, 2962–2966. [CrossRef]
30. Archer, J.E.; Baird, C.; Gardner, A.; Rushton, A.B.; Heneghan, N.R. Evaluating Measures of Quality of Life in Adult Scoliosis: A Systematic Review and Narrative Synthesis. *Spine Deform* **2022**, *10*, 991–1002. [CrossRef]
31. Luce, R.D.; Tukey, J.W. Simultaneous Conjoint Measurement: A New Type of Fundamental Measurement. *J. Math. Psychol.* **1964**, *1*, 1–27. [CrossRef]
32. Caronni, A.; Picardi, M.; Scarano, S.; Tropea, P.; Gilardone, G.; Bolognini, N.; Redaelli, V.; Pintavalle, G.; Aristidou, E.; Antoniotti, P.; et al. Differential Item Functioning of the Mini-BESTest Balance Measure: A Rasch Analysis Study. *Int. J. Environ. Res. Public Health* **2023**, *20*, 5166. [CrossRef]

Disclaimer/Publisher's Note: The statements, opinions and data contained in all publications are solely those of the individual author(s) and contributor(s) and not of MDPI and/or the editor(s). MDPI and/or the editor(s) disclaim responsibility for any injury to people or property resulting from any ideas, methods, instructions or products referred to in the content.

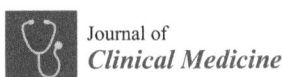

Article

Vertebral Rotation in Functional Scoliosis Caused by Limb-Length Inequality: Correlation between Rotation, Limb Length Inequality, and Obliquity of the Sacral Shelf

Martina Marsiolo [1,*], Silvia Careri [1], Diletta Bandinelli [1], Renato Maria Toniolo [1] and Angelo Gabriele Aulisa [1,2]

1 U.O.C. of Orthopaedics and Traumatology, Bambino Gesù Children's Hospital, Istituto di Ricerca e Cura a Carattere Sceintifico (IRCCS), 00165 Rome, Italy; silvia.careri@opbg.net (S.C.); diletta.bandinelli@opbg.net (D.B.); renatom.toniolo@opbg.net (R.M.T.); agabriele.aulisa@opbg.net (A.G.A.)
2 Department of Human Sciences, Society and Health, University of Cassino and Southern Lazio, 03043 Cassino, Italy
* Correspondence: martina.marsiolo@opbg.net; Tel.: +39-3066-8594-873

Abstract: Background: Scoliosis is a structured rotatory deformity of the spine defined as >10° Cobb. Functional scoliosis (FS) is a curve < 10° Cobb, which is non-rotational and correctable. FS is often secondary to leg length inequality (LLI). To observe vertebral rotation (VR) in functional scoliosis due to LLI, one must demonstrate a correlation between LLI, sacral shelf inclination (SSI), and VR and discover a predictive value of LLI capable of inducing rotation. Methods: We studied 89 patients with dorso-lumbar or lumbar curves < 15° Cobb and radiographs of the spine and pelvis. We measured LLI, SSI, and VR. The patients were divided into VR and without rotation (WVR) groups. Statistical analysis was performed. Results: The mean LLI value was 6.5 ± 4.59 mm, and the mean SSI was 2.8 ± 2.53 mm. The mean value of LLI was 5.2 ± 4.87 mm in the WVR group and 7.4 ± 4.18 mm in the VR group. The mean SSI value for WVR was 1.4 ± 2.00 and that for VR was 3.9 ± 2.39. For each mm of LLI, it was possible to predict 0.12° of rotation. LLI ±5 mm increased the probability of rotation (R2.08 $p < 0.0016$), while this was ±2 mm for SSI (R2 0.22 $p < 0.01$). Each mm of LLI corresponded to 0.3 mm of SSI (R2 0.29, $p < 0.01$). Conclusions: FS secondary to LLI can cause VR, and 5 mm of LLI can cause SSI and rotation.

Keywords: scoliosis; vertebral rotation; limb inequality; limb discrepancy; sacral shelf obliquity; functional scoliosis; sacral shelf inclination

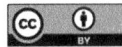

1. Introduction

The term scoliosis, first used by Galen, derives from the Greek word "crooked". In 1741, André used the crooked spine as his symbol for orthopedics [1]. Scoliosis is a structured deformity of the spine that is expressed in three dimensions of space: a curve in the frontal plane (which is the most evident manifestation) is associated with vertebral rotation in the transverse plane (which is the characteristic element) and a deformity in the sagittal plane. The term "structured" means that one cannot spontaneously correct the curve. Scoliosis can be classified according to its etiology, the location of the curve, and the extent of angular deviation. The most frequent type of pathology is idiopathic scoliosis, with a prevalence of 0.47–5.2%. The prevalence and curve severity are higher for girls than for boys, and the female-to-male ratio increases with increasing age among children. The ratio is 1.5:1 for the mild forms, while it increases by 10:1 for the more severe forms (>30° Cobb). A diagnosis of idiopathic scoliosis is made if a non-idiopathic form has been excluded [2]. Clinically, a patient with scoliosis will present with an asymmetry of the shoulder line, an asymmetry of the size triangles between the line of the arms and that of the hips, and a hump in the anterior bending test. Clinical suspicion should be confirmed based on the presence of a curve of the spine on radiographic examination. The Report of the Terminology Committee of the Scoliosis Research Society, which is the international body responsible for regulating and standardizing the terminology and classifications of vertebral deformities, states that "scoliosis is a lateral curvature of the spine". According to this definition, deviations of the spine in the frontal plane are generically defined as scoliosis. In the literature, it is universally accepted that for a curve to be defined as scoliosis it must be greater than 10° Cobb in the frontal plane, but there is no agreement on the pathogenesis of idiopathic scoliosis. Various theories have been posited to explain the pathogenesis of idiopathic scoliosis; these can be classified into the following groups to provide a better understanding of the multifactorial pathogenesis of AIS: genetics, mesenchymal stem cells, tissues, spine biomechanics, neurology, hormones, biochemistry, environment, and lifestyle [3–6]. Despite much research, the mechanism underlying the onset of idiopathic scoliosis remains unknown. Furthermore, the official terminology distinguishes another type of scoliosis in addition to the structured one mentioned above, namely, unstructured scoliosis, also called scoliotic attitude or "functional scoliosis". This is a mild, non-structural, and steady lumbar curve often secondary to limb length inequality without vertebral rotation. The major skeletal reactions or adaptations to leg length discrepancy are pelvic obliquity and scoliosis [7–9]. Leg length inequality (LLI) or discrepancy is a difference between the length of the legs and is a common orthopedic condition with a prevalence rate of 90% in the general population, and it is more frequently observed among the pediatric population [10]. Leg length discrepancy can be measured clinically by measuring the length from the anterior superior iliac spine to the medial malleolus and calculating the difference between the two lower limbs. Another method of measurement is to calculate the difference in length between the two malleoli in the supine position. A more precise method is to measure the difference in length on a radiograph of the lower extremities under load. It is possible to measure the length by calculating the difference in the height of the iliac crest or the femoral heads on a radiograph of the pelvis or by measuring the lengths of the tibia and femur. The femur is measured from the top of the greater trochanter to the most distal point of the lateral condyle. The tibia is measured from the most proximal point to the most distal point at the ankle joint line.

Length differences are typically less than 10 mm, asymptomatic, and develop as a momentary condition during growth. In some rare cases, children are born with leg discrepancies, while other causes are acquired (fractures, tumors, radiation, infections). LLI is classified as mild (0–2.5 cm), moderate (2.5–6 cm), and severe (>6 cm) [11] and can be categorized etiologically as structural or functional. Structural or anatomical LLI is due to the physical shortening or lengthening of a unilateral lower extremity, while functional LLD refers to the apparent asymmetry of the lower extremity, without the physical shortening or lengthening of the osseous components of the lower limb. A functional leg length discrepancy (LLD) refers to a situation where one leg appears longer than the other due to factors such as pelvic tilt, muscular imbalances, or poor alignment, rather than an actual difference in bone length. Unlike a structural LLD, where there is a measurable difference in the bones' length, a functional LLD is often temporary and can be corrected with proper intervention. If the pelvis is tilted or rotated, it can affect the apparent leg lengths. This can occur due to muscle imbalances, joint issues, or posture problems. Tightness or weakness in the hip, thigh, or calf muscles can lead to altered alignment and functional LLD. Tightness in soft tissues, such as ligaments and fascia, can contribute to uneven alignment of the pelvis and legs. Unlike structural LLD, functional LLD cannot be corrected with a lift, but it requires physical therapy to assess posture, muscle imbalances, and alignment so as to develop a personalized exercise program that addresses the underlying causes of functional LLD [7]. The effects of LLD on the spine vary depending on the cause and size of the difference. The correlation between LLI, the alignment of the spine, and pelvic imbalance has been assessed in various ways, even methods based on simulating LLI [12] and studying its consequences for trunk, spinal, and pelvic posture [13–15]. These parameters regress with the equalization of LLI [16]. Scoliosis due to LLD is referred to as functional scoliosis, and it totally or partially regresses when the LLD is eradicated.

The pattern of scoliosis associated with LLD is described as compensatory, non-structural, and non-progressive, but it has been suggested that LLD can produce structural changes in the spine over time.

LLD can also occur secondary to scoliosis, particularly in the case of compensatory scoliosis. In these cases, LLD appears as the result of an asymmetrical load on the lower extremities. However, the factors associated with variations in LLD and its relationship with pelvic obliquity are unknown [9]. Moreover, the literature provides discordant results on the degree of LLI that can cause vertebral misalignment. Some authors believe that an LLD of 5 mm or less has real significance for mechanically related dysfunctions around the hips, pelvis, and spine, while other investigators believe that an LLD of less than 1 cm is not significant and has no pathological implication [11–17].

No study has ever investigated the specific relationship between LLI, sacral inclination, and vertebral rotation in patients of growing age with functional scoliosis (Cobb < 10°). As previously mentioned, the most frequent type of scoliosis is "adolescent idiopathic scoliosis (AIS)". Its cause is unknown, and the prognostic factors linked to curve progression are still debated. Prognosis can vary widely depending on factors such as the severity of the curvature, the age of onset, the underlying cause, and the patient's overall health.

The severity of the curvature (degree of spinal curvature measured based on the Cobb angle on radiograph) is a crucial factor in predicting the prognosis. Mild curves (less than 20–25 degrees) are generally considered as less likely to progress significantly, while more severe curves may have a higher likelihood of progression.

Age of onset can influence prognosis. Early onset scoliosis, occurring before puberty, tends to have higher potential for progression due to growth spurts during adolescence. Skeletal maturity is another important prognostic factor; once growth is complete, the progression of scoliosis usually slows down significantly. The greater the stage of skeletal maturity is, the less likely the curvature will progress.

Curve pattern and location: The location and pattern of the curves can impact prognosis, as can gender; in general, girls are more likely to experience scoliosis progression than boys, especially during growth spurts. This is particularly true for idiopathic scoliosis.

Family history: A family history of scoliosis might increase the likelihood of progression, suggesting a genetic predisposition. It is not known which has the greatest influence on prognosis.

Recently, many studies have demonstrated the importance of vertebral rotation. Indeed, the maintenance of the viscous–elastic property of the intervertebral disc depends on this aspect, which is directly linked, together with the Cobb degree, to the distribution of forces on the spine. In children, especially, the spine is in a state of dynamic equilibrium; the entire spine is subject to elastic deformation during movement and has the ability to return to its primitive configuration. It has been demonstrated that when the column starts in an altered condition, it imposes alterations of movement followed by a change in elastic return, which can lead to structural changes over time [18]. These alterations have a great impact on the evolution of the scoliotic curve. The resetting of vertebral rotation has been shown to change the progression of the curve once conservative treatment has ended [19]. Based on these premises, we decided to focus our attention on vertebral rotation in curves of less than 15 degrees in patients of growing age with LLI.

The aim of this study was to research the presence of vertebral rotation in functional scoliosis caused by limb length inequality (LLI). In addition, we aimed to examine the correlation between LLI, sacral inclination, and vertebral rotation to discover whether there is a quantitative measure of LLI in which the risk of vertebral body rotation increases.

2. Materials and Methods

2.1. Design of the Study

This study was a retrospective analysis of 343 consecutive patients (male and female) who underwent view-standing X-rays of the whole spine in our hospital from September 2022 to November 2022. We only selected X-rays from our hospital database, featured in our Carestream program (Figure 1).

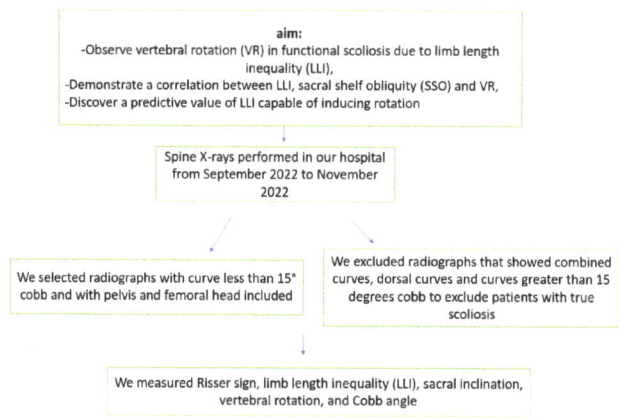

Figure 1. Flow chart of the study design.

2.2. Population

The inclusion criteria were a Cobb angle < 15°, primary scoliosis, the absence of thoracic curve, sacral shelf, femoral heads visible on X-ray, and age less than 16 years old. The exclusion criteria were curves secondary to other pathologies, thoracic curves, or combined curves, curves with a Cobb angle > 15°, sacral shelf, and femoral heads that were not visible. From among 343 patients, we found 89 patients meeting the inclusion criteria. In the X-ray of the spine in two projections, we measured the presence of a vertebral rotation seat of the curve, as well as the entity of the curve using the Cobb degree, observed the Risser degree, and determined whether the scoliosis was primary or secondary to bone causes (Figure 2A,B). We also measured limb length inequality (LLI) and sacral shelf inclination. The femoral horizontal reference line was defined as a horizontal line tangent to the top of the highest part of the femoral head. The height between the right and left femoral horizontal reference lines was defined as the size of the LLI. The inclination of the sacral shelf was measured by drawing a horizontal line at the level of the first two foramina or the sacroiliac joint, while vertebral rotation was evaluated using a Perdriolle's torsionmeter (Figure 3). To render the measurements more precise, in addition to the X-ray grid reference, we double-checked the measurement using a ruler placed on the computer screen. During the visit of the patient with suspected scoliosis, we evaluated the symmetry of the sacral shelf and measured the length of the lower limbs. It is important to observe the change in the alignment of the spine by applying a lift below the limb, showing a measure inferior to the contralateral limb (Figure 4).

All measurements were performed by a single operator.

2.3. Statistical Analysis

The statistical analysis was performed using STATA (Stata, College Station, TX, USA), and a p value less than 0.05 was considered statistically significant.

The Shapiro–Francia test was used to check the normality of each variable. Pearson's correlation coefficient and the logistic regression type ($r2$) were calculated for the correlation between pelvic inclination, vertebral rotation, and limb length inequality (LLI).

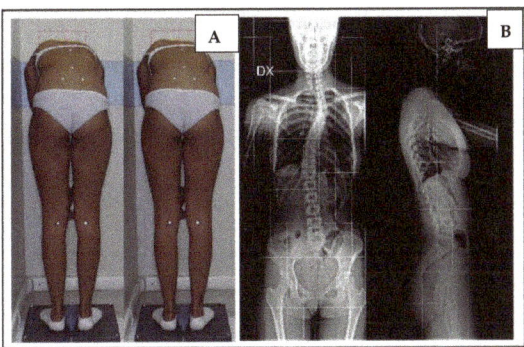

Figure 2. (**A**) Clinical aspects of scoliosis; (**B**) Radiological aspects of scoliosis.

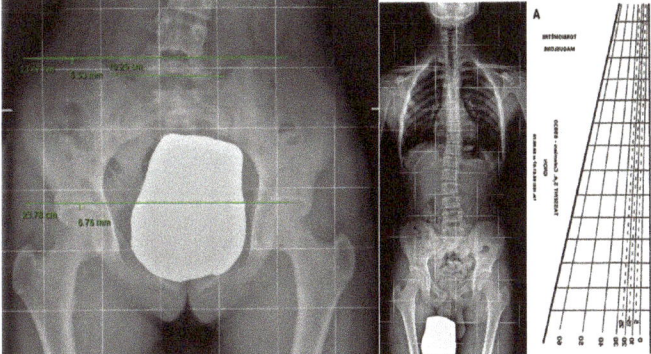

Figure 3. These figures show how the measurements were taken. A: Pedriolle's Torsionometer.

The correlation of pelvic obliquity (SSI) and LLI was calculated for the whole group (N = 89 subjects) and divided by vertebral rotation (Perdriolle 0° group N = 38; Perdriolle 5–15° group N = 51).

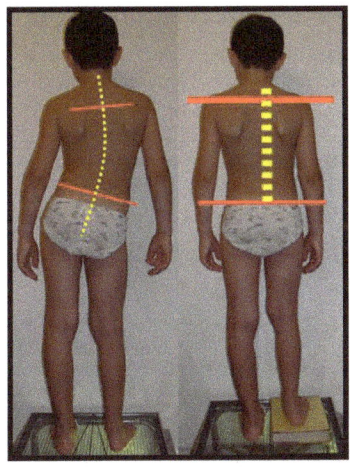

Figure 4. Clinical aspects of functional scoliosis.

3. Results

Fifty-seven out of eighty-nine patients had vertebral rotation (51% of cases) of the apical vertebrae. Most cases involved L2 (21 out of 57 cases). The Risser sign was 1.8 ± 1.9 (mean ± SD). A total of 33 patients had a left lumbar curve, 36 had a left dorso-lumbar curve, 3 had a right lumbar curve, and 17 had a right dorso-lumbar curve (Table 1).

Table 1. Curve location and n° of patients.

Curve Location	n° Patients
Left lumbar	33
Left dorso-lumbar	36
Right lumbar	3
Left dorso-lumbar	17

In these patients, vertebral rotation ranged from 5 to 15 Peridiolle's degrees. In total, 25 showed 5 degrees of rotation, 27 showed 10 degrees of rotation, and 5 showed 15 degrees of rotation (Table 2). Seven patients did not show lower limb inequality, and of these, only one showed vertebral rotation.

Table 2. Perdriolle's value and n° of patients.

Perdriolle	N° Patients
5	25
10	27
15	5

Fifty-eight patients had between 5 mm and 24 mm of LLI, while the remaining patients had a lower degree of LLI. Of these 58 patients, only 15 did not show vertebral rotation, while among the 24 patients with LLI of less than 5 mm, 14 not show vertebral rotation (Table 3).

Table 3. LLI, n° of patients and rotation.

	LLI 5–24	LLI < 5 mm	LLI 5–24 with Rotation	LLI < 5 mm with Rotation
N° Patients	58	24	43	10

The mean LLI value of the whole group was 6.5 ± 4.59 mm. Splitting the patients into two subgroups, those without rotation and those with rotation, the mean LLI value was 5.2 ± 4.87 mm for the first group and 7.4 ± 4.18 mm for the second group.

The mean value of sacral shelf inclination (SSI) for the whole group was 2.8 ± 2.53 mm, with a value of 1.4 ± 2.00 mm for patients without rotation and 3.9 ± 2.39 mm for patients with Perdriolle ranging from 5 to 15°. The correlation between sacral inclination and LLI showed a $p > 0.001$ in both subgroups, with rotation and without rotation (Table 4).

Table 4. Mean values of lower limb inequality (LLI) and sacral shelf inclination (SSI) in the whole group and in patients with and without rotation.

	LLI (Lower Limb Inequality) Mean ± SD	SSI (Sacral Shelf Inclination) Mean ± SD	Cohen d	p Value
Total sample	6.5 ± 4.59	2.8 ± 2.53	0.97	$p < 0.001$
With Rotation	7.4 ± 4.18	3.9 ± 2.39	1.03	$p < 0.01$
Without rotation	5.2 ± 4.87	1.4 ± 2.00	0.94	$p < 0.001$

The correlation between the inclination of the sacral shelf and vertebral rotation, variables in a statistical relationship of the logistic regression type, showed an R2 value of 0.22 and a $p < 0.001$; both were statistically significant (Figure 5A).

Furthermore, we found a predictive probability according to which, for each millimeter of inclination of the sacrum, it is possible to predict a rotation of the vertebral body of 0.58 degrees, and we found that with a threshold value of 2 mm of inclination, the probability of developing a rotation exponentially increases.

Moreover, the predictive probability of vertebral rotation is 0.23 in the absence of obliquity of the sacral shelf, while it is 0.99 for 11 mm of sacral inclination (Figure 5B).

Instead, the relationship between LLI and vertebral rotation, also variables in a statistical relationship of the logistic regression type, showed an R2 of 0.08, a statistically significant value but one that is smaller than that of the relationship between the sacral shelf and vertebral rotation, for which the p value was 0.0016. This value is statistically significant but lower than that of the previous correlation (Figure 6A).

We found that 5 mm is the value of LLI that increases the risk of vertebral rotation. Moreover, the probability of being in the patient group without spinal rotation was 0.38 for patients without heterometry, whereas it increased to 0.93 in the case of heterometry equal to 26 mm (Figure 6B).

The correlation between sacral inclination and LLI was a linear-regression-type statistical relationship and showed a value of $p < 0.001$ (Figure 7).

We found that every mm of length leg inequality corresponds to 0.3 mm of sacral shelf inclination; therefore, vertebral rotation is very likely to occur when LLI reaches a threshold of 5 mm.

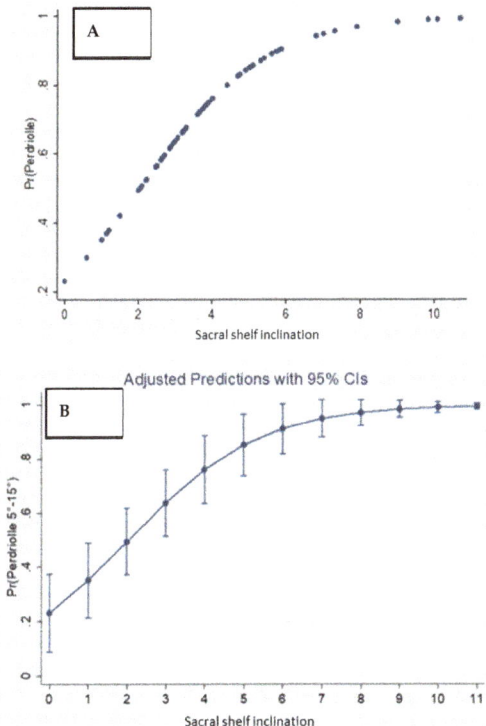

Figure 5. (**A**) Relationship between sacral shelf inclination and vertebral rotation. (**B**) Predictive probability of vertebral rotation correlated with sacral shelf inclination.

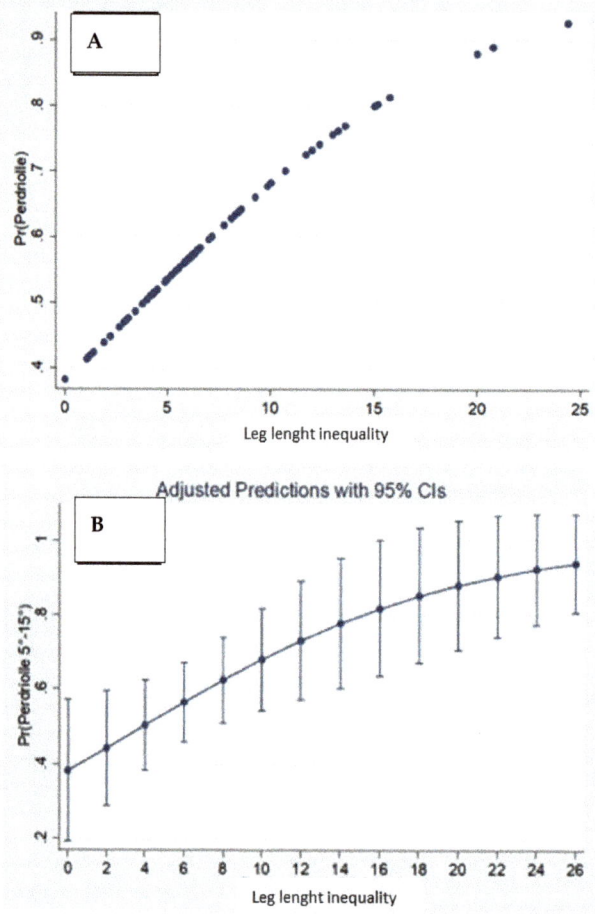

Figure 6. (**A**) Relationship between LLI and vertebral rotation. (**B**) Probability of being in the patient group without or with vertebral rotation based on LLI.

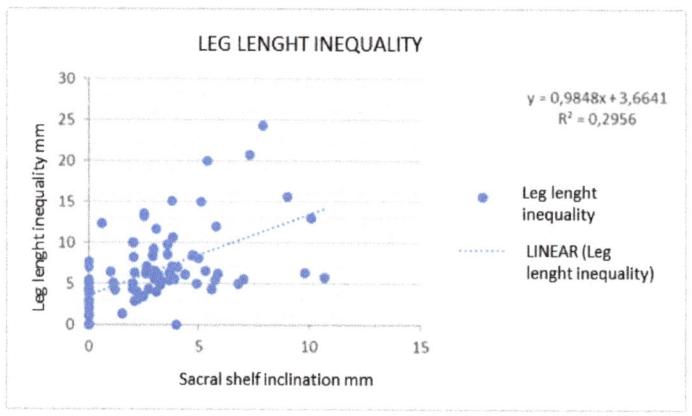

Figure 7. Relationship between LLI and sacral shelf inclination.

4. Discussion

According to the literature, to define a curve as "scoliosis", the deformity in the coronal plane must be greater than 10° Cobb, and it must present vertebral rotation in the transverse plane [20–23]. Instead, there is a consensus that "functional scoliosis" is an asymmetry in the coronal plane without evidence of a thoracic hump or lumbar asymmetry based on Adam's test. Often, this alteration is due to limb length discrepancy; it is not progressive and can be corrected without weight bearing [4–24]. The results of the present study demonstrated the presence of vertebral rotation in patients with functional scoliosis caused by LLI, and it was correlated with 5 mm of LLI, which will create changes in vertebral and sacral alignment. Previous studies investigated the relationship between LLI and spinal posture with conflicting findings. To the best of our knowledge, this is the first study focusing on vertebral rotation in pediatric patients with functional scoliosis determined by LLI. Moreover, we demonstrated a correlation between LLI, SSI, and vertebral rotation. These results are important, enabling us to better understand the role of vertebral rotation, a parameter related to the progression of this disease [12–25].

Hoikka et al. [12], in a study of 100 patients with an average leg length inequality of 5 mm and a main age of 47 years, found a correlation between LLI and sacral inclination but no relationship between LLI and the Cobb degree. Specht et al., in a retrospective study of 106 consecutive routine diagnostic X-ray procedures, found that 60% of the patients had LLI > 3 mm, 40% had LLI > 6 mm, 50% of the latter had lumbar scoliosis, and only 30% of the first group had lumbar scoliosis [26]. Gibson et al. [27], in a study of patients with LLI ranging from 15 to 55 mm due to a femoral shaft fracture sustained after skeletal maturity, observed that functional scoliosis resolved nearly completely after correction of the leg length discrepancy. However, in this study, the patients showed a contradictory increase in lateral flexion of the column to the shortest leg, although the spine returned to symmetry after LLD correction. This finding contradicts the study of Papaioannou et al., which only included patients who had LLI since childhood (the patients were young adults, and their LLI ranged from 1.2 to 5.2 cm) [28]. These results suggest that a long period of functional scoliosis may result in permanent biomechanical changes in the lumbar spine. The period for which the spine is subjected to functional scoliosis also seems to affect the risk of degenerative changes. Manganiello et al. conducted two different studies to analyze the impact of LLI on the lumbar column, and they even suggested that low LLI can induce high desalination of the lumbar region with respect to major LLI (>2 cm) [29,30]. They also proposed that LLI could be the primum movens for the onset of structured scoliosis. These findings supplemented those of the aforementioned studies demonstrating that changes in spinal alignment can form over time, suggesting a possible structuring of vertebral rotation over time secondary to the difference in length of the lower limbs. Although the recent literature has shown a relationship between the LLI and lumbar scoliosis, Grivas et al. analyzed patients with LLI ranging from 0.5 cm to 2 cm and found that LLI was significantly correlated with the 4DF (4D Formetric DIERS apparatus) reading of pelvis rotation, pelvic tilt, and surface rotation, while it was not correlated with the scoliosis angle or the scoliometer reading at the lumbar level [31]. Instead, Betsch et al. simulated LLI > 2 cm in 100 volunteers (53 females and 47 males) with a mean age of 34 years, finding a correlation between LLI, pelvic inclination, surface rotation, and lateral inclination (all parameters were investigated with raster stereography). In a previous study, the authors did not observe postural impairment for LLI < 2 cm [13,14].

Furthermore, a relationship between leg length inequality and adolescent idiopathic scoliosis (AIS) was also demonstrated. In a recent study published in the *Asian Spine Journal*, Kobayashi et al. [9] demonstrated a direct relationship between LLI, the Cobb angle, and vertebral rotation in 23 patients with AIS. A correlation was found between LLI and vertebral rotation, but compared to our study, the number of patients was small and included scoliosis patients with a Cobb angle between 10 and 30 degrees and LLI > 2 cm. Sekiya et al. [32] found a correlation between functional LLI, pelvic obliquity, and the Cobb angle of the lumbar region, but they suggested that in this case, LLI was secondary to AIS. This study revealed that patients with AIS have functional LLD but not significant structural LLD. The authors reported that the relationship between the lumbar Cobb angle and functional LLD indicates that the lumbar curve contributes to functional LLD; thus, the difference between functional and structural LLDs represents a compensatory mechanism involving the extension and flexion of the lower limbs. None of these studies specifically focused on the consequences of LLI for both the alignment of the sacral shelf and the lumbar spine, exploring how these affects vertebral rotation. Moreover, patients affected by idiopathic AIS show a rotation of the pelvis and the sacrum in addition to an inclination, and it has been demonstrated that these pathologies can arise because of an LLI. In the radiographs of patients affected by scoliosis, the right ilium often appears to be wider than the left ilium in patients with major thoracic curves, while the left ilium often appears to be wider than the right ilium in patients with major thoracolumbar/lumbar curves. Gum et al. also noted this phenomenon and interpreted it as the result of transverse pelvic rotation. They suggested that the transverse plane pelvic position that accompanies major thoracic curves is the fourth transverse plane compensation. The direction of transverse pelvic rotation is the same as that for the main thoracic curve in most patients with a compensatory thoracolumbar/lumbar curve [15–34]. These studies can, therefore, explain the relationship that we found in our study between leg length inequality, sacral shelf, and vertebral rotation.

Our study was limited by the difficulty of undertaking a differential diagnosis between structured scoliosis and functional scoliosis due to LLI when there is vertebral rotation, because most lumbar curves are not progressive and the prognostic factors and causes of AIS are not yet known.

Our future objectives will be to follow these patients up to skeletal maturity, to observe the evolution of functional scoliosis due to LLI, and to understand the role of vertebral rotation. Another interesting point to evaluate is whether the use of a custom foot orthosis with sole lift would be useful in cases of a discrepancy starting from 5 mm to avoid the onset of a possible rotation that could not be reduced over time.

5. Conclusions

Functional scoliosis due to leg length inequality can involve vertebral rotation with a direct correlation between leg length inequality, sacral shelf inclination, and vertebral rotation. A limb length inequality greater than 5 mm can be considered as the threshold value above which the sacral shelf could tilt, causing a rotation of the spine.

Author Contributions: A.G.A. and M.M. participated in the conception, design and coordination, acquisition of data, analysis, and interpretation of data, drafted the manuscript, and performed the statistical analysis. S.C., D.B. and R.M.T. helped to draft the manuscript. All authors have read and agreed to the published version of the manuscript.

Funding: This work was supported by the Italian Ministry of Health with "Current Research funds". No benefits in any form have been or will be received from a commercial party related directly or indirectly to the subject of this manuscript. The manuscript submitted does not contain information about medical device(s)/drug(s).

Institutional Review Board Statement: Considering the retrospective nature of the analysis, the current study did not require the approval of the local ethics committee according to current legislation, but a notification was sent. The study was conducted by the Declaration of Helsinki and approved by the ethics committee of Bambino Gesù Children Hospital, Rome. Etihic code RAP-2023-0008 Approved 12 June 2023.

Informed Consent Statement: Written informed consent to participate in this study was provided by the participants. The participants provided written consent for the publication of data.

Data Availability Statement: Datasets generated and/or analyzed during the current study are available from the corresponding author upon reasonable request.

Conflicts of Interest: The authors declare no conflict of interest.

References

1. *L'orthopédie ou l'art de Prevenir et de Corriger dans les Enfans, les Difformités du Corps*; Alix: New York, NY, USA, 1741; Volume 2.
2. Konieczny, M.R.; Senyurt, H.; Krauspe, R. Epidemiology of adolescent idiopathic scoliosis. *J. Child. Orthop.* **2013**, *7*, 3–9. [CrossRef] [PubMed]
3. Sarwark, J.F.; Castelein, R.M.; Maqsood, A.; Aubin, C.E. The Biomechanics of Induction in Adolescent Idiopathic Scoliosis: Theo-retical Factors. *J. Bone Jt. Surg. Am.* **2019**, *101*, e22. [CrossRef] [PubMed]
4. Peng, Y.; Wang, S.R.; Qiu, G.X.; Zhang, J.G.; Zhuang, Q.Y. Research progress on the etiology and pathogenesis of adolescent idiopathic scoliosis. *Chin. Med. J. Engl.* **2020**, *133*, 483–493. [CrossRef] [PubMed]
5. Lenz, M.; Oikonomidis, S.; Harland, A.; Fürnstahl, P.; Farshad, M.; Bredow, J.; Eysel, P.; Scheyerer, M.J. Scoliosis and Prognosis—A systematic review regarding patient-specific and radiological predictive factors for curve progression. *Eur. Spine J.* **2021**, *30*, 1813–1822. [CrossRef] [PubMed]
6. Janicki, J.A.; Alman, B. Scoliosis: Review of diagnosis and treatment. *Paediatr. Child. Health* **2007**, *12*, 771–776. [CrossRef]
7. Brady, R.J.; Dean, J.B.; Skinner, T.M.; Gross, M.T. Limb Length Inequality: Clinical Implications for Assessment and Intervention. *J. Orthop. Sports Phys. Ther.* **2003**, *33*, 221–234. [CrossRef]
8. Negrini, S.; Donzelli, S.; Aulisa, A.G.; Czaprowski, D.; Schreiber, S.; De Mauroy, J.C.; Diers, H.; Grivas, T.B.; Knott, P.; Kotwicki, T.; et al. 2016 SOSORT guidelines: Orthopaedic and rehabilitation treatment of idiopathic scoliosis during growth. *Scoliosis Spinal Disord.* **2018**, *13*, 3. [CrossRef] [PubMed]
9. Kobayashi, K.; Ando, K.; Nakashima, H.; Machino, M.; Morozumi, M.; Kanbara, S.; Ito, S.; Inoue, T.; Yamaguchi, H.; Mishima, K.; et al. Scoliosis Caused by Limb-Length Discrepancy in Children. *Asian Spine J.* **2020**, *14*, 801–807. [CrossRef]
10. Gordon, J.E.; Davis, L.E. Leg length discrepancy: The natural history (and what do we trulyreally know). *J. Pediatr. Orthop.* **2019**, *39* (Suppl. S1), S10–S13. [CrossRef]
11. Reid, D.; Smith, B. Leg length discrepancy assessment: Accuracy and precision in five clinical methods of evaluation. *Physiother. Can.* **1984**, *36*, 177–182.
12. Hoikka, V.; Ylikoski, M.; Tallroth, K. Leg-length inequality has poor correlation with lumbar scoliosis. A radiological study of 100 patients with chronic low-back pain. *Arch. Orthop. Trauma Surg.* **1989**, *108*, 173–175. [CrossRef]
13. Betsch, M.; Rapp, W.; Przybylla, A.; Jungbluth, P.; Hakimi, M.; Schneppendahl, J.; Thelen, S.; Wild, M. Determination of the amount of leg length inequality that alters spinal posture in healthy subjects using rasterstereography. *Eur. Spine J.* **2013**, *22*, 1354–1361. [CrossRef]
14. Betsch, M.; Wild, M.; Große, B.; Rapp, W.; Horstmann, T. The effect of simulating leg length inequality on spinal posture and pelvic position: A dynamic rasterstereographic analysis. *Eur. Spine J.* **2012**, *21*, 691–697. [CrossRef]
15. Young, R.S.; Andrew, P.D.; Cummings, G.S. Effect of simulating leg length inequality on pelvic torsion and trunk mobility. *Gait Posture* **2000**, *11*, 217–223. [CrossRef] [PubMed]
16. Rannisto, S.; Okuloff, A.; Uitti, J.; Paananen, M.; Rannisto, P.-H.; Malmivaara, A.; Karppinen, J. Leg-length discrepancy is associated with low back pain among those who must stand while working. *BMC Musculoskelet. Disord.* **2015**, *16*, 110. [CrossRef] [PubMed]
17. Lupparelli, S.; Pola, E.; Pitta, L.; Mazza, O.; De Santis, V.; Aulisa, L. Biomechanical factors affecting progression of structural scoliotic curves of the spine. *Stud. Health Technol. Inform.* **2002**, *91*, 81–85. [CrossRef] [PubMed]
18. Aulisa, A.G.; Guzzanti, V.; Falciglia, F.; Galli, M.; Pizzetti, P.; Aulisa, L. Curve progression after long-term brace treatment in ado-lescent idiopathic scoliosis: Comparative results between over and under 30 Cobb degrees—SOSORT 2017 award winner. *Scoliosis Spinal Disord.* **2017**, *12*, 36. [CrossRef] [PubMed]
19. Vialle, R.; Thévenin-Lemoine, C.; Mary, P. Neuromuscular scoliosis. *Orthop. Traumatol. Surg. Res.* **2013**, *99*, S124–S139. [CrossRef]
20. Rothschild, D.; Ng, S.Y.; Ng, Y.L.E. Indications of sole lift and foot orthoses in the management of mild idiopathic scoliosis-a review. *J. Phys. Ther. Sci.* **2020**, *32*, 251–256. [CrossRef]
21. *Lovell and Winter's Pediatric Orthopaedics, Level 1 and 2*, 7th ed.; Lippincott Williams & Wilkins: Philadelphia, PA, USA, 2006.
22. Cheng, J.C.; Castelein, R.M.; Chu, W.C.; Danielsson, A.J.; Dobbs, M.B.; Grivas, T.B.; Gurnett, C.A.; Luk, K.D.; Moreau, A.; Newton, P.O.; et al. Adolescent idiopathic scoliosis. *Nat Rev Dis Primers*. **2015**, *1*, 15030. [CrossRef]
23. Troy, M.J.; Miller, P.E.; Price, N.; Talwalkar, V.; Zaina, F.; Donzelli, S.; Negrini, S.; Hresko, M.T. The "Risser+" grade: A new grading system to classify skeletal maturity in idiopathic scoliosis. *Eur. Spine J.* **2019**, *28*, 559–566. [CrossRef] [PubMed]
24. Cummings, G.M.; Scholz, J.P.; Barnes, K.B. The Effect of Imposed Leg Length Difference on Pelvic Bone Symmetry. *Spine* **1993**, *18*, 368–373. [CrossRef] [PubMed]
25. Aulisa, A.G.; Guzzanti, V.; Falciglia, F.; Giordano, M.; Galli, M.; Aulisa, L. Brace treatment of Idiopathic Scoliosis is effective for a curve over 40 degrees, but is the evaluation of Cobb angle the only parameter for the indication of treatment? *Eur J Phys Rehabil Med.* **2019**, *55*, 231–240. [CrossRef] [PubMed]
26. Specht, D.L.; De Boer, K.F. Anatomical leg length inequality, scoliosis and lordotic curve in unselected clinic patients. *J. Manip. Physiol. Ther.* **1991**, *14*, 368–375.
27. Gibson, P.H.; Papaioannou, T.; Kenwright, J. Theinfluence on the spine of leg-length discrepancy after femoral fracture. *J Bone Joint Surg Br.* **1983**, *65*, 584–587. [CrossRef]
28. Papaioannou, T.; Stokes, I.; Kenwright, J. Scoliosis associated with limb-length inequality. *J. Bone Jt. Surg.* **1982**, *64*, 59–62. [CrossRef]

29. Manganiello, A. Rilievi radiologici nelle scoliosi idiopatiche. Interpretazione etiopatogenetica [Radiologic findings in idiopathic scoliosis. Etiopathogenetic interpretation]. *Radiol Med.* **1987**, *73*, 271–276. (In Italian)
30. Manganiello, A.; Scapin, F. Differenza di lunghezza degli arti inferiori e scoliosi. Studio clinico-radiologico [Lower extremity length inequality and scoliosis. Clinical and radiological study (author's transl)]. *Radiol Med.* **1980**, *66*, 911–914. (In Italian)
31. Grivas, T.B.; Angouris, K.; Chandrinos, M.; Kechagias, V. Truncal changes in children with mild limb length inequality: A surface topography study. *Scoliosis* **2018**, *13*, 27. [CrossRef]
32. Sekiya, T.; Aota, Y.; Yamada, K.; Kaneko, K.; Ide, M.; Saito, T. Evaluation of functional and structural leg length discrepancy in patients with adolescent idiopathic scoliosis using the EOS imaging system: A prospective comparative study. *Scoliosis* **2018**, *13*, 7. [CrossRef]
33. Qiu, X.-S.; Zhang, J.-J.; Yang, S.-W.; Lv, F.; Wang, Z.-W.; Chiew, J.; Ma, W.-W.; Qiu, Y. Anatomical study of the pelvis in patients with adolescent idiopathic scoliosis. *J. Anat.* **2012**, *220*, 173–178. [CrossRef] [PubMed]
34. Gum, J.L.; Asher, M.A.; Burton, D.C.; Lai, S.M.; Lambart, L.M. Transverse plane pelvic rotation in adolescent idiopathic scoliosis: Primary or compensa-tory? *Eur. Spine J.* **2007**, *16*, 1579–1586. [CrossRef] [PubMed]

Disclaimer/Publisher's Note: The statements, opinions and data contained in all publications are solely those of the individual author(s) and contributor(s) and not of MDPI and/or the editor(s). MDPI and/or the editor(s) disclaim responsibility for any injury to people or property resulting from any ideas, methods, instructions or products referred to in the content.

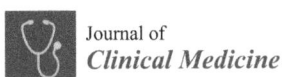

Article

Is Thoracic Kyphosis Relevant to Pain, Autonomic Nervous System Function, Disability, and Cervical Sensorimotor Control in Patients with Chronic Nonspecific Neck Pain?

Ibrahim M. Moustafa [1,2,3], Tamer Shousha [1,2,3], Ashokan Arumugam [1,2,4] and Deed E. Harrison [5,*]

1. Department of Physiotherapy, College of Health Sciences, University of Sharjah, Sharjah 27272, United Arab Emirates
2. Neuromusculoskeletal Rehabilitation Research Group, RIMHS–Research Institute of Medical and Health Sciences, University of Sharjah, Sharjah 27272, United Arab Emirates
3. Faculty of Physical Therapy, Cairo University, Giza 12613, Egypt
4. Sustainable Engineering Asset Management Research Group, RISE-Research Institute of Sciences and Engineering, University of Sharjah, Sharjah 27272, United Arab Emirates
5. CBP Nonprofit (A Spine Research Foundation), Eagle, ID 83616, USA
* Correspondence: drdeedharrison@gmail.com

Abstract: There is great interest in thoracic kyphosis, as it is thought to be a contributor to neck pain, neck disability, and sensorimotor control measures; however, this has not been completely investigated in treatment or case control studies. This case control design investigated participants with non-specific chronic neck pain. Eighty participants with a defined hyper-kyphosis (>55°) were compared to eighty matched participants with normal thoracic kyphosis (<55°). Participants were matched for age and neck pain duration. Hyper-kyphosis was further categorized into two distinct types: postural kyphosis (PK) and Scheuermann's kyphosis (SK). Posture measures included formetric thoracic kyphosis and the craniovertebral angle (CVA) to assess forward head posture. Sensorimotor control was assessed by the following measures: smooth pursuit neck torsion test (SPNT), overall stability index (OSI), and left and right rotation repositioning accuracy. A measure of autonomic nervous system function included the amplitude and latency of skin sympathetic response (SSR). Differences in variable measures were examined using the Student's t-test to compare the means of continuous variables between the two groups. One-way ANOVA was used to compare mean values in the three groups: postural kyphosis, Scheuermann's kyphosis, and normal kyphosis group. Pearson correlation was used to evaluate the relationship between participant's thoracic kyphosis magnitude (in each group separately and as an entire population) and their CVA, SPNT, OSI, head repositioning accuracy, and SSR latency and amplitude. Hyper-kyphosis participants had a significantly greater neck disability index compared to the normal kyphosis group ($p < 0.001$) with the SK group having greatest disability ($p < 0.001$). Statistically significant differences between the two kyphosis groups and the normal kyphosis group for all the sensorimotor measured variables were identified with the SK group having the most decreased efficiency of the measures in the hyper-kyphosis group, including: SPNT, OSI, and left and right rotation repositioning accuracy. In addition, there was a significant difference in neurophysiological findings for SSR amplitude (entire sample of kyphosis vs. normal kyphosis, $p < 0.001$), but there was no significant difference for SSR latency ($p = 0.07$). The CVA was significantly greater in the hyper-kyphosis group ($p < 0.001$). The magnitude of the thoracic kyphosis correlated with worsening CVA (with the SK group having the smallest CVA; $p < 0.001$) and the magnitude of the decreased efficiency of the sensorimotor control measures and the amplitude and latency of the SSR. The PK group, overall, showed the greatest correlations between thoracic kyphosis and measured variables. Participants with hyper-thoracic kyphosis exhibited abnormal sensorimotor control and autonomic nervous system dysfunction compared to those with normal thoracic kyphosis.

Keywords: thoracic spine; neck pain; kyphosis; sensorimotor control; posture

Citation: Moustafa, I.M.; Shousha, T.; Arumugam, A.; Harrison, D.E. Is Thoracic Kyphosis Relevant to Pain, Autonomic Nervous System Function, Disability, and Cervical Sensorimotor Control in Patients with Chronic Nonspecific Neck Pain? *J. Clin. Med.* **2023**, *12*, 3707. https://doi.org/10.3390/jcm12113707

Received: 16 April 2023
Revised: 21 May 2023
Accepted: 25 May 2023
Published: 27 May 2023

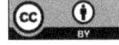

Copyright: © 2023 by the authors. Licensee MDPI, Basel, Switzerland. This article is an open access article distributed under the terms and conditions of the Creative Commons Attribution (CC BY) license (https://creativecommons.org/licenses/by/4.0/).

1. Introduction

Neck pain is the fourth leading cause of long-term disability with an annual prevalence exceeding 30%, most often in females [1]. Neck pain is a common condition with several proposed biomechanical and psycho-social contributing factors [2]. While the mechanical causes of neck pain are not completely understood, they are thought to be linked to the interconnected functions of anatomical components of the cervical spine [2]. Neck discomfort can be caused by any incident that alters joint mechanics or muscle function via alterations and increases in general loading and load sharing of the various tissues [2–4]. For instance, several studies have demonstrated the impact of thoracic spine abnormalities on the kinematics of the cervical spine and overall neck mobility [5–7]. In particular, studies have demonstrated a link to movement coordination between the cervical and thoracic spines [3,5,6,8]. While the prevalence of neck disorders is greater in older persons, who also have a higher prevalence of thoracic hyper-kyphosis [6], neck pain is also one of the most common musculoskeletal disorders in young adult populations, with a reported 12-month prevalence ranging from 42 to 67% [9–11]. An explanation for such a high rate of neck pain in young and older populations is possible concomitant impairments in the thoracic spine leading to a dysfunction of the cervico-thoracic musculature such as the serratus anterior, levator scapulae, and trapezius [12,13].

Since changes in sagittal thoracic alignment have been reported to alter the mechanical loading of the cervical spine [14,15], this may subtly or overtly impair proprioceptive afferentation from spine ligaments, muscles, and discs, which are considered to be major components of sensorimotor control supplying the essential neurophysiological information for feedforward and feedback responses via linkages to the vestibular, visual, and central nervous systems [16–18]. Sensorimotor control is altered in neck pain populations compared to healthy controls, where slower reaction times in visual acuity, cervical movement, and inefficient motor control in general has been reported [19,20]. It is unclear if the altered sensorimotor control is causative of neck pain and disability or a result due to kinesiophobia (fear-based movement variables) [21]; however, it is clear that inefficient sensorimotor control is part of the cycle of chronicity and likely influences recovery [16–21]. In addition to sensorimotor control influences, several studies show that the cervical receptors and the sympathetic nervous system have direct interactions [22–24]. However, there is limited evidence suggesting that the autonomic nervous system is sensitive to alterations in articular afferent input driven by thoracic hyper-kyphosis and joint dysfunction [22,23,25].

It is known that thoracic hyper-kyphosis is related to a patients' pain, disability, shoulder kinematics, and general health status [26–31]. The threshold for hyper-kyphosis has been reported to be 45° on x-rays (T4-T12 and T5-T12) for pain and disability [26,27], while the 60° value has been reported to be the threshold for more severe disability as in adult spine deformity cases [28,29]. The assumption that a normal thoracic alignment and normal cervical kinematics are important for a better afferentation process has some preliminary evidence [5–8,12–14]. However, studies have not fully investigated the relationship between hyper-kyphosis, forward head posture, and the correlation (if any) on sensorimotor control measurements and the autonomic nervous system.

In general, there is a lack of studies assessing the effect of the thoracic spine sagittal alignment on cervical pain, autonomic nervous system function, disability, and sensorimotor control. Therefore, the purpose of this study was to investigate the correlation in sensorimotor control, neck disability index, and autonomic dysfunction in chronic nonspecific neck patients with a thoracic hyper-kyphosis compared to a matched group of normal kyphosis participants but also having chronic nonspecific neck pain. We hypothesized that patients with chronic neck pain and a thoracic hyper-kyphosis would have impaired sensorimotor control and autonomic dysfunction compared to those chronic neck pain patients with a normal thoracic alignment. Secondarily, we hypothesized that the magnitude of thoracic kyphosis would be correlated to the measures of sensorimotor control and autonomic nervous system function as performed herein.

2. Materials and Methods

In this cross-sectional study, we compared 80 young adults over the age of 18 years with chronic nonspecific neck pain and thoracic hyper-kyphosis to 80 matched individuals with chronic nonspecific neck pain who had a normal thoracic kyphotic alignment. Participants were considered matched if their age difference was within 2 years and if their duration of neck pain was of a similar length of time. When the pain duration varied by less than two months, participants were deemed to be matched. Participants were patients recruited from a specialized pain and rehabilitation unit at the Farouk Hospital, Cairo, Egypt from January to August 2022. All cases received a thorough examination in the pain clinic, and all hyper-kyphotic cases underwent radiological assessment. Ethical approval was obtained from the Research and Ethics Committee at Cairo University (CA-REC-22-5-20), with informed consent obtained from all participants prior to data collection in accordance with relevant guidelines and regulations. A flow chart of the recruitment process is shown in Figure 1.

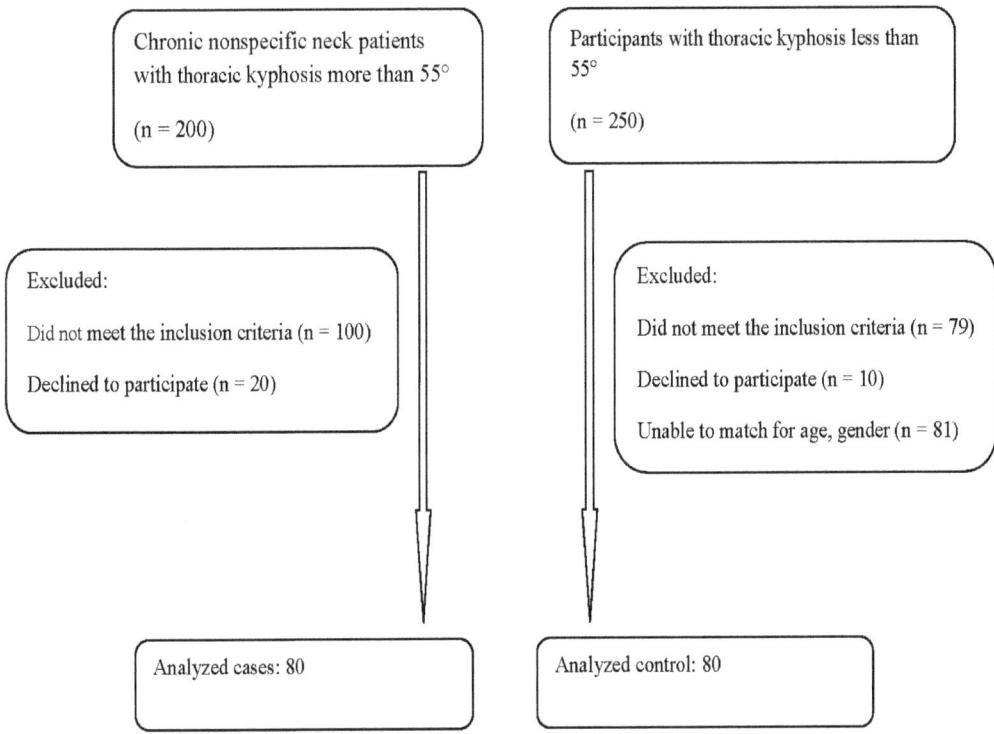

Figure 1. Participant study flow chart for group inclusion and exclusion.

2.1. Participant Inclusion and Exclusion Criteria

2.1.1. Inclusion

All participants had to have the diagnosis of chronic non-specific neck pain (CNSNP) with reduced cervical spine range of motion. Thoracic hyper-kyphotic participants were screened with a thorough examination by an orthopedic surgeon, including spine radiography, to rule out serious spine pathologies. However, participants with mild to moderate Scheuermann's kyphosis (SK) (SK participants were diagnosed via radiography and clinical examination with the orthopedic surgeon) were permitted in the hyper-kyphotic sample, though SK participants were also analyzed as a subgroup of hyper-kyphosis to identify any possible differences. See the results section for details. Participants with normal kyphosis did not receive thoracic spine radiographic imaging, as there was no clinical rationale for imaging in these participants; thus, an external measurement of thoracic kyphosis was chosen to make comparisons in all participants. Prior to inclusion, participants were evaluated by measuring the sagittal thoracic *kyphotic angle ICT-ITL (max)* using the 4D formetric system (note it is a 4D system, as it allows for a time variable to capture any sagittal shift and sway over 60 s) where ICT-ITL (max) is measured between tangents from the cervicothoracic junction (ICT-T1) and that of the thoracolumbar junction (ITL-T12). The reproducibility of results is excellent, making this non-invasive system appropriate for clinical assessment, as the reliability of thoracic kyphosis measurement is excellent with coefficients of variation of approximately 7% (3.5 degrees) for angulations [32,33]. Figure 2 depicts this measurement. Hyper-kyphosis participants were included if the *ICT-ITL (max)* angle measured more than 55°. Normal kyphosis participants were defined as the ICT-ITL (max) angle being less than 55° [33]. There is good correlation between the formetric vs. Cobb angle of thoracic kyphosis, but formetric measurements consistently overestimates kyphosis by an average of 5–7°, indicating that the radiographic kyphosis would be approximately 48–50°, which is the upper end of normal and the cutoff value for where thoracic kyphosis begins to be associated with pain and disability [26,27,30,31,33–35].

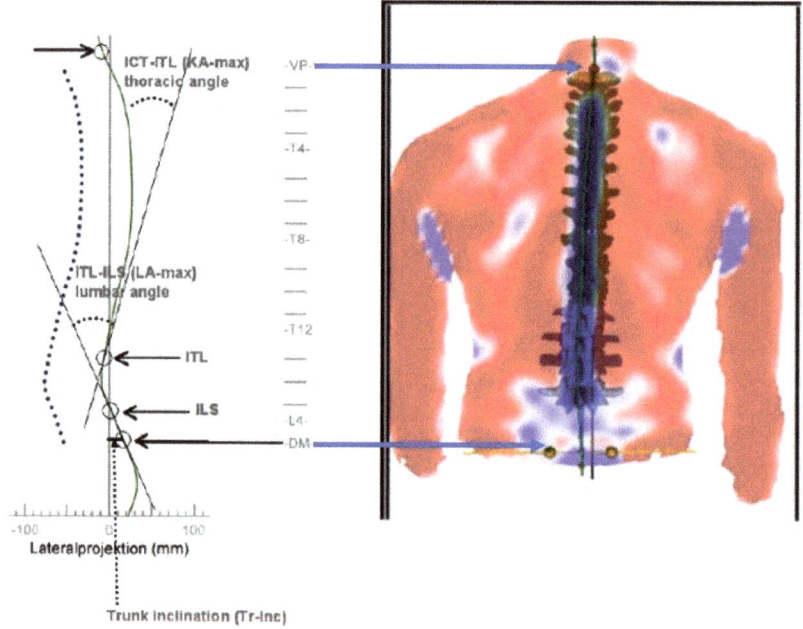

Figure 2. 4D formetric device measurement of thoracic kyphosis and trunk inclination where *kyphotic angle ICT-ITL (max)* is measured between tangents of cervicothoracic junction (ICT) and of thoracolumbar junction (ITL). ICT: inflectional points from cervical to thoracic spine. ITL: inflectional points from thoracic to lumbar spine. KA: kyphosis angle. LA: lordosis angle. VP: vertebra prominence. DM: dimple.

2.1.2. Exclusion

Exclusion criteria included the presence of any signs or symptoms of medical "red flags", a history of previous spine surgery, vertebral fracture, signs or symptoms of upper motor neuron disease, vertebrobasilar insufficiency, amyotrophic lateral sclerosis, and bilateral upper extremity radicular symptoms. Detailed exclusions were:

- Neck pain associated with whiplash injury;
- Neck pain with bilateral cervical radiculopathy;
- Fibromyalgia syndrome;
- Surgery in the neck area, regardless of the cause;
- Neck pain accompanied by vertigo caused by vertebra-basilar insufficiency or accompanied with non-cervicogenic headaches;
- Recent or recurrent middle ear infections or any hearing impairment requiring the use of a hearing aid;
- Visual impairment not corrected by glasses;
- Any disorder of the central nervous system.

2.2. Measurement Procedures

2.2.1. ICT-ITL (Max)

The thoracic posture was measured in a neutral position to ensure consistency between repeated images captured in the same session; also, this would aid comparison with other studies that measured Cobb's angle for thoracic kyphosis in radiographic studies. Each participant was positioned 2 m from the measurement system in front of a black background screen, and a valid and reliable formetric system [32,33,35] was used to analyze 3D body posture displacements (DIERS Medical Systems, Chicago, IL, USA). The column height was aligned to move the relevant parts of the patient's back into the center of the control monitor by using the column up/down button of the control unit. A permanent mark fixed with a tape on the floor was used to ensure the best lateral and longitudinal position of the patient. The participant's back (including the upper gluteal region) was uncovered to allow better imaging of the back. The participants' hair was tied up (when needed) to allow visualization of the vertebral prominences. The system was ready for image recording when the participant was correctly positioned in the participant's perception of their neutral resting, relaxed posture position, being defined as the relaxed upright stance, with feet hip width apart and barefooted, where the participant was instructed to:

- look straight ahead in a relaxed breathing state with their head in a neutral position, not being twisted or bent;
- relax their shoulders, do not hunch them or rotate them forward;
- keep their upper arms, elbows and hands comfortably at their sides;
- stand with their legs straight, but with knees relaxed, not locked back (preventing hyperextension).

Thoracic kyphosis was measured as the maximum kyphosis between tangents from the cervicothoracic junction (ICT-T1) and that of the thoracolumbar junction (ITL-T12). This would be considered a total thoracic kyphosis from T1–T12 vertebral levels. Kyphotic participants were included if the angle measured 55° or more and normal kyphosis if the angle measured less than 55° [26,27,30,33–35]. There is a good correlation between the formetric measurement and Cobb angle of thoracic kyphosis, but the former one consistently overestimates kyphosis by an average of 5–7° [33,35].

2.2.2. Craniovertebral Angle (CVA)

To assess the influence of thoracic kyphosis on forward head posture (FHP), we measured the craniovertebral angle (CVA) in both groups. The CVA is constructed using C7 spinous process and drawing a line from it to the tragus of the ear. Next, a horizontal line is drawn through C7 spinous, where the CVA is the acute angle between the two lines. Typically, when the CVA is less than 50°, then a participant is classified as having significant forward head posture [36,37]. The CVA has excellent reliability to assess forward head posture [36,37]. Figure 3 presents the CVA.

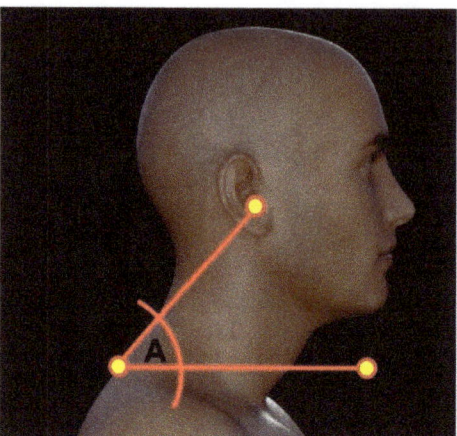

Figure 3. Measurement of the craniovertebral angle (CVA). Two markers are utilized and placed at the level of the C7 spinous process and the tragus of the ear; then a line is constructed connecting these two points. Finally, a horizontal line is drawn using the C7 marker as the reference, and the CVA is measured as angle A between the two lines [36,37].

2.2.3. Numerical Rating Score (NRS)

Neck pain average intensity over the previous week was assessed using a 0–10 NRS score ranging from 0 = no pain to 10 = bed ridden and incapacitated. The reliability and validity of the NRS has been found to be good to high [38].

2.2.4. Neck Disability Index

The neck disability index (NDI) to assess activities of daily living impact was administered. The NDI has good reliability, validity, and responsiveness to change [39].

2.2.5. Sensorimotor Control Measures

There is a detailed interplay between proprioception and postural control, such that normal posture alignment is likely a major component driving the afferentation process leading to improved sensorimotor integration and motor control. To assess the effects of thoracic kyphosis and forward head posture on the sensorimotor system, we measured three common measures of sensorimotor control herein, including the assessment of the following: (a) cervical joint position sense testing, (b) head and eye movement control, and (c) evaluation of postural stability.

a. Cervical Joint Position Sense Testing

Head repositioning accuracy (HRA) was assessed with the cervical range of motion (CROM) device as previously described in the literature (CROM deluxe device by Frabication: https://www.amazon.com/Fabrication-12-1156-Crom-Deluxe/dp/B00BRCGCNO, accessed on 19 May 2023). We followed the protocol of Loudon et al., as this is reliable and valid [40]. The CROM was placed on the participants' head while they were seated upright on a stool without a backrest, with both feet supported on the floor with knees flexed to ≈90°. The participant was asked to sit upright in a neutral, non-slouched, and comfortable thoracic posture attempting to keep the thoracic spine perpendicular to the plane of the stool. The neutral head position (NHP) was considered as the starting and reference position, where the CROM was adjusted to zero for the primary plane of rotational movement. Patients were instructed to close their eyes, memorize the starting position, actively rotate their head to 30° about the vertical axis, and reposition their head to the starting position with no restrictions for speed; only repositioning accuracy was encouraged. HRA was defined as the difference in degrees between the starting and the return positions [41]. Three repetitions were performed within 60 s for both the left and right directions; for a total of six sets. The test is reported as error in degrees (°), where less than 10% or 3° is normal [40,41].

b. Head and eye movement control: smooth pursuit neck torsion test (SPNT)

Assessment of disturbances in eye movement control by the electro-oculography was adopted from Tjell et al. [42]. The test was performed with the participant's head and trunk in a neutral straight ahead position and then two trunk rotation positions (head neutral, trunk in 45° rotation to each side). Patients were asked to blink three times (for recognition and elimination in data analysis) and then follow the path of a light as closely as possible with their eyes. The SPNT test value was defined as the difference between the average gain in the neutral and torsion positions for left vs. right rotation. Findings are reported as a percentage (%) of error of corrective saccades (eye movements), where 100% is perfect (0% error), 10–20% error is normal, and greater than 20% error is abnormal. The videonystagmography system VisualEyes™ 525 by Interacoustics A/S in Denmark was utilized to conduct the SPNT test.

c. Postural stability

The Biodex Balance System SD (Biodex Medical Systems, Inc., Shirley, NY, USA) was used to assess postural stability. Dynamic balance was assessed by simulating displacements in both anterior/posterior (AP) and medial/lateral (ML) directions by changing the device platform level of stability. The platform provides an objective assessment of balance using three indices: the overall stability index (OSI), an anteroposterior stability index (APSI), and a mediolateral stability index (MLSI). These indices are calculated according to the degree of platform oscillation. Smaller values indicate a good stability level of the participants. The reported inter-examiner reliability coefficients range between 0.77 and 0.99 [43,44]. Balance indices were calculated over three 10 s trials, with 20 s rest between trials. The average of three trials was recorded. The balance system was set to a dynamic position of 4 out of 8.

2.2.6. Sympathetic Skin Response (SSR)

On the day of the study, patients were asked to avoid using medicated lotions and cosmetics (on the hands), not to engage in physical activity, and avoid smoking, eating, and drinking coffee two hours prior to the recordings. To acclimatize patients to the experimental environment, all participants spent 20 min in a room with a temperature of 22–24 °C just before the measurements were taken.

The EMG was used to measure the SSR. Room temperature was maintained at 26 °C in order to maintain a stable skin temperature [45,46]. The active surface electrodes were attached on the palmar side, and the references were placed on the dorsum of the hand. The stimulus was given at the wrist contralateral to the recording side. Measurements were taken from both left and right sides. An intensity of 20–30 mA with an irregular interval of more than one minute was applied to prevent habituation. When habituation occurred, stimulation was delayed for about three or four minutes. Skin potentials were recorded for a 10 s analysis period. The latency and peak-to-peak amplitude SSR were determined. Mean values of three trials were used for each parameter. Sweep speed was 500 ms/div.

SSR was considered absent if there was no response after 10 stimuli [47]. In the SSR trace, the latency and amplitude character points markers placement was corrected manually if the ones automatically generated by the EMG software were inaccurately placed. Latencies were measured from the stimulation artifact to the initiation of the response which is defined as the earliest point where the amplitude begins to increase. The amplitude is measured from the peak of the first deflection to the peak of the next one (peak-to-peak) [48].

2.3. Sample Size Determination

A priori sample size calculation based on a pilot study conducted for 10 patients indicated that 70 participants per each group would be required to detect an effect size of 0.6. Pain was used as the outcome measure for this calculation. To insure robust data, the sample size was increased by 14% in order to attain 80 participants per group.

2.4. Statistical Analysis

The one-sample Kolmogorov–Smirnov normality test was used to determine whether the data were normally distributed, and homogeneity of variance assumption was assessed by the Levene statistic. Descriptive data were presented as mean ± standard deviation. The Student's *t*-test was used to compare the means of continuous variables, and the Chi-squared test for categorical variables was used to assess any differences between the two groups, the entire hyperkyphotic and normal groups. When separating the hyper-kyphosis sample into the two subgroups, the one-way ANOVA was used to compare the mean values in the three groups: postural kyphosis, Scheuermann's kyphosis, and normal kyphosis group. Post hoc Tukey's analysis was performed to determine differences between groups, when ANOVA revealed a significant difference.

A p-value < 0.05 was considered statistically significant. Correlations (Pearson's r) were used to examine the relationships between the ICT-ITL (KA-max) in both groups and the measured variables: SSR amplitude and latency, OSI, left and right rotation repositioning accuracy, NDI, SPNT, and NRS. The minimal clinically important difference (MCID) of the of the SSR and NDI outcomes were compared to the existing literature [45,46]. Whereas the MCID of the sensorimotor control variables were not available in the literature to our knowledge thus, effect sizes for all variables were measured using Cohen's d, where d ≈ 0.2 is limited effect, d ≈ 0.5 is a moderate effect, and d ≈ 0.8 is a large effect with very significant clinical relevance. Correlations were investigated for each group (postural kyphosis, Scheuermann's kyphosis, and normal kyphosis) separately and then as an entire sample of 160 participants to identify possible differences. SPSS version 20.0 software (SPSS Inc., Chicago, IL, USA) was used for analyzing data with normality and equal variance assumptions ensured before the analysis.

3. Results

3.1. Participant Demographics and Characteristics

Descriptive data for the demographic and clinical variables for the entire sample of 80 hyper-kyphotic and the 80 normal kyphosis participants are presented in Table 1. No statistically significant differences between the hyper-kyphotic group and the normal kyphosis group were found at baseline for their demographic and clinical variables. No data were missing for any of measured variables in any of the participants in this study. We separated the hyper-kyphotic participants into two groups: 35 postural kyphosis and 45 Scheuermann's kyphosis categories, and Table 2 presents this demographic and clinical data. No statistically significant baseline differences for the clinical and demographic variables was found for these two subgroups of thoracic hyper-kyphosis.

Table 1. Baseline participant demographics. The statistical significance between groups is shown. Here both the postural and Scheuermann's kyphosis group are combined into an entire kyphotic sample. The Student's *t*-test to compare the continuous variables and the Chi-squared test for categorical variables were used. Values are expressed as means ± standard deviation where indicated.

Variables	Entire Kyphotic (n = 80)	Normal (n = 80)	*p* Value
Age (years)	25.1 ± 3	24 ± 4.6	0.07
Weight (kg)	66 ± 10	60 ± 9	0.9

Table 1. *Cont.*

Variables	Entire Kyphotic (n = 80)	Normal (n = 80)	p Value
Sex			
Male	38	32	0.2
Female	42	48	
Marital status			
Single	61	59	
Married	19	21	0.3
Separated, divorced, or widowed	0	0	
Pain duration (months)	18 ± 4	17 ± 5	0.16
Smoking			
Light smoker	29	32	
Heavy smoker	14	15	0.4
No Smoker	37	33	

Table 2. Participant demographics of the hyper-kyphotic group separated by type of kyphosis with either a postural kyphosis or a Scheuermann's kyphosis. Statistical significance was tested using the ANOVA test to compare continuous variables, and the Chi-squared test for categorical variables. Values are expressed as means ± standard deviation. * is a statistically significant difference.

Variables	Postural Kyphosis N = 35	Scheuermann's kyphosis N = 45	Normal (n = 80)	p Value
Age (years)	25 ± 3.2	25.3 ± 3	24 ± 4.6	0.16
Weight (kg)	65 ± 11	67 ± 9	60 ± 9	0.6
Sex				
Male	18	20	32	0.5
Female	17	25	48	
Marital status				
Single	27	33	59	
Married	8	12	21	0.6
Separated, divorced, or widowed	0	0	0	
Pain duration (months)	17 ± 3	18.7 ± 4.5	17 ± 5	0.1
Smoking				
Light smoker	15	14	32	
Heavy smoker	8	6	15	0.15
No Smoker	12	25	33	
Kyphotic angle	66.5 ± 3	67.5 ± 4.9	49 ± 3	<0.001 *

3.2. Between Group Analysis

3.2.1. ICT-ITL (Max)

Box and whisker plots of the ICT-ITL (max) in the two hyper-kyphotic groups compared to the normal group are presented in Figure 4. As designed by our inclusion criteria, both hyper-kyphotic groups had the largest ICT-ITL (max) angles indicating an exaggerated kyphotic posture (entire hyper-kyphotic group, 67° ± 4; postural kyphosis group, 66.5° ± 3; and Scheuermann's kyphosis group, 67.5° ± 4.9). The normal kyphosis group had the smallest ICT-ITL (max) angles (normal kyphosis, 49° ± 3). As can be seen in Figure 4, there was no overlap between the kyphotic angles of the normal and kyphotic groups. Those with thoracic hyper-kyphosis were well above the threshold of 55°, thus eliminating any overlap within the standard error of measurement of the formetric system.

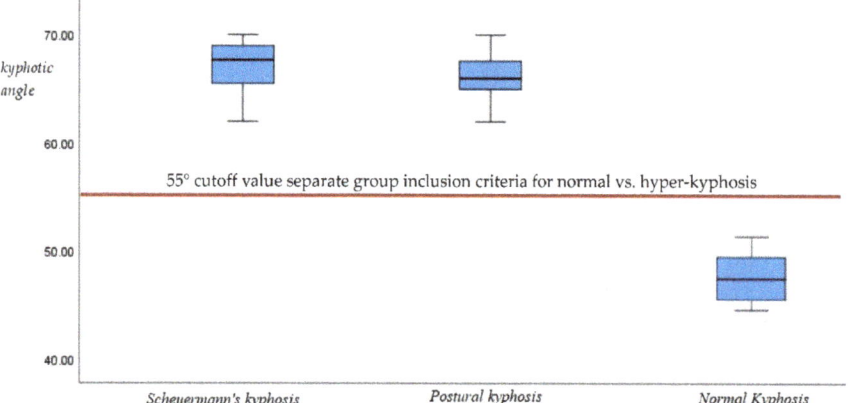

Figure 4. Box and whisker plots shown of the magnitude of thoracic kyphosis, ICT-ITL (max), in both hyper-kyphotic groups (postural kyphosis, 66.5° ± 3; Scheuermann's kyphosis; 67.5° ± 4.9) and the normal kyphosis (49° ± 3) groups. A statistically significant difference for these variables between normal kyphosis and total hyper-kyphosis (but not for hyper-kyphosis type) was forced by study design, where 55° (shown as red-dashed line) was the absolute cutoff for kyphosis between groups.

3.2.2. NRS and NDI

For pain level on the NRS, we found no statistically significant differences in pain intensity between groups ($p > 0.05$). However, the entire sample of the hyper-kyphotic group showed an increase in neck disability (NDI) scores compared to the normal kyphosis group ($p < 0.001$). When separating the hyper-kyphosis sample into the two subgroups, we identified a statistically significant difference in the NDI, where the Scheuermann's kyphosis group had a higher disability. Tables 3 and 4 presents these results.

Table 3. Between-group comparisons of pain and disability outcomes.

Variables	Entire Kyphotic Group (n = 80)	Normal Group (n = 80)	Cohen's d Effect Size	p Value (95% CI)
NDI	37.3 ± 4.1	29.8 ± 2.4	2.2	<0.001 * [−8.5, −6.45]
Pain intensity	5.3 ± 2.0	4.9 ± 1.8	0.20	0.18 [−0.99, 0.19]

CI = confidence interval; NDI = neck disability index; Pain intensity is 0–10 where 0 is no pain and 10 is incapacitated; all values are expressed as means ± standard deviation. * = statistically significant.

Table 4. Results of one-way-ANOVA and post hoc (Tukey) test. * = statistically significant.

	Postural Kyphosis N = 35	Scheuermann's Kyphosis N = 45	Normal Group (n = 80)	F-Value/ p-Value	Post Hoc
NDI	35.2 ± 2.4	39.1 ± 4.5	29.8 ± 2.4	132.67/ <0.001 *	Group 1 vs. Group 2: Diff = 3.9, 95% CI = 2.22 to 5.57, $p < 0.001$ * Group 1 vs. Group 3: Diff = −5.4, 95% CI = −6.90 to −3.89, $p < 0.001$ * Group 2 vs. Group 3: Diff = −9.3, 95% CI = −10.68 to −7.91, $p < 0.001$ *
Pain intensity	4.6 ± 1.4	5.9 ± 2.3	4.9 ± 1.8	2.68/0.07	

3.2.3. Sensorimotor Control Variables

The unpaired *t*-test analysis showed that there were statistically significant differences in the hyper-kyphotic group versus the normal kyphosis group for the sensorimotor control variables. For OSI, we found significant abnormality (less stability) in dynamic stability for the hyper-kyphotic group compared to the normal kyphosis group ($p < 0.001$); smaller values indicate a good stability level of the participants. Larger errors were evident for right and left rotation repositioning accuracy ($p < 0.001$) in the hyper-kyphotic group as well; results are reported as error in degrees (°) where less than 10% or 3° is normal. For SPNT, we found a significant difference between the two groups with a larger average gain for the hyper-kyphotic group; results are reported as a percentage (%) of error of corrective saccades, where 100% is perfect (0% error), 10–20% error is normal, and greater than 20% error is abnormal. Table 5 presents this data.

Table 5. Between group comparisons of the entire sample of the kyphotic group vs. normal group for sensorimotor control and CVA outcomes.

Variables	Kyphotic Group	Normal Group	Cohen's d Effect Size	*p* Value [95% CI]
CVA (°)	41 ± 5	53 ± 4	2.65	<0.001 * [10.6, 13.4]
Smooth pursuit neck torsion test (% error)	0.41 ± 0.17	0.31 ± 0.14	0.6	<0.001 * [−0.15, −0.05]
** Overall stability index (refer to methods)	0.62 ± 0.2	0.42 ± 0.1	1.26	<0.001 * [−0.05, −0.14]
Head repositioning accuracy (°) Right	4.0 ± 1.5	3.0 ± 1.2	0.74	<0.001 * [−0.57, −1.42]
Head repositioning accuracy (°) Left	4.3 ± 1.8	3.3 ± 1.5	0.6	<0.001 * [−0.45, −1.58]
Sympathetic skin resistance Amplitude	2.9 ± 0.9	2.1 ± 0.7	0.87	<0.001 * [−0.54, −1.05]
Sympathetic skin resistance Latency	1.2 ± 0.4	1.3 ± 0.3	0.2	0.07 [−0.01, 0.21]

* Denotes statistically significant differences. ** These indices are calculated according to the degree of platform oscillation; smaller values indicate a good stability level of the participants. CVA = craniovertebral angle. All values are expressed as means ± standard deviation. CI [] = 95% confidence interval.

Between group comparisons for the postural kyphosis, Scheuermann's kyphosis and normal groups are presented separately for sensorimotor control variables and the CVA in Table 6. Overall, the Scheuermann's kyphosis group is shown to have statistically and clinically significant worse sensorimotor control variables. Similarly, the Scheuermann's kyphosis group has a statistically significant reduction in the CVA indicating more forward head posture; $p < 0.001$, Table 6.

Table 6. Results of one-way-ANOVA and post hoc (Tukey) test. * = statistically significant.

Variables	Postural Kyphosis N = 35	Scheuermann's Kyphosis N = 45	Normal Group N = 80	F-Value/ *p*-Value	Post Hoc
CVA (°)	44 ± 4	38.5 ± 4.5	53 ± 4	187.4/ <0.001 *	Group 1 vs. Group 2: Diff = −5.5, 95% CI = −8.58 to −2.4, *p* = 0.0002 * Group 1 vs. Group 3: Diff = 9, 95% CI = 5.7 to 12.27, *p* < 0.001 * Group 2 vs. Group 3: Diff = 14.5, 95% CI = 11.3 to 17.6, *p* < 0.001 *

Table 6. Cont.

Variables	Postural Kyphosis N = 35	Scheuermann's Kyphosis N = 45	Normal Group N = 80	F-Value/ p-Value	Post Hoc
Smooth pursuit neck torsion test (% error)	0.34 ± 0.13	0.48 ± 0.18	0.31 ± 0.14	19.1/<0.001 *	Group 1 vs. Group 2: Diff = 0.14, 95% CI = 0.059 to 0.22, p = 0.0002 * Group 1 vs. Group 3: Diff = −0.03, 95% CI = −0.10 to 0.04, p = 0.5 Group 2 vs. Group 3: Diff = −0.17, 95% CI = −0.24 to −0.10, p < 0.001 *
** Overall stability index (refer to methods)	0.56 ± 0.2	0.68 ± 0.3	0.42 ± 0.1	25.7/<0.001 *	Group 1 vs. Group 2: Diff = 0.12, 95% CI = 0.015 to 0.23, p = 0.02 * Group 1 vs. Group 3: Diff = −0.14, 95% CI = −0.23 to −0.045, p = 0.0017 * Group 2 vs. Group 3: Diff = −0.26, 95% CI = −0.35 to −0.17, p < 0.001 *
Head repositioning accuracy (°) Right	3 ± 0.7	4.8 ± 1.6	3.0 ± 1.2	33.84/ <0.001 *	Group 1 vs. Group 2: Diff = 1.8, 95% CI = 1.14 to 2.5, p < 0.001 * Group 1 vs. Group 3: Diff = 0.0, 95% CI = −0.59 to 0.59, p = 0.99 Group 2 vs. Group 3: Diff = −1.8, 95% CI = −2.34 to −1.25, p < 0.001 *
Head repositioning accuracy (°) Left	3.8 ± 2	4.7 ± 1.6	3.3 ± 1.5	10.39/0.04 *	Group 1 vs. Group 2: Diff = 0.9, 95% CI = 0.02 to 1.77, p = 0.04 * Group 1 vs. Group 3: Diff = −0.5, 95% CI = −1.29 to 0.29, p = 0.29 Group 2 vs. Group 3: Diff = −1.4, 95% CI = −2.12 to −0.67, p < 0.001 *
Sympathetic skin resistance Amplitude	2.4 ± 0.6	3.3 ± 1	2.1 ± 0.7	34.68/<0.001 *	Group 1 vs. Group 2: Diff = 0.9, 95% CI = 0.48 to 1.31, p < 0.001 * Group 1 vs. Group 3: Diff = −0.3, 95% CI = −0.67 to 0.07, p = 0.14 Group 2 vs. Group 3: Diff = −1.2, 95% CI = −1.54 to −0.85, p < 0.001 *
Sympathetic skin resistance Latency	1.3 ± 0.3	1.2 ± 0.5	1.3 ± 0.3	1.19/0.3	NA

* Denotes statistically significant differences. ** These indices are calculated according to the degree of platform oscillation; smaller values indicate a good stability level of the participants. CVA = craniovertebral angle. All values are expressed as means ± standard deviation.

3.2.4. SSR Latency and Amplitude

For neurophysiological variables, we found an increase in SSR amplitude in the entire hyper-kyphotic group compared to the normal kyphosis group ($p < 0.001$). In contrast, no such difference was evident for in SSR latency ($p = 0.07$) as presented in Table 5. Between group comparisons for the postural kyphosis, Scheuermann's kyphosis, and normal groups are presented for SSR latency and amplitude in Table 6. SSR data show a statistically significant increased amplitude and a faster latency for the Scheuermann's kyphosis; however, the latency difference is a rather weak clinically and non-significant (effect size 0.2; $p = 0.29$). See Table 5.

3.3. Correlations

Pearson r correlations between the magnitude of thoracic kyphosis are presented in Table 7 for both subgroups of thoracic hyper-kyphosis, the normal kyphosis group, and the entire sample of 160 participants. The kyphotic angle showed a moderate positive correlation for all sensorimotor control variables (SPNT, OSI, and right and left rotation repositioning accuracy) with the postural kyphosis group showing significantly greater correlations than the other groups. We found a moderate positive correlation between the thoracic kyphotic angle and SSR amplitude for the entire sample of 180 participants ($r = 0.69$, $p < 0.001$), indicating as the kyphotic angles increased, the SSR amplitude increased in our population. Again, the strongest correlation was found for the postural kyphosis group. In contrast, we found a low negative correlation between the kyphotic angle and SSR latency for the entire sample of 180 participants ($r = -0.49$, $p < 0.001$), with the smallest correlation found in the postural kyphosis group. Additionally, pain and disability scores were moderately linearly correlated to the magnitude of kyphosis in the entire sample (NRS: $r = 0.53$, $p < 0.001$; NDI: $r = 0.67$; $p < 0.001$) with the postural kyphosis group showing slightly stronger correlations than the other participants. Table 7 presents this data in detail.

Table 7. Correlations (Pearson's r) between the postural kyphosis, the Scheuermann's kyphosis, the normal group, and the entire sample for all measured outcomes.

Correlation between Variables	Postural Kyphosis r (p Value) N = 35	Scheuermann's Kyphosis r (p Value) N = 45	Normal Group r (p Value) N = 80	Entire Sample r (p Value) N = 160
CVA	−0.7 (<0.001)	−0.6 (<0.001)	−0.51 (<0.001)	−0.61 (<0.001)
NDI	0.58 (<0.001)	0.50 (<0.001)	0.51 (<0.001)	0.67 (<0.001)
Pain intensity (NRS)	0.5 (<0.001)	0.35 (0.03)	0.34 (0.043)	0.53 (<0.001)
Smooth pursuit neck torsion test	0.54 (<0.001)	0.50 (<0.001)	0.50 (<0.001)	0.58 (<0.001)
Overall stability index	0.61 (<0.001)	0.49 (<0.001)	0.52 (<0.001)	0.59 (<0.001)
Head repositioning accuracy (Right)	0.7 (<0.001)	0.54 (<0.001)	0.61 (<0.001)	0.74 (<0.001)
Head repositioning accuracy (Left)	0.67 (<0.001)	0.52 (<0.001)	0.61 (<0.001)	0.71 (<0.001)
Sympathetic skin resistance amplitude	0.7 (<0.001)	0.56 (<0.001)	0.61 (<0.001)	0.69 (<0.001)
Sympathetic skin resistance latency	−0.2 (0.05)	−0.5 (<0.001)	−0.36 (<0.001)	−0.49 (<0.001)

CVA = Craniovertebral angle; NDI = neck disability index; NRS = numerical rating scale.

Craniovertebral Angle (CVA)

Box and whisker plots of the CVA in both hyper-kyphosis groups (postural kyphosis and Scheuermann's kyphosis) and the normal kyphosis group are presented in Figure 5. Overall, the Scheuermann's kyphosis group had the smallest CVA indicating greater forward head posture than the other two groups; CVA 38.5° ± 4.5. The normal kyphosis group had the greatest CVA indicating a more neutral sagittal head posture; CVA 53° ± 4. These results were statistically significant ($p < 0.001$). Lastly, the CVA is negatively correlated with the magnitude of thoracic kyphosis in all groups, with the strongest correlation found in the posture kyphosis group, indicating that as the magnitude of thoracic kyphosis increases, the CVA decreases and forward head posture increases (entire sample r = −0.061, p < 0.001). See Table 7.

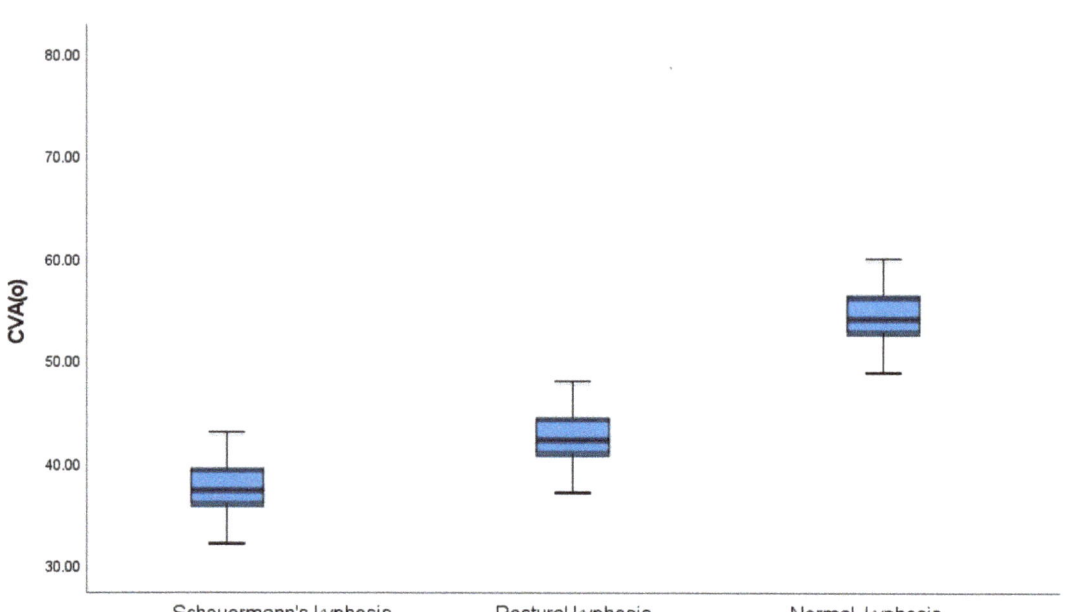

Figure 5. Box and whisker plots of the craniovertebral angle measured in degrees (CVA°) in the postural kyphosis groups (CVA, 44° ± 4), the Scheuermann's kyphosis group (CVA, 38° ± 4.5), and the normal kyphosis (CVA, 53° ± 4) groups.

4. Discussion

The results of the current study demonstrate that the sensorimotor control, disability, and autonomic nervous system function of patients with chronic nonspecific neck pain and thoracic kyphosis are distinctly different compared to those patients with normal thoracic alignment. Thus, our study's primary hypotheses are confirmed by these findings. As far as we know, this is the first study to provide objective evidence that these specific outcomes are differently affected by altered sagittal thoracic alignment. These differences cannot be explained in the context of the proposed different pain intensity or pain duration differences among groups, as the between group analysis revealed a non-significant difference between groups for both these variables. Most importantly, the difference between groups appear of clinical importance, as reflected by their effect sizes (d > 0.5) and the mean differences between groups, which are greater than the minimal clinically important difference (2.77 × SEM) for the SSR and the NDI outcomes [49–51].

4.1. Thoracic Kyphosis

Thoracic hyper-kyphosis represents one of the top four spine abnormalities associated with adult spine deformity (ASD), a world-wide, known set of spine deformities and associated disabilities affecting adults over the age of 18 years [28,29]. For example, Pellise et al. [28] identified that patients with radiographically determined thoracic hyper-kyphosis ≥60° had significantly lower health-related quality of life scores compared to patients afflicted with four other major health disorders (type II diabetes, rheumatoid arthritis, heart disease, or pulmonary disease). There are currently different proposed cut-off values that distinguish between normal and hyper-kyphosis. For example, 50° is suggested by some studies as a cut-point for thoracic hyper-kyphosis [30,31], while other investigations have identified that the cut-point between those with pain, lower self-image, and decreased function is 45° [26,27,52]. In the current investigation, we used a 4-D formetric scanner to evaluate the external measurement of thoracic kyphosis, and in the hyper-kyphosis group our average participants' kyphosis was 67°, while it was 49° in the normal kyphosis group. For comparison, it is known that the formetric and inclinometry measures of external thoracic kyphosis overestimate the radiographic determined thoracic kyphosis by approximately 5–7° and maybe more depending on the unique patient population [33,35,53,54]. Using this information, we estimate that our hyper-kyphosis group had a radiographic measured thoracic kyphosis averaging 60° (depending on the vertebral levels of measurement) meaning that this group would be at the threshold for ASD and that they would certainly be classified as an abnormal spine deformity group [28,29].

4.2. CVA, Pain, Disability, and Sensorimotor Control

In Table 7, we separated our study's findings into four separate correlation analyses: postural kyphosis, Scheuermann's kyphosis, normal kyphosis, and the entire population. This was chosen due to the possibility of identifying a stronger correlation between a specific variable within the hyper-kyphosis groups compared to the normal group. In this regard, most variables showed stronger correlations within the postural hyper-kyphosis group compared to the other two populations. It is unclear what this means in terms of chronic neck pain and neck disability in our study, but it may prove significant in future investigations. Between group differences in sensorimotor control and neck disability scores were identified, while there were no differences in pain intensity and duration between groups. The relationship between pain intensity and thoracic alignment has been detailed in several studies, where some investigations have reported significant positive associations, while other studies demonstrated no association between the two variables [14,55–57]. One such investigation concluded that neck pain was positively associated with hyper-kyphosis during a functional typing task [58]. These conflicting results might be due to multiple factors, such as the severity of chronic pain determined by a variety of other physical and psychosocial contributing factors [59]. Therefore, it is difficult to predict any linear relationship between thoracic kyphosis and neck pain intensity. Since the differences in disability and sensorimotor control found between our hyper-kyphosis and normal groups are not due to differences in pain intensity or pain duration, we propose the possible mechanism driving these changes might be dysafferentation mediated by abnormal forward head malalignment and increased thoracic kyphosis.

Increased thoracic kyphosis leads to the anterior shift of the trunk mass through an alteration of the thoracic spine loading, thereby resulting in forward head posture of the cervical spine as a direct compensation [14]. This has been confirmed in the current study by the fact that the mean CVA for the kyphotic group was significantly lower than that of the control (non-kyphotic) group indicating considerably larger forward head posture in the kyphotic group. Sustained forward head posture is implicated in the alteration of cervical motor control and the development of myofascial dysfunction. The assumption that abnormal forward head posture alignment is important for the afferentation process has some preliminary evidence. For instance, two modeling studies have predicted that as forward head posture increases, increased stress and strain are placed upon the muscles and ligaments of the cervical and thoracic region [60–62]. Increased forward head posture results in altered cervical spine alignment and shoulder joint position, causing abnormal kinematics and neurophysiologic afferent input (the so-called dysafferentation) [63–65]. We suggest that this information is consistent with and may partially explain the findings from Stanton and colleagues [66], where chronic idiopathic neck populations were identified to have an abnormal ability to return the cervical spine to the neutral position (altered sensorimotor control).

In the current investigation, it is difficult to discern between the effects of increased forward head posture (the CVA) versus increased thoracic kyphosis on the variables we have assessed, and conflicting results have been reported in the literature regarding the significance of sensorimotor control measures in neck pain populations. For example, in a recent systematic review with meta-analysis, it was found that increased forward head posture is associated with the presence of neck pain in adults [67,68]. However, Pacheco and colleagues [68] found that forward head posture was not different between young collegiate adults with "subclinical neck pain" compared to asymptomatic controls. This later investigation [69] used a very different participant population in both age (college students only 18–22 years) and a non-clinically relevant pain condition (treatment was not sought) as compared to our current investigation (significantly older and participants were seeking intervention from our pain clinic); thus, we believe our results to be more in line with the two recent systematic reviews with meta-analysis [67,68].

A significant negative correlation was found in the current study between the magnitude of thoracic kyphosis and a participant's CVA. This finding was previously reported in the study by Quek et al. [13]. Moreover, a multitude of biomechanics analysis have revealed that increased forward head posture along with thoracic hyper-kyphosis is associated with mobility limitations in the cervical spine [15]. Given the preliminary evidence for the significant role of normal sagittal configuration in normalizing the afferentation processes, it is not surprising that there was a considerable between group difference in the sensorimotor control variables. The current study's findings of increased disability and more disturbed sensorimotor control add credence to the above biomechanics and clinical investigations detailing the effects of thoracic spine abnormalities on the cervical spine. The relationship between increased forward head posture, that is, a smaller CVA, and thoracic kyphosis has been investigated in previous studies [14,15]. Lau et al. [14] reported a smaller CVA in participants with neck pain compared to a healthy control group. Lau et al. [14] suggested that a smaller CVA and upper thoracic angle were thought to be predictors of neck pain and disability in terms of their participants pain intensity. However, in the current study, it was not surprising that there were no significant variations in pain intensity between our two groups, because pain is a multidimensional phenomenon affected by many factors other than sagittal alignment. Moreover, symptoms caused by abnormal spine biomechanics likely appear after the consequences of mechanical distortions have progressed to the point where the body's adaptive ability has been overcome (as is the case with heart disease, cancer, hypertension, etc.). Since the participants in our study were much younger than those in the other study [14], the age differences between the two studies could explain the disparity in pain intensity findings. Interestingly, although the different postural alignments between our groups had no effect on pain intensity, it had a significant impact on the other measurement outcomes, as shown by the strong correlation between spinal alignment and those outcomes (disability, sensorimotor control measures, and sympathetic skin resistance). Our finding is consistent with that of Moustafa et al., who found that even in asymptomatic individuals with a forward head posture, there are significant abnormal neurophysiological responses, including prolonged central conduction time and abnormal sensorimotor integration [70].

4.3. SSR

Our choice of the sympathetic skin response (SSR) as an indicator for autonomic nervous system (ANS) function in the current study instead of other measures such as heart rate variability (HRV) measurement might by questioned. HRV is a commonly used and standardized method for assessing ANS function, as it provides separate metrics for sympathetic and parasympathetic functions through the low-frequency (LF) and high-frequency (HF) spectral components of HRV. However, recent studies have shown that the traditional HRV framework established in the 1980s has limitations in dealing with the evidence accumulated over the past half-century. As pointed out by Hayano and Yuda [71], using HRV without criticism may lead to incorrect conclusions or judgments. Moreover, a study by Ke et al. [72] has shown that both SSR and HRV parameters are sensitive in determining ANS dysfunction. Therefore, we chose SSR as an alternative and easily assessed measure for ANS function in our study. We acknowledge that HRV may provide additional information about ANS function, and future studies should use this to assess the influence of thoracic kyphosis and increasing FHP on HRV. However, our current findings using SSR highlight the potential clinical value of this measure in assessing ANS dysfunction.

We believe that a significant between group difference in SSR indicates the considerable role of spinal sagittal alignment in maintaining the normal function of the autonomic nervous system. Oakley et al. [73] detailed information indicating that restoring normal posture and spine alignment has important influences on neurophysiology, sensorimotor control, and autonomic nervous system function. There is limited but high-quality research identifying that sagittal spine alignment restoration plays an important role in improving neurophysiology, sensorimotor control, and autonomic nervous system function [73,74]. Disturbances in the afferentation process may be the possible explanation underpinning spine-related autonomic dysfunction. An adverse mechanical tension acting on the brainstem and cranial nerves 5–12, specially the 10th cranial nerve, may be one of the fundamental mechanisms that explain the autonomic dysfunction in the kyphotic group compared to the control group.

4.4. Clinical Relevance

Clinically, our study findings would implicate the thoracic hyper-kyphosis as a contributing factor in the disability levels reported in chronic non-specific neck pain disorders. We identified that increased FHP (a decreased CVA) is corelated to the magnitude of thoracic kyphosis. Since it is known that increasing FHP causes a simultaneous increased loading of the upper thoracic and lower cervical spine, it would be logical that this increased loading affects the ability of a person's cervical spine to perform complex and simple tasks that create further functional demands on the spine tissues [60,61]. Furthermore, increased FHP alters both the total range of motion and segmental kinematics of the cervical spine during movements, and this would further exacerbate cervical spine pain and create limits to functional movements as a result [13–15]. Similarly, the general results of our sensorimotor control assessments indicate that participants with increased thoracic kyphosis have a generally poorer ability to perform efficient tasks requiring stability (balance), movement accuracy (HRA), and ocular motor control (SPENT). The findings of inefficient sensorimotor control would have significant implications for continued injury (increased and altered stresses and strains on various spine tissues) of a participants cervical spine tissues, where a vicious cycle is set up of spine tissue damage due to inefficient motor control or coordination of movement. In general, our findings would suggest that structural rehabilitation (rehabilitation aimed at improving spine alignment) of the hyper-kyphotic spine should be a primary goal of patient treatment procedures. In fact, in a recent randomized trial, it was identified that structural rehabilitation of the thoracic hyper-kyphosis had positive effects on improving chronic non-specific neck pain, disability, and sensorimotor control as compared to standard rehabilitative care that did not improve the alignment of the thoracic hyper-kyphosis [74].

4.5. Limitations

The current study has limitations to consider which should lead to future investigations. First, the outcome measures used to verify if thoracic kyphosis affects sensorimotor control, pain, and disability may not be the only ones or the ideal assessment for chronic neck pain outcomes. Additionally, we measured the thoracic kyphosis using an external posture assessment device, and this does not provide the same quantitative data as radiographic or other imaging methods used for the measurement of thoracic kyphosis. Similarly, although the CVA is a valid and reliable method for measuring forward head alignment [14,36,37], it might not adequately describe the actual sagittal cervical vertebral alignment. Using the sagittal radiological profile would thus give further insights into exact rotation and translation displacements of individual vertebral and overall cervical curvature geometry and magnitude. Furthermore, our study did not include a true normal control group without chronic non-specific neck pain and a normal thoracic kyphosis; thus, comparison to populations without chronic non-specific neck pain cannot be made. Finally, although we demonstrated that increasing kyphotic magnitudes of the thoracic spine are correlated with sensorimotor control measurements and the autonomic nervous system function, it must be emphasized that correlation does not imply causation. Future investigations that are prospective and longitudinal in design along with randomized interventional trials are needed to confirm the relationship between the magnitude of thoracic hyper-kyphosis and the measures reported herein.

5. Conclusions

This case control on a chronic non-specific neck pain population identified that those with thoracic hyper-kyphosis also have an increased forward head posture (reduced CVA) and that this is related to abnormal autonomic nervous system function. Furthermore, increased thoracic kyphosis is correlated to disturbances of a variety of sensorimotor control measures. Our findings may have important implications for the assessment and rehabilitation of these populations of patients with hyper-kyphosis of the thoracic spine, increased forward head posture, and chronic non-specific neck pain.

Author Contributions: Conceptualization, I.M.M., T.S., A.A., D.E.H.; methodology, I.M.M., T.S., A.A., D.E.H.; software, I.M.M., T.S., A.A.; validation, I.M.M., T.S., A.A., D.E.H.; formal analysis, I.M.M., T.S., A.A., D.E.H.; investigation, I.M.M., T.S., A.A.; resources, I.M.M., T.S., A.A.; data curation, I.M.M., T.S., A.A.; writing—I.M.M., T.S., A.A., D.E.H.; I.M.M., T.S., A.A., D.E.H.; visualization, I.M.M., T.S., A.A., D.E.H.; supervision, I.M.M., T.S., A.A.; project administration, I.M.M., T.S., A.A. All authors have read and agreed to the published version of the manuscript.

Funding: This research received no external funding.

Institutional Review Board Statement: The study was conducted in accordance with the Declaration of Helsinki. Ethical approval was obtained from the Research and Ethics Committee at Cairo University (CA-REC-22-5-20), with informed consent obtained from all participants prior to data collection in accordance with relevant guidelines and regulations.

Informed Consent Statement: Written informed consent was obtained from all subjects involved in the study.

Data Availability Statement: Data supporting reported results can be ascertained by emailing the lead author of this study: Professor Ibrahim Moustafa at iabuamr@sharjah.ac.ae.

Conflicts of Interest: Dr. Deed Harrison (DEH) lectures to health care providers on rehabilitation methods and is the CEO of a company that sells products to physicians for patient care to aid in improvement of postural and spine ailments as described in this manuscript. All other authors declare no conflict of interest related to this project.

References

1. Cohen, S.P. Epidemiology, diagnosis, and treatment of neck pain. In *Mayo Clinic Proceedings*; Elsevier: Amsterdam, The Netherlands, 2015; pp. 284–299.
2. Oxland, T.R. Fundamental biomechanics of the spine-What we have learned in the past 25 years and future directions. *J. Biomech.* **2016**, *49*, 817–832. [CrossRef] [PubMed]
3. Kaya, F.; Celenay, S. An investigation of sagittal thoracic spinal curvature and mobility in subjects with and without chronic neck pain: Cut-off points and pain relationship. *Turk. J. Med. Sci.* **2017**, *47*, 891–896. [CrossRef] [PubMed]
4. Bergmann, T.F.; Peterson, D.H. *Chiropractic Technique Principles and Procedures*; Elsevier: Amsterdam, The Netherlands, 2011.
5. Norlander, S.; Gustavsson, B.; Lindell, J.; Nordgren, B. Reduced mobility in the cervico-thoracic motion segment: A risk factor for musculoskeletal neck-shoulder pain: A two-year prospective follow-up study. *Scand. J. Rehabil. Med.* **1997**, *29*, 167–174. [PubMed]
6. Norlander, S.; Aste-Norlander, U.; Nordgren, B.; Sahlstedt, B. Mobility in the cervico-thoracic motion segment: An indicative factor of musculo-skeletal neckshoulder pain. *Scand. J. Rehabil. Med.* **1996**, *28*, 183–192.
7. Fernández-de-las-Peñas, C.; Fernández-Carnero, J.; Fernández, A.P.; Lomas-Vega, R.; Miangolarra-Page, J.C. Dorsal manipulation in whiplash injury treatment. *J. Whiplash Relat. Disord.* **2004**, *3*, 55–72. [CrossRef]

8. Tsang, S.M.H.; Szeto, G.P.Y.; Lee, R.Y.W. Normal kinematics of the neck: The interplay between the cervical and thoracic spines. *Man. Ther.* **2013**, *18*, 431–437. [CrossRef]
9. Garni, A.D.; Al-Saran, Y.; Al-Moawi, A.; Bin Dous, A.; Al-Ahaideb, A.; Kachanathu, S.J. The prevalence of and factors associated with neck, shoulder, and low-back pains among medical students at university hospitals in central Saudi Arabia. *Pain Res. Treat.* **2017**, *2017*, 1235706.
10. Alshagga, M.A.; Nimer, A.R.; Yan, L.P.; Ibrahim, I.A.; Al-Ghamdi, S.S.; Radman Al-Dubai, S.A. Prevalence and factors associated with neck, shoulder and low back pains among medical students in a Malaysian medical college. *BMC Res. Notes* **2013**, *6*, 244. [CrossRef]
11. Almhdawi, K.A.; Mathiowetz, V.; Al-Hourani, Z.; Khader, Y.; Kanaan, S.F.; Alhasan, M. Musculoskeletal pain symptoms among allied health professions' students: Prevalence rates and associated factors. *J. Back Musculoskelet. Rehabil.* **2017**, *30*, 1291–1301. [CrossRef]
12. Cleland, J.; Selleck, B.; Stowell, T. Short-term effects of thoracic manipulation on lower trapezius muscle strength. *J. Man. Manip. Ther.* **2004**, *12*, 82–90. [CrossRef]
13. Quek, J.; Pua, Y.H.; Clark, R.A.; Bryant, A.L. Effects of thoracic kyphosis and forward head posture on cervical range of motion in older adults. *Man. Ther.* **2013**, *18*, 65–71. [CrossRef] [PubMed]
14. Lau, K.T.; Cheung, K.Y.; Chan kwok, B.; Chan, M.H.; Lo, K.Y.; Wing Chiu, T.T. Relationships between sagittal postures of thoracic and cervical spine, presence of neck pain, neck pain severity and disability. *Man. Ther.* **2010**, *15*, 457–462. [CrossRef] [PubMed]
15. Joshi, S.; Balthillaya, G.; Neelapala, Y.V.R. Thoracic posture and mobility in mechanical neck pain population: A review of the literature. *Asian Spine J.* **2019**, *13*, 849–860. [CrossRef] [PubMed]
16. Artz, N.J.; Adams, M.A.; Dolan, P. Sensorimotor function of the cervical spine in healthy volunteers. *Clin. Biomech.* **2015**, *30*, 260–268. [CrossRef]
17. Treleaven, J. Sensorimotor disturbances in neck disorders affecting postural stability, head and eye movement control. *Man. Ther.* **2008**, *13*, 2–11. [CrossRef]
18. Kristjansson, E.; Treleaven, J. Sensorimotor function and dizziness in neck pain: Implications for assessment and management. *J. Orthop. Sport. Phys. Ther.* **2009**, *39*, 364–377. [CrossRef]
19. Röijezon, U.; Jull, G.; Blandford, C.; Daniels, A.; Michaelson, P.; Karvelis, P.; Treleaven, J. Proprioceptive disturbance in chronic neck pain: Discriminate validity and reliability of performance of the clinical cervical movement sense test. *Front. Pain. Res.* **2022**, *3*, 908414. [CrossRef]
20. Sittikraipong, K.; Silsupadol, P.; Uthaikhup, S. Slower reaction and response times and impaired hand-eye coordination in individuals with neck pain. *Musculoskelet. Sci. Pract.* **2020**, *50*, 102273. [CrossRef]
21. Asiri, F.; Reddy, R.S.; Tedla, J.S.; ALMohiza, M.A.; Alshahrani, M.S.; Govindappa, S.C.; Sangadala, D.R. Kinesiophobia and its correlations with pain, proprioception, and functional performance among individuals with chronic neck pain. *PLoS ONE* **2021**, *16*, e0254262. [CrossRef]
22. Hellström, F.; Roatta, S.; Thunberg, J.; Passatore, M.; Djupsjöbacka, M. Responses of muscle spindles in feline dorsal neck muscles to electrical stimulation of the cervical sympathetic nerve. *Exp. Brain Res.* **2005**, *165*, 328–342. [CrossRef]
23. Corneil, B.D.; Olivier, E.; Munoz, D.P. Neck muscle responses to stimulation of monkey superior colliculus. II. Gaze shift initiation and volitional head movements. *J. Neurophysiol.* **2002**, *88*, 2000–2018. [CrossRef] [PubMed]
24. Bolton, P.S.; Kerman, I.A.; Woodring, S.F.; Yates, B.J. Influences of neck afferents on sympathetic and respiratory nerve activity. *Brain Res. Bull.* **1998**, *47*, 413–419. [CrossRef] [PubMed]
25. Budgell, B.S. Reflex effects of subluxation: The autonomic nervous system. *J. Manip. Physiol. Ther.* **2000**, *23*, 104–106. [CrossRef]
26. Petcharaporn, M.; Pawelek, J.; Bastrom, T.; Lonner, B.; Newton, P.O. The relationship between thoracic hyperkyphosis and the scoliosis research society outcomes instrument. *Spine* **2007**, *32*, 2226–2231. [CrossRef]
27. Nissinen, M.; Heliövaara, M.; Seitsamo, J.; Poussa, M. Left handedness and risk of thoracic hyperkyphosis in prepubertal schoolchildren. *Int. J. Epidemiol.* **1995**, *24*, 1178–1181. [CrossRef]
28. Pellisé, F.; Vila-Casademunt, A.; Ferrer, M.; Domingo-Sàbat, M.; Bagó, J.; Pérez-Grueso, F.J.S.; Alanay, A.; Mannion, A.F.; Acaroglu, E.; European Spine Study Group; et al. Impact on health related quality of life of adult spinal deformity (ASD) compared with other chronic conditions. *Eur. Spine J.* **2015**, *24*, 3–11. [CrossRef] [PubMed]
29. Bess, S.; Line, B.; Fu, K.M.; McCarthy, I.; Lafage, V.; Schwab, F.; Shaffrey, C.; Ames, C.; Akbarnia, B.; Jo, H.; et al. The health impact of symptomatic adult spinal deformity: Comparison of deformity types to United States population norms and chronic diseases. *Spine* **2016**, *41*, 224–233. [CrossRef]
30. McDaniels-Davidson, C.; Davis, A.; Wing, D.; Macera, C.; Lindsay, S.P.; Schousboe, J.T.; Nichols, J.F.; Kado, D.M. Kyphosis and incident falls among community-dwelling older adults. *Osteoporos Int.* **2018**, *29*, 163–169. [CrossRef] [PubMed]
31. Van Der Jagt-Willems, H.C.; De Groot, M.H.; Van Campen, J.P.C.M.; Lamoth, C.J.C.; Lems, W.F. Associations between vertebral fractures, increased thoracic kyphosis, a flexed posture and falls in older adults: A prospective cohort study. *BMC Geriatr.* **2015**, *15*, 34. [CrossRef] [PubMed]
32. Lason, G.; Peeters, L.; Vandenberghe, K.; Byttebier, G.; Comhaire, F. Reassessing the accuracy and reproducibility of Diers formetric measurements in healthy volunteers. *Int. J. Osteopath. Med.* **2015**, *18*, 247–254. [CrossRef]

33. Knott, P.; Sturm, P.; Lonner, B.; Cahill, P.; Betsch, M.; McCarthy, R.; Kelly, M.; Lenke, L.; Betz, R. Multicenter comparison of 3D spinal measurements using surface topography with those from conventional radiography. *Spine Deform.* **2016**, *4*, 98–103. [CrossRef]
34. Harrison, D.E.; Janik, T.J.; Harrison, D.D.; Cailliet, R.; Harmon, S.F. Can the thoracic kyphosis be modeled with a simple geometric shape. *J. Spinal Disord. Technol.* **2002**, *15*, 2130220. [CrossRef] [PubMed]
35. Krott, N.L.; Wild, M.; Betsch, M. Meta-analysis of the validity and reliability of rasterstereographic measurements of spinal posture. *Eur. Spine J.* **2020**, *29*, 2392–2401. [CrossRef] [PubMed]
36. Yip, C.H.T.; Chiu, T.T.W.; Poon, A.T.K. The relationship between head posture and severity and disability of patients with neck pain. *Man Ther.* **2008**, *13*, 148–154. [CrossRef]
37. Van Niekerk, S.M.; Louw, Q.; Vaughan, C.; Grimmer-Somers, K.; Schreve, K. Photographic measurement of upper-body sitting posture of high school students: A reliability and validity study. *BMC Musculoskelet Disord.* **2008**, *9*, 113. [CrossRef] [PubMed]
38. Lundeberg, T.; Lund, I.; Dahlin, L.; Borg, E.; Gustafsson, C.; Sandin, L.; Rosén, A.; Kowalski, J.; Eriksson, S.V. Reliability and responsiveness of three different pain assessments. *J. Rehabil. Med.* **2001**, *33*, 279–283. [CrossRef]
39. MacDermid, J.C.; Walton, D.M.; Avery, S.; Blanchard, A.; Etruw, E.; McAlpine, C.; Goldsmith, C.H. Measurement properties of the neck disability index: A systematic review. *J. Orthop. Sports Phys. Ther.* **2009**, *39*, 400–417. [CrossRef]
40. Loudon, J.K.; Ruhl, M.; Field, E. Ability to reproduce head position after whiplash injury. *Spine* **1997**, *22*, 865–868. [CrossRef]
41. Treleaven, J.; Jull, G.; Sterling, M. Dizziness and unsteadiness following whiplash injury: Characteristic features and relationship with cervical joint position error. *J. Rehabil. Med.* **2003**, *35*, 36–43. [CrossRef]
42. Tjell, C.; Rosenhall, U. Smooth pursuit neck torsion test: A specific test for cervical dizziness. *Am. J. Otol.* **1998**, *19*, 76–81.
43. Arnold, B.L.; Schmitz, R.J. Examination of balance measures produced by the biodex stability system. *J. Athl. Train.* **1998**, *33*, 323.
44. Schmitz, R.; Arnold, B. Intertester and intratester reliability of a dynamic balance protocol using the biodex stability system. *J. Sport Rehabil.* **1998**, *7*, 95–101. [CrossRef]
45. Elie, B.; Guiheneuc, P. Sympathetic skin response: Normal results in different experimental conditions. *Electroencephalogr. Clin. Neurophysiol.* **1990**, *76*, 258–267. [CrossRef] [PubMed]
46. On, A.Y.; Colakoglu, Z.; Hepguler, S.; Aksit, R. Local heat effect on sympathetic skin responses after pain of electrical stimulus. *Arch. Phys. Med. Rehabil.* **1997**, *78*, 1196–1199. [PubMed]
47. Kucera, P.; Goldenberg, Z.; Kurca, E. Sympathetic skin response: Review of the method and its clinical use. *Bratisl. Lek Listy.* **2004**, *105*, 108–116.
48. Chroni, E.; Argyriou, A.A.; Polychronopoulos, P.; Sirrou, V. The effect of stimulation technique on sympathetic skin responses in healthy subjects. *Clin. Auton. Res.* **2006**, *16*, 396–400. [CrossRef]
49. Wyrwich, K.W.; Tierney, W.M.; Wolinsky, F.D. Further evidence supporting an SEM-based criterion for identifying meaningful intra-individual changes in health-related quality of life. *J. Clin. Epidemiol.* **1999**, *52*, 861–873. [CrossRef]
50. Wolinsky, F.D.; Wan, G.J.; Tierney, W.M. Changes in the SF-36 in 12 months in a clinical sample of disadvantaged older adults. *Med. Care* **1998**, *36*, 1589–1598. [CrossRef] [PubMed]
51. McHorney, C.A.; Tarlov, A.R. Individual-patient monitoring in clinical practice: Are available health status surveys adequate? *Qual. Life Res.* **1995**, *4*, 293–307. [CrossRef]
52. González-Gálvez, N.; Gea-García, G.M.; Marcos-Pardo, P.J. Effects of exercise programs on kyphosis and lordosis angle: A systematic review and meta-analysis. *PLoS ONE* **2019**, *14*, e0216180. [CrossRef]
53. Bezalel, T.; Carmeli, E.; Levi, D.; Kalichman, L. The effect of Schroth therapy on thoracic kyphotic curve and quality of life in Scheuermann's patients: A randomized controlled trial. *Asian Spine J.* **2019**, *13*, 490–499. [CrossRef] [PubMed]
54. Hunter, D.J.; Rivett, D.A.; McKiernan, S.; Weerasekara, I.; Snodgrass, S.J. Is the inclinometer a valid measure of thoracic kyphosis? A cross-sectional study. *Braz. J. Phys. Ther.* **2018**, *22*, 310–317. [CrossRef] [PubMed]
55. Tsunoda, D.; Iizuka, Y.; Iizuka, H.; Nishinome, M.; Kobayashi, R.; Ara, T.; Yamamoto, A.; Takagishi, K. Associations between neck and shoulder pain (called katakori in Japanese) and sagittal spinal alignment parameters among the general population. *J. Orthop. Sci.* **2013**, *18*, 216–219. [CrossRef] [PubMed]
56. Szeto, G.P.Y.; Straker, L.M.; O'Sullivan, P.B. A comparison of symptomatic and asymptomatic office workers performing monotonous keyboard work - 2: Neck and shoulder kinematics. *Man. Ther.* **2005**, *10*, 281–291. [CrossRef]
57. Cross, K.M.; Kuenze, C.; Grindstaff, T.; Hertel, J. Thoracic spine thrust manipulation improves pain, range of motion, and self-reported function in patients with mechanical neck pain: A systematic review. *J. Orthop. Sports Phys. Ther.* **2011**, *41*, 633–643. [CrossRef]
58. Nejati, P.; Lotfian, S.; Moezy, A.; Nejati, M. The study of correlation between forward head posture and neck pain in Iranian office workers. *Int. J. Occup. Med. Environ. Health* **2015**, *28*, 295–303. [CrossRef]
59. Smart, K.M.; Blake, C.; Staines, A.; Doody, C. Clinical indicators of "nociceptive", "peripheral neuropathic" and "central" mechanisms of musculoskeletal pain. A delphi survey of expert clinicians. *Man Ther.* **2010**, *15*, 80–87. [CrossRef] [PubMed]
60. Harrison, D.E.; Jones, E.W.; Janik, T.J.; Harrison, D.D. Evaluation of axial and flexural stresses in the vertebral body cortex and trabecular bone in lordosis and two sagittal cervical translation configurations with an elliptical shell model. *J. Manip. Physiol. Ther.* **2002**, *25*, 391–401. [CrossRef]
61. Patwardhan, A.G.; Khayatzadeh, S.; Havey, R.M.; Voronov, L.I.; Smith, Z.A.; Kalmanson, O.; Ghanayem, A.J.; Sears, W. Cervical sagittal balance: A biomechanical perspective can help clinical practice. *Eur. Spine J.* **2018**, *27* (Suppl. S1), 25–38. [CrossRef]

62. Smith, J.S.; Lafage, V.; Ryan, D.J.; Shaffrey, C.I.; Schwab, F.J.; Patel, A.A.; Brodke, D.S.; Arnold, P.M.; Riew, K.D.; Traynelis, V.C.; et al. Association of myelopathy scores with cervical sagittal balance and normalized spinal cord volume: Analysis of 56 preoperative cases from the AOSpine North America myelopathy study. *Spine* **2013**, *38* (Suppl. S1), S161–S170. [CrossRef]
63. Fernández-de-las-Peñas, C.; Alonso-Blanco, C.; Cuadrado, M.; Pareja, J. Forward head posture and neck mobility in chronic tension-type headache. *Cephalalgia* **2006**, *26*, 314–319. [CrossRef] [PubMed]
64. Khayatzadeh, S.; Kalmanson, O.A.; Schuit, D.; Havey, R.M.; Voronov, L.I.; Ghanayem, A.J.; Patwardhan, A.G. Cervical spine muscle-tendon unit length differences between neutral and forward head postures: Biomechanical study using human cadaveric specimens. *Phys. Ther.* **2017**, *97*, 756–766. [CrossRef]
65. Thigpen, C.A.; Padua, D.A.; Michener, L.A.; Guskiewicz, K.; Giuliani, C.; Keener, J.D.; Stergiou, N. Head and shoulder posture affect scapular mechanics and muscle activity in overhead tasks. *J. Electromyogr. Kinesiol.* **2010**, *20*, 701–709. [CrossRef] [PubMed]
66. Stanton, T.R.; Leake, H.B.; Chalmers, K.J.; Moseley, G.L. Evidence of impaired proprioception in chronic, idiopathic neck pain: Systematic review and meta-analysis. *Phys. Ther.* **2016**, *96*, 876–887. [CrossRef] [PubMed]
67. Mahmoud, N.F.; Hassan, K.A.; Abdelmajeed, S.F.; Moustafa, I.M.; Silva, A.G. The relationship between forward head posture and neck pain: A systematic review and meta-analysis. *Curr. Rev. Musculoskelet. Med.* **2019**, *12*, 562–577. [CrossRef] [PubMed]
68. Rani, B.; Paul, A.; Chauhan, A.; Pradhan, P.; Dhillon, M.S. Is neck pain related to sagittal head and neck posture? A systematic review and meta-analysis. *Indian J. Orthop.* **2023**, *57*, 371–403. [CrossRef]
69. Pacheco, J.; Raimundo, J.; Santos, F.; Ferreira, M.; Lopes, T.; Ramos, L.; Silva, A.G. Forward head posture is associated with pressure pain threshold and neck pain duration in university students with subclinical neck pain. *Somat. Mot. Res.* **2018**, *35*, 103–108. [CrossRef]
70. Moustafa, I.M.; Diab, A.A.; Hegazy, F.; Harrison, D.E. Demonstration of central conduction time and neuroplastic changes after cervical lordosis rehabilitation in asymptomatic subjects: A randomized, placebo-controlled trial. *Sci. Rep.* **2021**, *11*, 15379. [CrossRef]
71. Hayano, J.; Yuda, E. Pitfalls of Assessment of Autonomic Function by Heart Rate Variability. *J. Physiol. Anthropol.* **2019**, *38*, 3. [CrossRef]
72. Ke, J.Q.; Shao, S.M.; Zheng, Y.Y.; Fu, F.W.; Zheng, G.Q.; Liu, C.F. Sympathetic Skin Response and Heart Rate Variability in Predicting Autonomic Disorders in Patients with Parkinson Disease. *Medicine* **2017**, *96*, e6523. [CrossRef] [PubMed]
73. Oakley, P.A.; Moustafa, I.M.; Harrison, D.E. The influence of sagittal plane spine alignment on neurophysiology and sensorimotor control measures: Optimization of function through structural correction. In *Therapy Approaches in Neurological Disorders*; Bernardo-Filho, M., Ed.; IntechOpen: London, UK, 2021. [CrossRef]
74. Moustafa, I.M.; Shousha, T.M.; Walton, L.M.; Raigangar, V.; Harrison, D.E. Reduction of thoracic hyper-kyphosis improves short and long term outcomes in patients with chronic nonspecific neck pain: A randomized controlled trial. *J. Clin. Med.* **2022**, *11*, 6028. [CrossRef] [PubMed]

Disclaimer/Publisher's Note: The statements, opinions and data contained in all publications are solely those of the individual author(s) and contributor(s) and not of MDPI and/or the editor(s). MDPI and/or the editor(s) disclaim responsibility for any injury to people or property resulting from any ideas, methods, instructions or products referred to in the content.

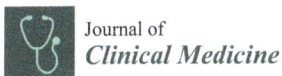

Journal of
Clinical Medicine

Article

An Investigation of the Association between 3D Spinal Alignment and Fibromyalgia

Amal Ahbouch [1], Ibrahim M. Moustafa [1,2,3], Tamer Shousha [1,2,3], Ashokan Arumugam [1,2], Paul Oakley [4,5,6] and Deed E. Harrison [4,*]

1. Department of Physiotherapy, College of Health Sciences, University of Sharjah, Sharjah 27272, United Arab Emirates
2. Neuromusculoskeletal Rehabilitation Research Group, RIMHS–Research Institute of Medical and Health Sciences, University of Sharjah, Sharjah 27272, United Arab Emirates
3. Faculty of Physical Therapy, Cairo University, Giza 12613, Egypt
4. CBP Nonprofit (a Spine Research Foundation), Eagle, ID 83616, USA
5. Private Practice, Newmarket, ON L3Y 8Y8, Canada
6. Kinesiology and Health Sciences, York University, Toronto, ON M3J 1P3, Canada
* Correspondence: drdeed@idealspine.com; Tel.: +1-775-340-4734

Abstract: Fibromyalgia syndrome (FMS) is a common condition lacking strong diagnostic criteria; these criteria continue to evolve as more and more studies are performed to explore it. This investigation sought to identify whether participants with FMS have more frequent and larger postural/spinal displacements in comparison to a matched control group without the condition of FMS. A total of 67 adults (55 females) out of 380 participants with FMS were recruited. Participants with FMS were sex- and age-matched with 67 asymptomatic participants (controls) without FMS. We used a three-dimensional (3D) postural assessment device (Formetric system) to analyze five posture variables in each participant in both groups: (1) thoracic kyphotic angle, (2) trunk imbalance, (3) trunk inclination, (4) lumbar lordotic angle, and (5) vertebral rotation. In order to determine whether 3D postural measures could predict the likelihood of a participant having FMS, we applied the matched-pairs binary logistic regression analysis. The 3D posture measures identified statistically and clinically significant differences between the FMS and control groups for each of the five posture variables measured ($p < 0.001$). For three out of five posture measurements assessed, the binary logistic regression identified there was an increased probability of having FMS with an increased: (1) thoracic kyphotic angle proportional odds ratio [Prop OR] = 1.76 (95% CI = 1.03, 3.02); (2) sagittal imbalance Prop OR = 1.54 (95% CI = 0.973, 2.459); and (3) surface rotation Prop OR = 7.9 (95% CI = 1.494, 41.97). We identified no significant probability of having FMS for the following two postural measurements: (1) coronal balance ($p = 0.50$) and (2) lumbar lordotic angle ($p = 0.10$). Our study's findings suggest there is a strong relationship between 3D spinal misalignment and the diagnosis of FMS. In fact, our results support that thoracic kyphotic angle, sagittal imbalance, and surface rotation are predictors of having FMS.

Keywords: fibromyalgia; posture; prediction; regression analysis; formetric analysis

Citation: Ahbouch, A.; Moustafa, I.M.; Shousha, T.; Arumugam, A.; Oakley, P.; Harrison, D.E. An Investigation of the Association between 3D Spinal Alignment and Fibromyalgia. *J. Clin. Med.* **2023**, *12*, 218. https://doi.org/10.3390/jcm12010218

Academic Editors: Hideaki Nakajima and Antonio Barile

Received: 7 October 2022
Revised: 5 December 2022
Accepted: 25 December 2022
Published: 28 December 2022

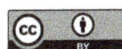

Copyright: © 2022 by the authors. Licensee MDPI, Basel, Switzerland. This article is an open access article distributed under the terms and conditions of the Creative Commons Attribution (CC BY) license (https://creativecommons.org/licenses/by/4.0/).

1. Introduction

Fibromyalgia syndrome (FMS) is a prevalent musculoskeletal condition that manifests with pain, stiffness, and tenderness of different body structures, such as muscles and tendons. Characteristic symptoms of FMS include general malaise with anxiety and depression, poor sleep, cognitive dysfunction, and disturbances in bowel functions [1,2]. FMS is underdiagnosed and undertreated due to the complexity of the multiple symptoms and comorbidities associated with it [3]. Despite the many efforts that have been made with specific diagnostic criteria for FMS, healthcare providers still find these criteria unclear, which causes a lack of confidence when using them [3,4]. In fact, these criteria have required multiple revisions as more and more data were made available. Despite elimination of the associated symptoms criterion in the 1990 classification and the tender points examination in the 2010/2011 revision, the 2016 revision included these two criteria [4].

Despite the debate around the FMS diagnostic criteria, it is well-established that pain is a centrally mediated phenomenon [2,4–6]. Currently, the evidence conceptualizes pain as the personal experience of a complex process compiling sources of input from joint mechano-receptors and information from the general environment, coupled with previous painful experiences and or memories of a painful event [6]. In fact, evidence has linked pain to posture and supported that moderation or elimination of pain can be achieved through improved posture [7,8]. While this association between pain and postural alignment has been questioned by other studies [9,10], the evidence supporting it is constantly growing [7]. For example, evidence supports a strong link between body misalignment and pain syndromes, many of which are found in FMS patients, including: tension-type and cervico-genic headaches [11,12], temporomandibular disorders [13–15], shoulder impingement [16,17], abnormal sagittal plane postures like protracted shoulders and forward head posture, respiratory dysfunction [18,19], back pain [20,21], impaired balance [22], FMS itself [23], and osteoporotic spinal deformity [24].

Determining objective postural assessment outcome measures could add another dimension to the diagnostic criteria of FMS, leaving less room for doubt for healthcare providers in diagnosis, and guiding more robust interventional treatments. The objective of the current investigation is to examine the potential relationship between FMS and postural misalignment, through detailed measurement of three-dimensional (3D) posture including kyphotic and lordotic angles, sagittal and coronal imbalance, and vertebral rotation. We designed a case control investigation to explore any postural diagnostic relationships that might predict cases with FMS versus those controls without FMS in an effort to help with diagnosing and treating this complex condition. The current study explores the hypothesis that 3D postural analysis will be able to accurately determine FMS participants compared to matched healthy controls.

2. Materials and Methods

We used a single-blind case control design to assess possible differences in 3D postural alignment among participants with chronic FMS in comparison to an age- and sex-matched asymptomatic control group. All ethical standards for use in human experimental research designs were followed in compliance with the Helsinki Declaration. Participant recruitment began following an approval from the Cairo University Ethics Committee (approval number: Cairo-PT.3-4561). Participants were recruited via advertisements posted on notice boards and relevant social media pages.

Initial inclusion criteria were assessed via a screening phone call for potential participants, and those with suspected FMS were then scheduled for and received a detailed evaluation with one of three neurologists working at our outpatient department to confirm their eligibility to participate. The asymptomatic control group comprised of volunteers who received the same examination and assessments using a therapist who was blind to the participants' possible group status (control vs. FMS). In order to be eligible for the control group, participants were required to be asymptomatic and could not report pain during the physical examination process. All participants signed informed consent forms prior to entering the investigation and also prior to data collection.

Sixty-seven adult participants with FMS ($\geq$18 years of age, 12 males and 55 females) out of 380 participants were enrolled after meeting the 2016 fibromyalgia diagnostic criteria [4]. All participants were screened for conditions that would affect their inclusion into our study: severe cardiopulmonary disease and hyper-tension, long-standing viral infections, a history of any significant medical condition, any moderate or severe scoliosis, and a history of spine surgery.

2.1. 3D Posture Measurement Using a Formetric System

The Formetric software system (DIERS Medical Systems, Chicago, IL, USA) was used to provide analysis of the following posture profiles in three planes: (1) sagittal plane parameters (kyphotic angle, lordotic angle, and sagittal imbalance); (2) frontal/coronal plane parameters (coronal imbalance); (3) and transverse plane parameters (vertebral rotation). This system is both valid and reliable for postural measurements as used herein [25,26]. We followed previously published standard protocols for patient positioning, measurements, and data acquisition for Formetric software analysis, and we refer the interested reader to this publication [12]. A sample Formetric system report is shown in Figure 1 and each of these measurement variables is described below.

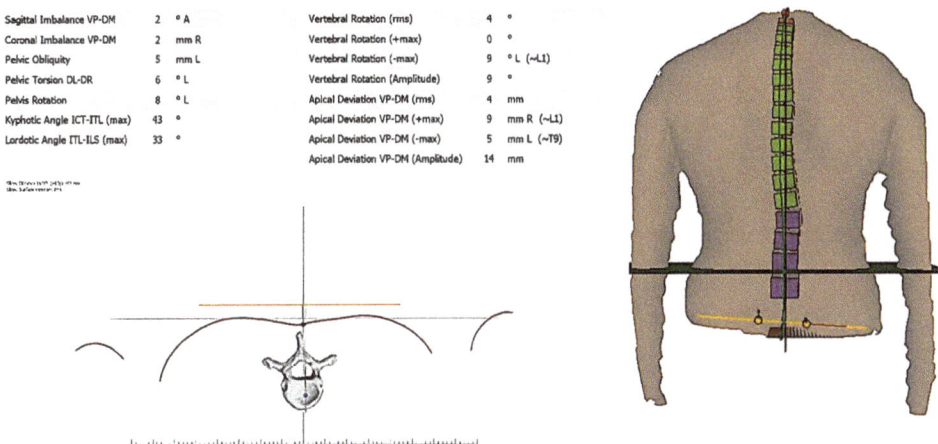

Figure 1. Illustrative example for the Formetric report.

2.2. Kyphotic Angle

The thoracic kyphotic angle (cervicothoracic transition point (ICT)- thoracolumbar transition point (ITL) max) was measured between tangents from the cervicothoracic junction (ICT-T1) and that of the thoracolumbar junction (ITL-T12). The cutoff value to determine hyper-kyphosis of our participants was set at an angle greater than or equal to 55° [25,27]. Formetric measurements of thoracic kyphosis over-estimate the actual radiographic measured kyphosis of the same person by a mean of 7–8°; however, a strong correlation between the two different measurement methods has been found (r = 0.79 to 0.872) [25,27]. Thus, a formetric value of 55° for thoracic kyphosis would approximate a 48° radiographic measurement value from T1–T12 (the upper end of normal in healthy middle-aged adults) [28].

2.3. Lordotic Angle

The lumbar lordotic angle was assessed between the intersection of two lines drawn tangent to: (1) a surface marker at the inflection point of the thoraco-lumbar junction (termed ITL) and (2) the point of inflection between the lumbar and sacral spines (termed ILS) and the maximum lumbar lordosis was thus termed ITL-ILS max. The Formetric measurement of lumbar lordosis is both reliable and valid with a good correlation (r > 0.70) to radiography and small measurement differences (8° difference from radiographic measurements) [25,27].

2.4. Sagittal Imbalance or Trunk Inclination

Sagittal imbalance was measured as a height difference between the vertebral prominence of C7 (VP) and dimple middle (DM), defined as the point lying on the center of the straight line connecting the left dimple to the right dimple, based on a vertical plane (sagittal section). When the VP is anterior relative to the DM, then the angle has a positive value, while if the VP is posterior to the DM, then the angle has a negative value.

2.5. Coronal Imbalance

The coronal imbalance of the trunk is measured as the left and right displacement of the VP relative to a DM lying in the center of a straight line that connects the left and right dimples. A positive shift is indicated by the VP offset to the right while a negative shift is directed to the left.

2.6. Vertebral Rotation

The vertebral rotation is measured as the root mean square (RMS) of the horizontal components of the surface normal relative to a line of symmetry.

2.7. Fibromyalgia Impact Questionnaire (FIQ)

Our primary outcome to determine the relationship between 3D posture displacements and FMS was whether or not posture displacements variables would correlate to the fibromyalgia impact questionnaire FIQ score of the FMS participants. The FIQ is a patient questionnaire designed to quantify the impact of FMS on a participant's current status, their progress or response to intervention. The FIQ is valid and reliable and has 10 subscales that include: physical, day missed from work, ability to perform job duties, well-being, pain intensity, fatigue or malaise, sleep quality, generalized stiffness, and depression and anxiety. The FIQ is scored from 0–100 with greater scores indicating more disability or impairment due to FMS [29].

2.8. Sample Size Determination

A pilot study consisting of 10 participants with FMS compared to 10 age- and sex-matched controls was performed, and this data was used to identify the sample size of participants needed for statistical findings. The mean differences and SD of the posture parameters; kyphotic angle, lordotic angle, sagittal imbalance, coronal imbalance; vertebral rotation were: kyphotic angle: −12 (SD 6.2), lordotic angle: -4 (SD 4.8), −sagittal imbalance: −5.2 (SD 2.1) coronal imbalance: -4 (SD 1.9), vertebral rotation: −3.9 (SD 1.8). We applied a Bonferroni correction to adjust the significance value for each of the primary outcomes. Using the largest value of the needed sample size estimate determined the final sample size for our trial. It was determined that 56 participants in each group (with a statistical power of 90%) was necessary herein; we increased the sample size by 20% to account for possible participant dropouts.

2.9. Data Analysis

In order to test normality of the distribution of our data, we used a one-sample Kolmogorov–Smirnov normality test. Where the data are normally distributed, they are presented as mean ± standard deviation (SD). Baseline participant demographics of age, weight, body mass index (BMI), highest education level completed, marital status, and pain duration, were compared between both groups using the independent t tests for continuous data and chi square tests of independence for categorical data. The Student's t-test was used to compare the means of continuous variables between the two groups. A p-value of < 0.05 was considered statistically significant. A matched-pairs binary logistic regression procedure for estimating odds ratios for a matched pairs case-control design determined whether the 3D posture parameters (kyphotic angle (ICT-ITL (max)), lordotic angle (ITL-ILS (max)), sagittal imbalance (VP-DM), coronal imbalance (VP-DM), and vertebral rotation (RMS)) demonstrated an association with the likelihood of experiencing FMS. Multiple regression was carried out to examine whether posture parameters could significantly predict FMS participants' FIQ scores. SPSS version 20.0 software was used for analyzing data (IBM SPSS Inc., Armonk, NY, USA).

3. Results

We screened by phone greater than 380 possible participants. The most often reason for participant exclusion was an uncontrolled medical condition such as diabetes mellitus, heart disease, renal failure, and so forth. A hierarchy of control group participant was applied whereby a control participant was only included after a FMS group participant of a similar age and gender had been recruited, thus, further exclusions occurred when matching was not possible. Included group participants were: (1) FMS (mean age 46.4 years, SD = 9; 12 males, 55 females) and (2) 67 sex and age matched controls (mean age = 46.5 years, SD = 9.1; 12 males, 55 female). Figure 2 demonstrates the participants' inclusion and exclusion flow chart for this study.

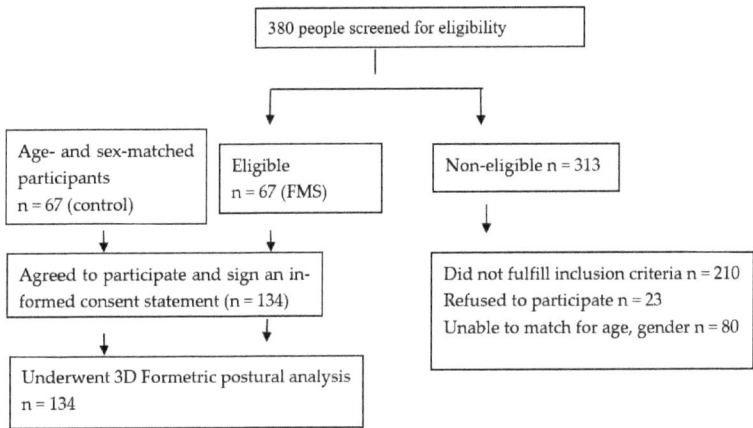

Figure 2. Participant flow chart.

3.1. Sample Characteristics

The baseline participant demographics are presented in Table 1. The FMS and control groups were statistically matched for each of the included demographic variables (Table 1).

Table 1. Baseline participant demographics.

Variable	Fibromyalgia Group (n = 67)	Control Group (n = 67)
Age (years)	46.4 ± 9	46.5 ± 9.1
Weight (kg)	75 ± 9	80 ± 10
Gender (%)		
Male	12	12
Female	55	55
Body mass index mean (SD), Kg/m^2		
Graduation		
Primary school	5 (7.5%)	2 (3%)
Secondary school	10 (14.9%)	8 (11.9%)
Advanced technical colleague certificate	10 (14.9%)	15 (22.4%)
University diploma	32 (47.8%)	30 (44.8%)
Others	10 (14.9%)	12 (17.9%)
Marital status (%)		
Single	5 (7.5%)	4 (6%)
Married	55 (82.1%)	57 (85%)
Separated, divorced, or widowed	7 (10.4%)	6 (9%)
Pain duration		
1–5 y	20 (29.9%)	Asymptomatic
>5 y	47 (70.1%)	Asymptomatic

There were no statistically significant differences between the FMS and control groups; $p > 0.05$ for all variables using the independent t test for continuous data and chi squared test of independence for categorical data. y: year.

3.2. Formetric Postural Variables between Group Differences

Each of the five postural variables were found to be statistically significant different between both groups: kyphotic ICT-ITL (max) ($p < 0.001$); lordotic angle ITL-ILS (max) ($p < 0.001$); sagittal imbalance ($p < 0.001$); coronal imbalance ($p < 0.001$); and vertebral rotation (rms) ($p < 0.001$). Table 2 reports the 3D Formetric data means and SD between the FMS and control groups.

Table 2. Means, standard deviation (SD), 95% confidence interval (CI) and statistical significance of the postural measurements between participants with FMS and controls.

3D Formetric Measurement		Mean	±SD	SEM	Cohen's d	95% CI	p-Value
Kyphotic angle ICT-ITL (max) (deg.)	FMS	74.1	4.75	0.58	6.8	[14.3–19.04]	<0.001
	Control	57.4	8.41	1.02			
Lordotic angle ITL-ILS (max) (deg.)	FMS	45.1	5.71	0.69	4.3	[1.9–4.9]	<0.001
	Control	41.5	2.46	0.30			
Sagittal imbalance (mm)	FMS	9.53	2.77	0.33	2.3	[4.1–5.7]	<0.001
	Control	4.5	1.89	0.23			
Coronal imbalance (mm)	FMS	8.04	3.19	0.39	2.4	[3.6–5.6]	<0.001
	Control	3.22	1.37	0.16			
vertebral rotation (rms) (deg.)	FMS	9.5	1.86	0.22	1.8	[3.5–4.7]	<0.001
	Control	5.3	1.75	0.21			

SEM: Std. Error of Mean; SD: standard deviation; CI: confidence interval; ICT-ITL: Cervico-thoracic inflection point-thoraco-lumbar inflection point; ITL-ILS: thoracic-lumbar inflection point- lumbo-sacral inflection point; rms: root mean square.

3.3. Binary Logistic Regressions

The binary logistic regression analysis identified a statistically significant increased probability of having FMS as the following postural variables become increasingly abnormal: (1) kyphotic angle ICT-ITL (max) ($p < 0.03$), (2) sagittal trunk imbalance ($p = 0.005$), and (3) vertebral rotation (rms) ($p = 0.015$). In contrast, no statistically significant differences were found for the two remaining postural displacement variables of coronal balance ($p = 0.50$) and lumbar lordotic angle (ITL-ILS (max); $p = 0.10$). See Table 3.

Table 3. Variables in the equation for logistic regression and odds ratio calculation.

Variables in the Equation							95% CI for EXP(B)	
	B	S.E.	Wald	df	Sig.	Exp(B)	Lower	Upper
Sagittal imbalance (mm)	0.437	0.236	3.409	1	0.005	1.547	0.973	2.459
vertebral rotation (rms) (degrees)	2.069	0.851	5.914	1	0.015	7.919	1.494	41.970
Kyphotic ICT−ITL (max) (degrees)	0.569	0.275	4.273	1	0.039	1.766	1.030	3.029
Coronal imbalance (mm)	−0.188	0.313	0.360	1	0.549	0.829	0.449	1.530
Lordotic angle (degrees)	0.472	0.326	2.105	1	0.147	1.604	0.847	3.035
Constant	−52.309	21.782	5.767	1	0.016	0.000		

Variable(s) entered on step 1: Sagittal imbalance, vertebral rotation, Kyphotic ICT-ITL (max), Coronal imbalance, Lordotic angle.

3.4. Odds Ratios between Having FMS and Posture Variables

Three of the five postural displacement variables were found to have statistically significant odds ratios identifying an increased risk of having FMS with increases in the magnitude of the abnormal posture. These three postural variables and their odds ratios were: (1) Thoracic kyphotic angle = 1.76 (95% CI = 1.03, 3.02) indicating that for each degree of increased angle, there was an approximate 76% increased likelihood of having FMS; (2) Sagittal imbalance = 1.54 (95% CI = 0.973, 2.459) indicating that for each degree increase of sagittal imbalance, there was an approximate 54% increased likelihood of having FMS; (3) Surface rotation = 7.9 (95% CI = 1.494, 41.97) indicating that with each 7 degrees increase in surface rotation, there was an approximate 90% increased likelihood of having FMS in this sample.

Similarly, multiple linear regression analysis identified that the 3 postural displacement variables (thoracic kyphotic angle, sagittal imbalance, and vertebral surface rotation) were statistically significant predictors of a participant's FMS impact questionnaire scores; $F = 104.4$, $p < 0.01$. The multiple-regression analysis revealed that 80% of the variance in the dependent variable FMS impact questionnaire scores could be explained by the independent variables (postural displacements). Table 4 presents these findings.

Table 4. Multiple linear regression for the fibromyalgia impact questionnaire score versus postural variables and their associated risk factors.

Model		Unstandardized Coefficients		Standardized Coefficients	t	Sig.	95.0% Confidence Interval for B	
		B	Std. Error	Beta			Lower Bound	Upper Bound
1	Constant	−2.043	0.214		−9.562	<0.001	−2.466	−1.620
	Kyphotic ICT−ITL (max) (deg.)	0.021	0.003	0.459	8.462	<0.001	0.016	0.026
	sagittal imbalance (mm)	0.024	0.009	0.166	2.739	0.005	0.007	0.042
	vertebral rotation (deg.)	0.078	0.011	0.430	7.197	<0.001	0.057	0.099
	Lordotic angle (deg.)	0.010	0.004	0.092	2.206	0.029	0.001	0.019
	Coronal imbalance (mm)	−0.007	0.010	−0.046	−0.688	0.493	−0.026	0.013

B: Unstandardized coefficients.

4. Discussion

This case control investigation sought to identify if 3D posture displacements can identify FMS participants versus a matched control group without overt signs and symptoms and no FMS. The results identified from this study show that there is a strong relationship between spinal 3D misalignment and the diagnosis of FMS. In fact, our results support that the outcome measures used to objectively assess thoraco-lumbar postural alignments could be used as strong predictors for the diagnosis of FMS. We believe that our investigation is the first study to seek and identify a predictive association between comprehensive 3D thoraco-lumbar postural alignments and FMS.

Some recent studies investigated spine posture in individuals, commonly women, with FMS [30–33]. Sempere-Rubio et al. [30] found that there is an altered trunk posture in women with FMS compared to a control group. These findings agree with those of the current study; both studies found differences in the same direction for one of the most common outcome measures; namely an increased kyphotic angle of the group with FMS [30]. However, our study offers other more objective outcome measures for the posture assessment by using the 3D Diers Formetric device. Another study by Sempere-Rubio et al. showed that women with FMS have an altered postural control compared to a healthy group, adding to the strong factors that should be considered in diagnosing and treating FMS [31].

The increased thoracic kyphosis in FMS populations has also been supported by Celenay et al. [33], who found that women with FMS had an increased thoracic kyphosis angle compared to the control group. However, the lumbar lordosis was not significantly different between groups while in our study the group with FMS had a slightly higher lumbar lordotic angle compared to the control group. This discrepancy for lumbar lordosis between investigations is likely explained by the fact that the compensation to an increased kyphotic angle (which is the confirmed common deviation in all the studies mentioned including our study) can be either an increased or a decreased lordotic angle depending on the general posture assumed by the individual [34]. The increased kyphosis in the kyphotic, flat-back and sway-back postures is linked to neutral lumbar spine, hypolordotic upper lumbar spine and a hyperlordotic lower lumbar spine in each of those three postures, respectively [34].

Although a normal clinical neurological examination is most often identified, FMS patients consistently report sensory deficits which has been confirmed on dynamic posturography [35,36]. Indeed, abnormalities of body posture in women suffering from FMS have been identified to be related to poor trunk position sense and balance instability [33]. Sempere-Rubio et al. identified that females with FMS have poorer postural control compared to a healthy group which further emphasizes including postural alignment in diagnosing and treating FMS [31]. Another study by Sempere-Rubio et al. reported that a decreased ability in maintaining sitting thoracic posture could predict a reduction in quality of life in women with FMS [32].

Previously, investigators have suggested that objective studies are needed to understand postural balance abnormalities in FMS populations and their relationship to different types of musculoskeletal abnormalities [37]. The relationship between FMS and postural misalignment has been investigated in several studies [7,38–40]. Moustafa and Diab speculated that sustained postural imbalances can result in the establishment of a state of continuous asymmetric loading [38]. If a significant maladaptive posture is sustained long enough, it will consequently affect the quality of life [41]. These speculations are supported by other authors [42,43] who discuss that biomechanical dysfunction causing a sustained asymmetrical loading and muscle imbalance leads to an increased stress and strain on body structures. For instance, Hiemeyer et al. linked poor flexed posture to the tender points characterizing FMS, most of which are in postural muscles [43]; restoring a correct posture diminished these tender points if not completely eliminated them [43,44].

The most intriguing finding was that the predictors of postural features included not only the sagittal profile, but also the abnormal transverse profile as indicated by surface rotation. This finding is not surprising as previously, Veldhuizen et al. [45] identified that alterations in transverse plane rotational alignment were positively correlated to sagittal alignment abnormalities. Similarly, other authors have reported the correlation between the sagittal and coronal and transverse spinal contours [46–48]. Incorrect posture and spinal abnormalities in sagittal and axial planes may modify the stability of this structure and its load distribution, which can generate abnormal stresses and strains, thus provoking a reduction in quality of life and an increased risk of FMS.

The present paper adds to the present body of FMS literature that supports an optimal alignment of upright human posture. Due to the significant relationships between the magnitude of the posture displacements as identified with the Formetric analysis and the odds of having FMS our findings indicate that postural displacements are predictive of not only who has fibromyalgia but also of the severity of the identified disability as measured with the FIQ. Our findings are in general agreement of the randomized trial by Moustafa where it was identified that correction of the cervical sagittal plane alignment was found to improve 3D posture and improve the short- and long-term pain and impairments of patients suffering from chronic FMS [44].

4.1. Limitations

Because this study was a cross-sectional, case-control investigation and not a treatment outcome trial, it is unknown how our findings may or may not influence patient treatment outcomes when postural rehabilitation is pursued. However, since the 3D postural analysis showed increased posture aberrations in the FMS group, we recommend that interventions designed to improve 3D posture should be implemented as part of a multi-modal treatment approach. Lastly, although the Formetric measurement of 3D posture is valid and reliable [25,27], it does not completely describe the actual sagittal and coronal spine alignment. In FMS participants, using sagittal and anterior-posterior radiological profiles would likely give further insights into exact rotation and translation displacements of individual vertebral and overall spine curvature geometry and magnitudes.

4.2. Conclusions

The results derived from this study identified that there is a strong relationship between spinal three-dimensional (3D) misalignment as measured with the Formetric system and the diagnosis of FMS. Our results support that the posture displacements of the thoracolumbar regions can be used as part of the clinical and diagnostic indicators to determine who has FMS and as possible outcomes of treatment interventions. Future trials should use 3D postures as an outcome measure to determine if posture rehabilitation impacts short- and long-term outcomes in FMS sufferers.

Author Contributions: A.A. (Amal Ahbouch), I.M.M., T.S. and A.A. (Ashokan Arumugam) conceived the research idea and participated in its design. A.A. (Amal Ahbouch), I.M.M., T.S., A.A. (Ashokan Arumugam), P.O. and D.E.H. all contributed to the statistical analysis. A.A. (Amal Ahbouch), I.M.M., T.S. and A.A. (Ashokan Arumugam) participated in the data collection and study supervision. I.M.M., P.O. and D.E.H. all contributed to the interpretation of the results and wrote the drafts. All authors have read and agreed to the published version of the manuscript.

Funding: This research received no external funding.

Institutional Review Board Statement: The study was conducted in accordance with the Declaration of Helsinki, and approved by the Ethics Committee of the Faculty of Physical Therapy, Cairo University; all participants signed informed consent prior to data collection. The IRB approval number is Cairo-PT.3-4561.

Informed Consent Statement: Not applicable.

Data Availability Statement: The datasets analysed in the current study are available from the corresponding author on reasonable request.

Conflicts of Interest: P.A.O. is a paid consultant for CBP NonProfit, Inc. D.E.H. teaches rehabilitation methods and distributes products for patient rehabilitation that use posture analysis similar to that used in this manuscript. All the other authors declare that they have no competing interests.

Abbreviations

3D	Three-dimensional
FMS	Fibromyalgia syndrome
ICT-ITL	Cervicothoracic transition point (ICT)-thoracolumbar transition point (ITL) max
ITL-ILS	Thoracic-lumbar inflection point (ITL)-lumbar-sacral inflection point (ILS) max
RMS	Root mean square

References

1. Apkarian, A.V. Definitions of Nociception, Pain, and Chronic Pain with Implications Regarding Science and Society. *Neurosci. Lett.* **2019**, *702*, 1–2. [CrossRef] [PubMed]
2. Chinn, S.; Caldwell, W.; Gritsenko, K. Fibromyalgia Pathogenesis and Treatment Options Update. *Curr. Pain Headache Rep.* **2016**, *20*, 25. [CrossRef] [PubMed]
3. Arnold, L.M.; Bennett, R.M.; Crofford, L.J.; Dean, L.E.; Clauw, D.J.; Goldenberg, D.L.; Fitzcharles, M.A.; Paiva, E.S.; Staud, R.; Sarzi-Puttini, P.; et al. AAPT Diagnostic Criteria for Fibromyalgia. *J. Pain* **2019**, *20*, 611–628. [CrossRef] [PubMed]
4. Wolfe, F.; Clauw, D.J.; Fitzcharles, M.A.; Goldenberg, D.L.; Häuser, W.; Katz, R.L.; Mease, P.J.; Russell, A.S.; Russell, I.J.; Walitt, B. 2016 Revisions to the 2010/2011 Fibromyalgia Diagnostic Criteria. *Semin. Arthritis Rheum.* **2016**, *46*, 319–329. [CrossRef] [PubMed]
5. Jahan, F.; Nanji, K.; Qidwai, W.; Qasim, R. Oman Medical Specialty Board Fibromyalgia Syndrome: An Overview of Pathophysiology, Diagnosis and Management. *Oman Med. J.* **2012**, *27*, 192. [CrossRef] [PubMed]
6. Cuyul-Vásquez, I.; Araya-Quintanilla, F.; Gutiérrez-Espinoza, H. Comment on Siracusa et al. Fibromyalgia: Pathogenesis, Mechanisms, Diagnosis and Treatment Options Update. *Int. J. Mol. Sci.* **2021**, *22*, 3891.
7. Makofsky, B.H.W.; Goldstein, L.B. The Role of Body Posture in Musculoskeletal Pain Syndromes. *Pract. Pain Manag.* **2011**, *3*, 31.

8. Lennon, J.; Shealy, N.; Cady, R.; Matta, W.; Cox, R.S.W. Postural and Respiratory Modulation of Autonomic Function, Pain and Health. *Am. J. Pain Manag.* **1994**, *4*, 36–39.
9. Cameron, M.H.; Monroe, L.G. *Physical Rehabilitation: Evidence-Based Examination, Evaluation, and Intervention*; Saunders Elsevier: St Louis, MO, USA, 2007; p. 953.
10. Raine, S.; Twomey, L. Attributes and qualities of human posture and their relationship to dysfunction or musculoskeletal pain. *Crit. Rev. Phys. Rehabil. Med.* **1994**, *6*, 409–437.
11. Fernandez-de-las-Penas, C.; Alonso-Blanco, C.; Cuadrado, M.L.; Gerwin, R.D.; Pareja, J.A. Trigger Points in the Suboccipital Muscles and Forward Head Posture in Tension-Type Headache. *Headache J. Head Face Pain* **2006**, *46*, 454–460. [CrossRef]
12. Moustafa, I.M.; Shousha, T.M.; Harrison, D.E. An investigation of 3D spinal alignment in cervicogenic headache. *Musculoskelet. Sci. Pract.* **2021**, *51*, 102284. [CrossRef] [PubMed]
13. Evcik, D.; Aksoy, O. Relationship Between Head Posture and Temporomandibular Dysfunction Syndrome. *J. Musculoskelet. Pain* **2010**, *12*, 19–24. [CrossRef]
14. Gonzalez, H.E.; Manns, A. Forward Head Posture: Its Structural and Functional Influence on the Stomatognathic System, a Conceptual Study. *Cranio* **1996**, *14*, 71–80. [CrossRef] [PubMed]
15. Wright, E.F.; Domenech, M.A.; Fischer, J.R. Usefulness of Posture Training for Patients with Temporomandibular Disorders. *J. Am. Dent. Assoc.* **2000**, *131*, 202–210. [CrossRef]
16. Ludewig, P.M.; Cook, T.M. Alterations in shoulder kinematics and associated muscle activity in people with symptoms of shoulder impingement. *Phys. Ther.* **2000**, *80*, 276–291. [CrossRef]
17. Bullock, M.P.; Foster, N.E.; Wright, C.C. Shoulder Impingement: The Effect of Sitting Posture on Shoulder Pain and Range of Motion. *Man. Ther.* **2005**, *10*, 28–37. [CrossRef]
18. McMaster, M.J.; Glasby, M.A.; Singh, H.; Cunningham, S. Lung Function in Congenital Kyphosis and Kyphoscoliosis. *J. Spinal Disord. Tech.* **2007**, *20*, 203–208. [CrossRef]
19. Kapreli, E.; Vourazanis, E.; Billis, E.; Oldham, J.A.; Strimpakos, N. Respiratory Dysfunction in Chronic Neck Pain Patients. A Pilot Study. *Cephalalgia* **2009**, *29*, 701–710. [CrossRef]
20. Christie, H.J.; Kumar, S.; Warren, S.A. Postural Aberrations in Low Back Pain. *Arch. Phys. Med. Rehabil.* **1995**, *76*, 218–224. [CrossRef]
21. Cacciatore, T.W.; Horak, F.B.; Henry, S. Improvement in Automatic Postural Coordination Following Alexander Technique Lessons in a Person with Low Back Pain. *Phys. Ther.* **2005**, *85*, 565. [CrossRef]
22. Nemmers, T. The Influence of the forward Head Posture on Balance, Fall Self-Efficacy, and Physical Activity Level in Community-Dwelling Women Age 60 and Older; and the Relationship of These Variables to Self-Reported Fall History. Ph.D. Thesis, Oklahoma State University, Stillwater, OK, USA, 2006. Available online: https://hdl.handle.net/11244/7521 (accessed on 29 October 2022).
23. Hiemeyer, K.; Lutz, R.; Menninger, H. Dependence of tender points upon posture: A key to the understanding of fibromyalgia syndrome. *J. Man. Med.* **1990**, *5*, 169–174.
24. Keller, T.S.; Harrison, D.E.; Colloca, C.J.; Harrison, D.D.; Janik, T.J. Prediction of Osteoporotic Spinal Deformity. *Spine* **2003**, *28*, 455–462. [CrossRef] [PubMed]
25. Tabard-Fougère, A.; Bonnefoy-Mazure, A.; Hanquinet, S.; Lascombes, P.; Armand, S.; Dayer, R. Validity and Reliability of Spine Rasterstereography in Patients with Adolescent Idiopathic Scoliosis. *Spine* **2017**, *42*, 98–105. [CrossRef] [PubMed]
26. Krott, N.L.; Wild, M.; Betsch, M. Meta-Analysis of the Validity and Reliability of Rasterstereographic Measurements of Spinal Posture. *Eur. Spine J.* **2020**, *29*, 2392–2401. [CrossRef] [PubMed]
27. Frerich, J.M.; Hertzler, K.; Knott, P.; Mardjetko, S. Comparison of Radiographic and Surface Topography Measurements in Adolescents with Idiopathic Scoliosis. *Open Orthop. J.* **2012**, *6*, 261–265. [CrossRef]
28. Harrison, D.D.; Harrison, D.E.; Janik, T.J.; Cailliet, R.; Haas, J. Do alterations in vertebral and disc dimensions affect an elliptical model of thoracic kyphosis? *Spine* **2003**, *28*, 463–469. [CrossRef] [PubMed]
29. El-Naby, M.A.; Hefny, M.A.; Fahim, A.E.; Awadalla, M.A. Validation of an adapted arabic version of fibromyalgia syndrome impact questionnaire. *Rheumatol. Int.* **2013**, *33*, 2561–2567. [CrossRef]
30. Sempere-Rubio, N.; Aguilar-Rodríguez, M.; Espí-López, G.V.; Cortés-Amador, S.; Pascual, E.; Serra-Añó, P. Impaired Trunk Posture in Women with Fibromyalgia. *Spine* **2018**, *43*, 1536–1542. [CrossRef]
31. Sempere-Rubio, N.; López-Pascual, J.; Aguilar-Rodríguez, M.; Cortés-Amador, S.; Espí-López, G.; Villarrasa-Sapiña, I.; Serra-Añó, P. Characterization of Postural Control Impairment in Women with Fibromyalgia. *PLoS ONE* **2018**, *13*, e0196575. [CrossRef]
32. Sempere-Rubio, N.; Aguilar-Rodríguez, M.; Inglés, M.; Izquierdo-Alventosa, R.; Serra-Añó, P. Physical Condition Factors That Predict a Better Quality of Life in Women with Fibromyalgia. *Int. J. Environ. Res. Public Health* **2019**, *16*, 3173. [CrossRef]
33. Toprak Celenay, S.; Mete, O.; Coban, O.; Oskay, D.; Erten, S. Trunk Position Sense, Postural Stability, and Spine Posture in Fibromyalgia. *Rheumatol. Int.* **2019**, *39*, 2087–2094. [CrossRef] [PubMed]
34. Czaprowski, D.; Stoliński, L.; Tyrakowski, M.; Kozinoga, M.; Kotwicki, T. Non-Structural Misalignments of Body Posture in the Sagittal Plane. *Scoliosis Spinal Disord.* **2018**, *13*, 6. [CrossRef] [PubMed]
35. Jones, K.D.; King, L.A.; Mist, S.D.; Bennett, R.M.; Horak, F.B. Postural Control Deficits in People with Fibromyalgia: A Pilot Study. *Arthritis Res. Ther.* **2011**, *13*, R127. [CrossRef] [PubMed]
36. Jones, K.D.; Horak, F.B.; Winters-Stone, K.; Irvine, J.M.; Bennett, R.M. Fibromyalgia Is Associated with Impaired Balance and Falls. *J. Clin. Rheumatol.* **2009**, *15*, 16–21. [CrossRef]

37. Moustafa, I.M.; Diab, A.A. The Addition of Upper Cervical Manipulative Therapy in the Treatment of Patients with Fibromyalgia: A Randomized Controlled Trial. *Rheumatol. Int.* **2015**, *35*, 1163–1174. [CrossRef]
38. Müller, A.; Hartmann, M.; Eich, W. Health Care Utilization in Patients with Fibromyalgia Syndrome (FMS). *Schmerz* **2000**, *14*, 77–83. [CrossRef]
39. Cramer, H.; Mehling, W.E.; Saha, F.J.; Dobos, G.; Lauche, R. Postural Awareness and Its Relation to Pain: Validation of an Innovative Instrument Measuring Awareness of Body Posture in Patients with Chronic Pain. *BMC Musculoskelet. Disord.* **2018**, *19*, 109. [CrossRef]
40. Mannerkorpi, K.; Ahlmén, M.; Ekdahl, C. Six- and 24-Month Follow-up of Pool Exercise Therapy and Education for Patients with Fibromyalgia. *Scand. J. Rheumatol.* **2002**, *31*, 306–310. [CrossRef]
41. Imagama, S.; Hasegawa, Y.; Matsuyama, Y.; Sakai, Y.; Ito, Z.; Hamajima, N.; Ishiguro, N. Influence of sagittal balance and physical ability associated with exercise on quality of life in middle-aged and elderly people. *Arch. Osteoporos.* **2011**, *6*, 13–20. [CrossRef]
42. Simons, D.G.; Travell, J.G.; Simons, L.S. *Travell, Simons & Simons' Myofascial Pain and Dysfunction: The Trigger Point Manual*, 2nd ed.; Hardcover; Lippincott Williams & Wilkins: Baltimore, MD, USA, 1998; p. 1056.
43. Hiemeyer, K.; Lutz, R.; Menninger, H. Generalisiertes Auftreten von Schmerzhaften Druckpunkten an Sehnen Und Muskeln Beim Habituellen Rundräcken Ein Beitrag Zur Diskussion Um Das Fibromyalgiesyndrom (FMS). *Aktuelle Rheumatol.* **1989**, *14*, 193–201. [CrossRef]
44. Moustafa, I.M. Does improvement towards a normal cerivcal sagittal configuration aid in the management of fibromyalgia syndrome. A randomized controlled trial. *Bull. Fac. Ph. Ther. Cairo Univers.* **2013**, *18*, 29–41.
45. Veldhuizen, A.G.; Wever, D.J.; Webb, P.J. The Aetiology of Idiopathic Scoliosis: Biomechanical and Neuromuscular Factors. *Eur. Spine J.* **2000**, *9*, 178–184. [CrossRef] [PubMed]
46. Rigo, M.; Quera-Salvá, G.; Villagrasa, M. Sagittal Configuration of the Spine in Girls with Idiopathic Scoliosis: Progressing Rather than Initiating Factor. *Stud. Health Technol. Inform.* **2006**, *123*, 90–94. [PubMed]
47. De Jonge, T.; Dubousset, J.F.; Illés, T. Sagittal Plane Correction in Idiopathic Scoliosis. *Spine* **2002**, *27*, 754–761. [CrossRef] [PubMed]
48. Dobosiewicz, K.; Durmala, J.; Jendrzejek, H.; Czernicki, K. Influence of Method of Asymmetric Trunk Mobilization on Shaping of a Physiological Thoracic Kyphosis in Children and Youth Suffering from Progressive Idiopathic Scoliosis. *Stud. Health Technol. Inform.* **2002**, *91*, 348–351.

Disclaimer/Publisher's Note: The statements, opinions and data contained in all publications are solely those of the individual author(s) and contributor(s) and not of MDPI and/or the editor(s). MDPI and/or the editor(s) disclaim responsibility for any injury to people or property resulting from any ideas, methods, instructions or products referred to in the content.

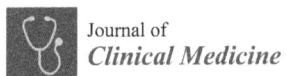

Article

Does Forward Head Posture Influence Somatosensory Evoked Potentials and Somatosensory Processing in Asymptomatic Young Adults?

Ibrahim M. Moustafa [1,2], Aliaa Attiah Mohamed Diab [1,3] and Deed E. Harrison [4,*]

1. Department of Physiotherapy, College of Health Sciences, University of Sharjah, Sharjah 27272, United Arab Emirates
2. Neuromusculoskeletal Rehabilitation Research Group, RIMHS—Research Institute of Medical and Health Sciences, University of Sharjah, Sharjah 27272, United Arab Emirates
3. Faculty of Physical Therapy, Cairo University, Giza 12613, Egypt
4. CBP Nonprofit (A Spine Research Foundation), Eagle, ID 83616, USA
* Correspondence: drdeedharrison@gmail.com or drdeed@idealspine.com

Abstract: The current investigation used somatosensory evoked potentials (SEPs) to assess differences in sensorimotor integration and somatosensory processing variables between asymptomatic individuals with and without forward head posture (FHP). We assessed different neural regions of the somatosensory pathway, including the amplitudes of the peripheral N9, spinal N13, brainstem P14, peak-to-peak amplitudes of parietal N20 and P27, and frontal N30 potentials. Central conduction time (N13–N20) was measured as the difference in peak latencies of N13 and N20. We measured these variables in 60 participants with FHP defined as a craniovertebral angle (CVA) < 50° and 60 control participants matched for age, gender, and body mass index (BMI) with normal FHP defined as CVA > 55°. Differences in variable measures were examined using the parametric t-test. Pearson's correlation was used to evaluate the relationship between the CVA and sensorimotor integration and SEP measurements. A generalized linear model (GLM) was used to compare the SEP measures between groups, with adjustment for educational level, marital status, BMI, and working hours per week. There were statistically significant differences between the FHP group and control group for all sensorimotor integration and SEP processing variables, including the amplitudes of spinal N13 ($p < 0.005$), brainstem P14 ($p < 0.005$), peak-to-peak amplitudes of parietal N20 and P27 ($p < 0.005$), frontal N30 potentials ($p < 0.005$), and the conduction time N13–N20 ($p = 0.004$). The CVA significantly correlated with all measured neurophysiological variables indicating that as FHP increased, sensorimotor integration and SEP processing became less efficient. FHP group correlations were: N9 ($r = -0.44$, $p < 0.001$); N13 ($r = -0.67$, $p < 0.001$); P14 ($r = -0.58$, $p < 0.001$); N20 ($r = -0.49$, $p = 0.001$); P27 ($r = -0.58$, $p < 0.001$); N30 potentials ($r = -0.64$, $p < 0.001$); and N13–N20 ($r = -0.61$, $p < 0.001$). GLM identified that increased working hours adversely affected the SEP measures ($p < 0.005$), while each 1° increase in the CVA was associated with improved SEP amplitudes and more efficient central conduction time (N13–N20; $p < 0.005$). Less efficient sensorimotor integration and SEP processing may be related to previous scientific reports of altered sensorimotor control and athletic skill measures in populations with FHP. Future investigations should seek to replicate our findings in different spine disorders and symptomatic populations in an effort to understand how improving forward head posture might benefit functional outcomes of patient care.

Keywords: forward head posture; cervical spine; somatosensory evoked potential

Citation: Moustafa, I.M.; Diab, A.A.M.; Harrison, D.E. Does Forward Head Posture Influence Somatosensory Evoked Potentials and Somatosensory Processing in Asymptomatic Young Adults? *J. Clin. Med.* 2023, 12, 3217. https://doi.org/10.3390/jcm12093217

Academic Editor: Hideki Murakami

Received: 23 February 2023
Revised: 12 April 2023
Accepted: 28 April 2023
Published: 29 April 2023

Copyright: © 2023 by the authors. Licensee MDPI, Basel, Switzerland. This article is an open access article distributed under the terms and conditions of the Creative Commons Attribution (CC BY) license (https://creativecommons.org/licenses/by/4.0/).

1. Introduction

Sensorimotor integration and central somatosensory processing are brain processes that allow for the execution of certain voluntary motor behaviors in response to specific demands of the environment [1]. In other words, it is the synergistic relationship between the sensory and motor systems [2]. Thus, the behavior pattern of healthy individuals and movement disorder patients depends on the sensorimotor integration process [3]. Alterations in sensorimotor integration and somatosensory processing may offer insights into differences in patient motor control abnormalities and disturbances seen in specific spinal disorders with neurologic components [4,5].

Chronic pain is a strong contributing factor triggering sensorimotor integration alterations [6–8]. It is known to alter specific regions of the brain functionally and structurally, such as the amygdala, the anterior cingulate cortex, the medial prefrontal cortex, and the primary somatosensory cortex. These alterations are considered maladaptive as they result in hyper-excitability and pathway re-organization [9,10]. Theoretically, altered afferent input is a likely explanation for the production and sustained occurrence of central neurophysiological processing dysfunctions [11–13]. The primary motor cortex (termed M1) is considered the central station where sensory input from the peripheral systems converges and is processed in order to execute proper and efficient voluntary motor tasks (sensorimotor integration). Sensorimotor integration also occurs in other regions of the brain (the parietal cortex, the supplementary motor area, the dorsal premotor cortex, the ventral premotor cortex, the basal ganglia, the cerebellum, and the thalamus, to name a few). These regions are known to alter and/or contribute to voluntary motor tasks as well. In simple terms, abnormalities of the peripheral (extremity) and central (spinal) tissues responsible for contributing to sensory input into the sensorimotor integration and somatosensory processing systems can cause disruption or dysfunction in the normal afferent input and processing in the M1 region, and thus, lead to inefficient motor control output [14,15].

There are many important questions regarding sensorimotor integration and somatosensory processing remaining to be addressed. For instance, the relevance of altered alignment of the sagittal cervical spine in symptomatic and asymptomatic persons to function/dysfunction in the sensorimotor integration and somatosensory processing systems remains understudied. It is known that the magnitude of forward head posture (FHP) is inversely correlated to the cervical spine range of motion [16]. Furthermore, FHP alters the length of the cervical spine through kinematic flexion/extension coupling and alters load sharing among the discs, ligaments, and muscles of the cervical spine [17,18]. Investigations on sustained cervical spine flexion have found changes in afferentation and abnormal feed-forward control due to mechanical viscoelastic changes to the cervical spine soft tissues that affect position sense repeatability [19]. Furthermore, straightening of the cervical spine lordotic curvature (as often occurs with FHP) has been found to significantly reduce the F-wave in the median nerve of the upper limbs of tested individuals, indicating a reduction in motor–Neuronal excitability [20]. Relatively few studies have addressed the relationship between FHP and inefficient sensorimotor integration and somatosensory processing [21,22].

Therefore, the purpose of the current investigation is to compare the sensorimotor integration and somatosensory processing at different neural regions of the somatosensory system, including central conduction time, in persons with and without forward head posture (FHP) and without overt symptomatology. The specific research questions to be addressed herein include: (1) Using somatosensory evoked potentials, is there a difference in sensorimotor integration and processing in asymptomatic participants without FHP compared to participants with FHP?; (2) Do persons with FHP have abnormal sensorimotor integration and at what region(s) does this occur?; (3) Is the possible alteration to somatosensory processing linearly related to the amount of FHP displacement?

2. Materials and Methods

Participants were collected as a convenience sample of asymptomatic individuals. Recruitment was obtained using both printed advertisements and social media. These advertisements were directed only to university-related communities, such as employees, alums, and students. All the participants were asymptomatic and had not received any physical therapy or any type of manual therapy treatment in the last year between November 2021 and July 2022. Ethics approval was obtained from our University (College of Health Sciences, University of Sharjah, UAE) (Ethical approval number: REC-21-03-11-03-S), and informed consent was provided to and obtained from all participants prior to data collection, in accordance with relevant guidelines and regulations.

2.1. Participants

Sixty participants with definite forward head posture (FHP) and sixty matched control participants without FHP were recruited for this study. Participants were matched for age, sex, demographics, and body mass index (BMI). In order for a participant to be categorized as having FHP, the craniovertebral angle (CVA) measurement was used, and published cutoff values were followed. Utilizing the data published by Yip et al. [23], FHP was classified as having a CVA < 50°; thus, participants were in the FHP group when CVA was <50°. Conversely, the control group was defined as having normal or no FHP when a participant's CVA was >55°. All FHP screening procedures were carried out by a physiotherapist with 15 years of clinical experience.

As standard practice, clinicians with 10 years of experience assessed all participants. Exclusion criteria for the current investigation were as follows: (i) any inflammatory joint disease; (ii) any systemic pathology; (iii) a history of significant injury or primary musculo-skeletal surgical interventions; (iv) deformity of the spine or extremities; and (v) any pain in the past 3-months involving the musculo-skeletal system. All participants were required to be pain-free. This was done in order to assess the potential effects of abnormal head posture without the presence of acute pain, as the presence of pain alone is known to induce a significant reduction in the post-central N20–P25 complex and a significant increase in the N18 wave [24].

2.2. Measurement Techniques

2.2.1. Craniovertebral Angle (CVA)

The CVA is reliable and valid for the assessment of FHP [25]. The CVA is measured as the angle of intersection between a horizontal line and a line bisecting the tragus of the ear and the C7 spinous process. We followed a previously published protocol for the measurement of the CVA in a neutral, relaxed sitting position [26]. Lateral photographs of each participant were taken with the instructions for them to be seated in a comfortable, relaxed, and neutral position. A tripod, with a mounted digital camera positioned 0.8 m from the sitting participant, was placed perpendicular to the sagittal plane of the participant. The height of the camera was set at the height of each person's seventh cervical vertebra. To identify the tragus of the ear and the 7th cervical spinous process, adhesive markers were fixed on these two landmarks, which then allowed the measurement of the CVA on the photographs. Figure 1 depicts the CVA measurement used with a representative participant with (a) normal head posture and (b) considerable forward head posture (FHP).

2.2.2. Evaluation of Sensorimotor Integration and Somatosensory Processing

Sensorimotor integration and somatosensory processing were assessed using the neurophysiological measured variables, including amplitudes of the following potentials: the peripheral N9; spinal N13; brainstem P14; parietal N20 and P27; and frontal N30. Differences in peak latencies between N13 and N20 were measured as the central conduction time (N13–N20). In order to assess the neurophysiological variables in this study, we used an electromyogram device (Neuropack S1 MEB-9400K, Nihon Koden, Japan). We followed the protocol previously reported in our earlier investigation and repeated key components herein for clarity of understanding [21]. The skin was cleaned, and the stimulating electrodes were placed on the skin overlying the median nerve 2–3 cm superiorly relative to the distal crease of the wrist. We used a bearable, painless stimulus intensity set at 3 times above the sensory level. No participant reported this as noxious or pain-causing [21].

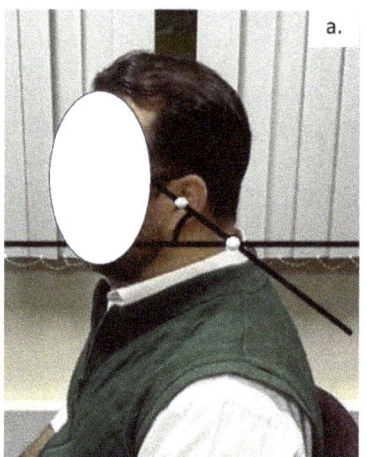 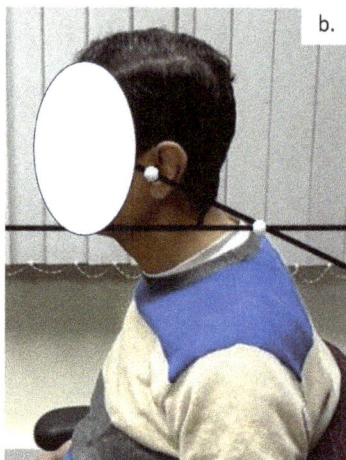

Figure 1. An example of the cranio-vertebral angle (CVA) measurement used with a representative participant with (**a**) normal head posture and (**b**) considerable forward head posture (FHP).

For recording, all somatosensory evoked potential (SEP) recording electrodes (7 mm Ag-AgCl disposable adhesive electrodes from Neurosoft) were placed according to the International Federation of Clinical Neurophysiologists' (IFCN) recommendations [21,27]. Careful attention was paid to cleaning and scarifying the skin before the attachment of the recording electrodes on the scalp. Using an impedance below 5 kΩ, recording electrodes were placed over the ipsilateral Erb's point, superficial to the sixth cervical vertebra spinous process (Cv6). Additional recording electrodes were placed at the frontal and parietal scalp regions contralateral to the side of stimulation at 2 cm posterior to the contralateral central and frontal scalp cites C3/4 and F3/4, which are referred to as Cc′, and Fc′, respectively. Frontal and partial recording electrodes were referenced to the ipsilateral earlobe [27]. The C6 spinous electrode was referenced to the anterior neck (tracheal cartilage). The Erb's point electrode was also referenced to the contralateral shoulder, as SEP components originating from subcortical regions are best recorded with a non-cephalic reference [21,28]. A ground electrode was attached to the forehead FPz. Figure 2 demonstrates this procedural setup.

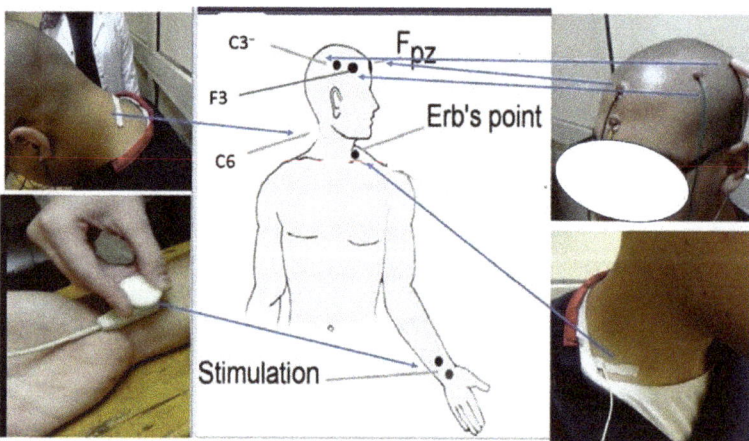

Figure 2. An illustrative example of sensorimotor integration and somatosensory processing measurement.

Our study protocol utilized previously published protocols [29–31]. The band was set between 5 and 1500 Hz, with a time of 100 ms and a bandwidth of 103 µs. Using an electrical square pulse stimulus with a duration of 0.2 ms, a total of 800 sweeps were performed and averaged. We repeated each test a minimum of two times, where the summated tracings were quantified for the amplitude and latency of the potentials [29–31]. The amplitude of the individual SEP components was measured from their peak to the preceding or succeeding trough according to the IFCN guidelines [27]. The following potentials were assessed and recorded:

1. The peripheral N9;
2. The spinal N13 potential to the succeeding positive trough [21,31];
3. The far-field P14–N18 complex [21];
4. The parietal N20 (P14–N20 and N20–P27 complexes) [32];
5. The frontal N30 (P22–N30 complex) [21,33]. The N30 potential reflects the functional connectivity of sensorimotor integration, which includes the thalamus, premotor area, basal ganglia, and primary motor cortex [33–36].

The amplitude of each respective peak represents the degree of activity of its neural structure. Alterations are believed to reflect alterations in the amount of activity of the same assumed neural structures [27]. Peak-to-peak amplitude potentials were measured. We used two different rates to process the different potentials: (1) the slower rate of 2.47 Hz was optimum for N30, while (2) a faster rate of 4.98 Hz was used to quantify the potentials for N13, P14, N20, and P27.

To assess central conduction time (N13–N20), median nerve stimulation at the wrist of each participant was performed and determined [37,38]. Differences in peak latencies between N13 and N20 waves function as a measure of the conduction time along the central and spinal somatosensory pathways. All neurophysiological measures were carried out by a physiotherapist with 20 years of experience in such measurement techniques. All measurements were conducted at the EMG research laboratory, University of Sharjah, UAE.

2.3. Sample Size Determination

We used data from our previous study [21] to estimate the sample size needed to identify differences in somatosensory integration measures between participants with and without FHP. The mean differences and standard deviation of the N30 potential were estimated to be 0.5 and 0.6, respectively, from this study. Accordingly, at least 60 participants per group, given a significance level of 5% and a statistical power of 80%, were needed in the current study [21].

2.4. Data Analysis

The normal distribution of all descriptive baseline variables was determined using the Kolmogorov–Smirnov test, where continuous data are noted as mean with standard deviation (SD) in the text and tables. Equality of variance was assessed with Levene's test, attaining a 95% confidence level, p-value < 0.05. Descriptive statistics (means ± SD unless otherwise stated) are listed at each time point. In order to identify if group equivalence was achieved for proper case-control analysis, a Student's t-test for continuous variables or Chi-squared for categorical variables test was performed for each demographic and clinical variable [21].

The Student's t-test was used to compare the means of continuous variables between the two groups. A p-value of less than 0.05 was considered statistically significant. The effect size was calculated using Cohen's d where d ≈ 0.2 indicates negligible clinical importance, d ≈ 0.5 indicates moderate clinical importance, and d ≈ 0.8 indicates high clinical importance [39]. Correlations (Pearson's r) were used to examine the relationships between the CVA (in the study and control groups) and the measured variables: amplitudes of the peripheral N9; spinal N13; brainstem P14; parietal N20 and P27; frontal N30 potentials; and the central somatosensory conduction time (N13–N20).

A generalized linear model was used to compare the neurophysiological scores between groups, with adjustment for potential confounding variables (educational level, marital status, BMI, and number of working hours per week). Multiple logistic regression models were used to assess the predictors of the neurophysiological outcomes (P14, N20, P27, N30, N13, and N13–N20). SPSS version 20.0 software was used for analyzing data (SPSS Inc., Chicago, IL) with normality and equal variance assumptions ensured before the analysis [21].

3. Results

Initially, 680 potential participants were screened. Neck pain and shoulder pain were the most common reasons for participant exclusion. Sixty participants with FHP (mean age 23.5 years, SD = 2; 35 males, 25 females) and sixty age-, BMI-, and sex-matched controls without FHP were recruited. Figure 3 shows the participant flow chart.

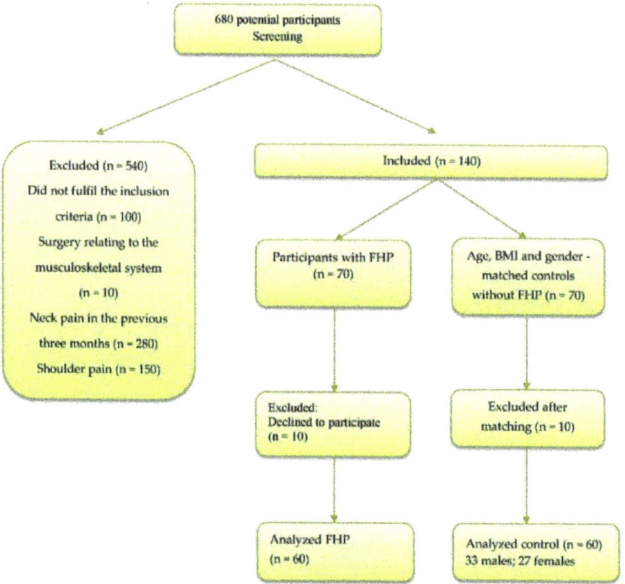

Figure 3. Participants' inclusion and exclusion flow chart.

3.1. Demographic Characteristics of the Participants

Descriptive data for baseline participant demographics are presented in Table 1. No statistically significant differences between the control and the FHP groups were found at baseline in any of their demographic variables; $p > 0.05$. The mean and distribution of craniovertebral angle for both groups are shown in Figure 4.

Table 1. Descriptive data for demographic variables. No statistically significant differences between the control group (CG) and forward head posture (FHP) groups ($p > 0.05$) were found. The independent *t*-test for continuous data and the Chi-squared test of independence for categorical data were used. Values are presented as mean and standard deviation (SD) for age and weight.

Variable	FHP (n = 60)	CG (n = 60)	*p*-Value
Age (years)	23.5 ± 2	25.9 ± 2	0.07
Weight (kg)	67.2 ± 3	69.2 ± 5	0.11

Table 1. *Cont.*

Variable	FHP (n = 60)	CG (n = 60)	*p*-Value
Gender (%)			
Male	35 (58%)	33 (55%)	0.3
Female	25 (42%)	27 (45%)	
Smoking			
Light smoker	18	16	0.2
Heavy smoker	0	0	
No Smoker	42	44	
Educational level			
Bachelor or Master	43	36	<0.005
High school or less	17	24	
Marital status			
Married	32	24	<0.005
Not married	28	36	
BMI			
Normal	45	26	<0.005
Obese	15	34	
Working hours			
Full-time	22	42	<0.005
Part-time	38	18	

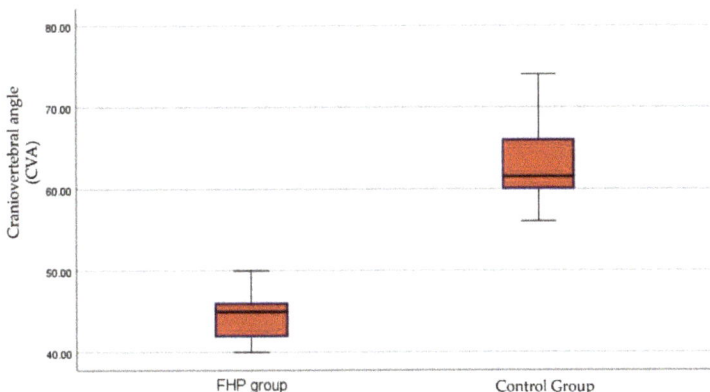

Figure 4. Box and whiskers for craniovertebral angle (CVA) between the forward head posture (FHP) and control groups.

3.2. Between Group Analysis

Statistically significant differences between the FHP and control groups for all measured neurophysiological variables were identified, including amplitude of spinal N13 ($p < 0.005$), brainstem P14 ($p < 0.005$), parietal N20 and P27 ($p < 0.005$), frontal N30 ($p < 0.005$), and N13–N20 interpeak latency as a measure of central conduction time (CCT) ($p = 0.004$). There was no significant difference between groups regarding the amplitudes of the peripheral potential N9 ($p = 0.07$). The effect size (Cohen's d) was moderate for only one variable (N13–N20) and of high clinical significance for the remaining variables. Table 2 and Figure 5 report these data. Figure 6 shows an example of the frontal, parietal, and cervical somatosensory findings for a representative participant with (a) normal head posture and (b) considerable forward head posture (FHP).

Table 2. Differences between the forward head posture group (FHP) and control group (CG) for each outcome measure of the DSSEPs for sensorimotor integration assessment. The amplitudes of the following potentials are reported: peripheral potential N9; spinal N13; brainstem P14; parietal N20 and P27; and frontal N30. Differences in peak latencies between N13 and N20 were measured as central conduction time (N13–N20). CI = confidence interval. (A) is a generalized linear model with adjustment for potential confounding variables, including educational level, marital status, BMI, and number of working hours per week.

Neurophysiological Outcome Measure	FHP Group	Control Group	Mean Difference between the Two Groups	(95% CI)/ Cohen's d	p Value	p Value (A)
N9	1.8 ± 0.2	1.7 ± 0.34	0.1	[0.07, 0.21]/0.1	=0.07	0.6
P14	1.67 ± 0.6	1.3 ± 0.63	0.37	[0.25, 0.49]/0.77	<0.005	0.02
N20	2.61 ± 0.61	2.1 ± 0.52	0.51	[0.33, 0.6]/0.9	<0.005	<0.005
P27	3.2 ± 0.7	2.7 ± 0.5	0.5	[0.41, 0.69]/0.8	<0.005	0.04
N30	2.91 ± 0.64	2.4 ± 0.58	0.51	[0.359, 0.69]/2.45	<0.005	0.003
N13	2 ± 0.5	1.6 ± 0.45	0.4	[0.11, 0.35]/0.8	<0.005	0.004
N13–N20	1.77 ± 0.46	1.5 ± 0.51	0.27	[0.07, 0.51]/0.56	=0.004	<0.005

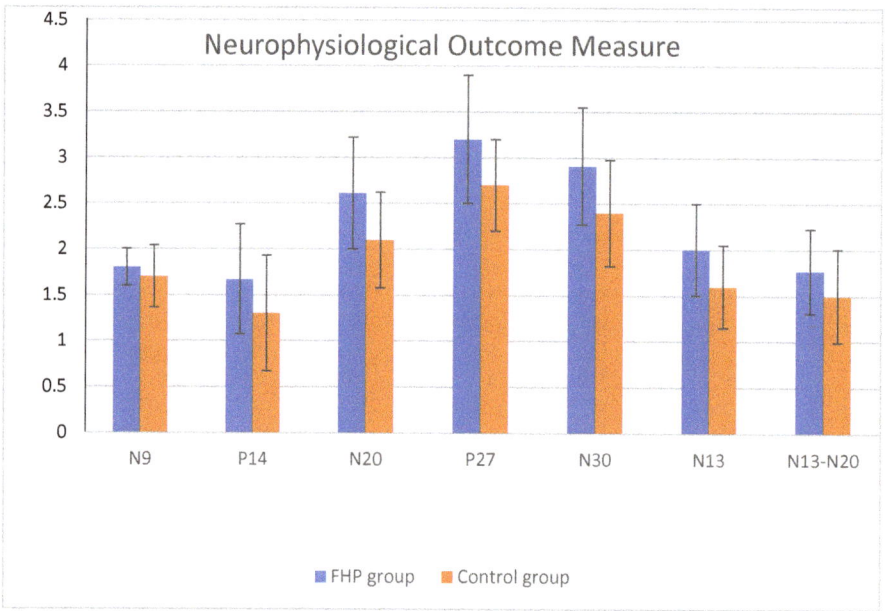

Figure 5. Neurophysiological outcomes for both groups. FHP = forward head posture and Control group = normal head posture group as measured with the CVA. Statistically significant differences between the FHP and control groups for all measured neurophysiological variables were identified, including amplitudes of spinal N13 ($p < 0.005$), brainstem P14 ($p < 0.005$), parietal N20 and P27 ($p < 0.005$), frontal N30 ($p < 0.005$), and N13–N20 interpeak latency as measures of central conduction time (CCT) ($p = 0.004$). There was no significant difference between both groups regarding the amplitudes of the peripheral potential N9 ($p = 0.07$).

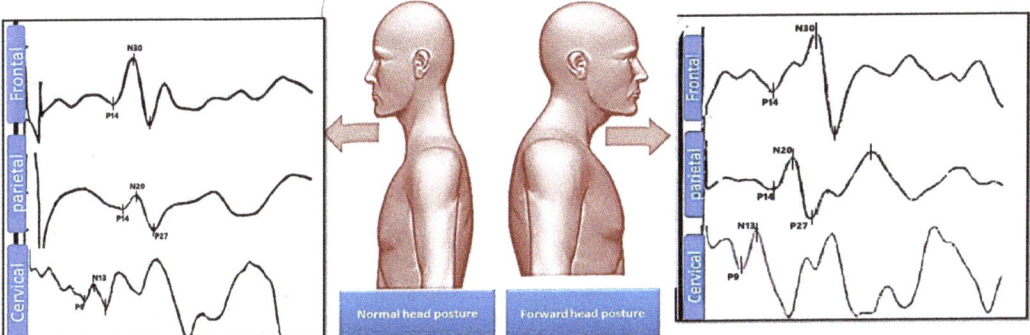

Figure 6. Shown is an example of the frontal N30, parietal N20 and P27, and cervical spinal N13 somatosensory findings for a representative participant with normal head posture on the left side and with considerable forward head posture (FHP) on the right side.

3.3. Correlation of Findings between Groups

For correlation findings, significant negative correlations were identified between the amount of CVA and the measured neurophysiological variables in both groups. Specific to the FHP group the correlations were: amplitudes of the peripheral N9 (r = −0.44, $p < 0.001$); spinal N13 (r = −0.67, $p < 0.001$); brainstem P14 (r = −0.58, $p < 0.001$); parietal N20 (r = −0.49, $p = 0.001$); P27 (r = −0.58, $p < 0.001$); frontal N30 potentials (r = −0.64, $p < 0.001$); and for central conduction time the correlation was N13–N20 (r = −0.61, $p < 0.001$). Table 3 reports these data.

Table 3. Correlations (Pearson's *r*) were used to examine the relationships between the cranial vertebral angle (CVA) in the forward head posture (FHP) group and control group (CG) and the following variables measured: amplitudes of peripheral potential N9; spinal N13; brainstem P14; parietal N20 and P27; and frontal N30 potentials; and central somatosensory conduction time (N13–N20).

Correlation	CVA FHP r (*p*-Value)	CVA CG r (*p*-Value)
N9	−0.44 <0.001	−0.5 <0.001
N13	−0.67 <0.001	−0.54 <0.001
P14	−0.58 <0.001	−0.57 <0.001
N20	−0.49 <0.001	−0.51 <0.001
P27	−0.58 <0.001	−0.6 <0.001
N30	−0.64 <0.001	−0.61 <0.001
N13–N20	−0.61 <0.001	−0.56 <0.001

3.4. Logistic Regession Modelling

Working hours and the CVA angle measures significantly affected the neurophysiological outcomes. Full-time work significantly increased the odds of having a higher amplitude of the neurophysiological potentials and slower N13–N20 conduction time when compared with part-time work; $p < 0.005$. Additionally, each 1-degree increase in the CVA measurement significantly decreased the amplitudes of all the potentials and resulted in a faster, more efficient N13–N20 conduction time; $p < 0.005$. Table 4 reports these data.

Table 4. Logistic regression models showing the predictors of the neurophysiological outcomes.

Predictors	P14 Odds ratios (p-value)	N20 Odds ratios (p-value)	P27 Odds ratios (p-value)	N30 Odds ratios (p-value)	N13 Odds ratios (p-value)	N13–N20 Odds ratios (p-value)
BMI (Obesity)	0.4 / 0.06	0.23 / 0.06	0.13 / 0.3	0.16 / 0.34	0.2 / 0.06	0.2 / 0.06
Educational level (Bachelor or Master)	1.2 / 0.4	3.2 / 0.08	2.3 / 0.3	1.2 / 0.4	2.4 / 0.32	1.5 / 0.42
Marital status (Not married)	1.54 / 0.2	1.54 / 0.2	1.3 / 0.3	1.3 / 0.3	1.5 / 0.2	1.8 / 0.09
Weekly working hours (Full-time)	13.1 / <0.005	12.4 / <0.005	19.5 / <0.005	25.9 / <0.005	28 / <0.005	19.4 / <0.005
CVA	0.41 / <0.005	0.3 / <0.005	0.3 / <0.005	0.57 / <0.005	0.23 / <0.005	0.34 / <0.005

4. Discussion

Using somatosensory evoked potentials, we investigated possible differences in sensorimotor integration and somatosensory processing variables between asymptomatic young adults with FHP and a control group with normal head posture. Our findings indicated that forward head posture, as measured with the CVA, has an impact on sensorimotor integration and somatosensory processing parameters. These findings confirmed our study's hypotheses. We believe this is the first investigation to provide clear evidence that the amount of FHP alignment influences these specific neurophysiological measures in asymptomatic persons. In our between-group analysis, the only non-significant finding (small effect size) was for N9, which reflects the peripheral nerve volley at the axilla. This finding ruled out peripheral nerve entrapment as a possible cause of any change. Using generalized linear modeling with adjustment for confounding variables, working hours per week and the CVA magnitude were found to affect the neurophysiological outcomes significantly. Surprisingly, full-time work was found to increase the odds of having a higher amplitude of the neurophysiological potentials and slower N13–N20 conduction time when compared with part-time work, indicating an adverse effect on somatosensory processing variables herein. In contrast, each 1-degree increase in the CVA measurement (indicating better posture) significantly decreased the amplitudes of all the potentials and resulted in a faster, more efficient N13–N20 conduction time.

4.1. Cortical, Subcortical, and Spinal Neural Changes

We identified sensorimotor integration differences and somatosensory processing changes between both groups occurring in different regions of the spinal and cortical regions. Previous investigations have identified results that are generally consistent with our findings [34–36,40,41]. Likewise, previous research using symptomatic populations has found that a general abnormal afferentation process is responsible for spinal, cortical, and subcortical reorganization [29,30]. Thus, reorganization of the somatosensory system is primarily driven by alterations to or modifications of sensory input, which, in turn, alters sensorimotor integration and generalized somatosensory processing [11–13,42].

The idea that increased and abnormal FHP is a primary mechanism having the ability to alter afferent input leading to disturbances in the sensorimotor and somatosensory processing system, is not without evidence. Sagittal plane cervical biomechanics studies have identified that tissue component (muscle, tendon, disc, bone) stress and strain are increased due to increasing FHP [17,18]. Further, it is known that as FHP increases, there is an influence on altered joint position, kinematics, and dysfunction that may lead to abnormal neurophysiologic afferent information (so-called dysafferentation). Furthermore, studies suggest that increased FHP may result in increased physical demands, resulting in premature and accelerated degenerative changes in the muscles, ligaments, bone, and neural tissues [5,43,44]. Additionally, abnormal head posture is associated with both a reduced range of movement and an altered segmental cervical spine kinematic pattern. Thus, non-neutral sagittal cervical spine alignment could potentially *lead to* altered sensorimotor integration through an altered afferent input from abnormal cervical spine movements, a change in the muscle-tendon length-tension relationships, and altered spine tissue load sharing [16–22]. This would seem to explain the findings of Moustafa et al. [21], where collegiate athletes with considerable FHP compared to a control group without FHP were found to be less efficient in athletic skill tests in both static and dynamic situations.

4.2. Central Somatosensory Conduction Time

The finding of a faster (more efficient) central condition time in the participants with normal head posture (control group) is likely multi-factorial in nature but may be largely explained by two mechanical phenomena: (1) FHP likely increases longitudinal stress and strain in the spinal cord tissues and (2) increased FHP alters and influences respiratory function. Regarding the former, spinal cord biomechanics, it is expected that participants without FHP or more normal posture alignment also have a more normal (deeper) cervical lordosis [5,45]. A proper cervical lordosis and reduced FHP have been found to reduce stress and strain on the spinal cord, brainstem, nerve roots, and cranial nerves 5–12 in both surgical and non-surgical rehabilitation investigations [4,5,46–49]. Furthermore, more normal FHP is linearly correlated with an increased overall cervical range of motion [16] because it is known that neural axoplasm has thixotropic properties [50]. It seems logical, therefore, that an increased viscosity (driven by impaired motion and increased spinal cord or neural strain) could alter neuronal transport mechanisms.

Likewise, FHP may act to reduce respiratory functions of both inspiration and expiration volume and strength, and thus, the maintenance of a more neutral sagittal head posture is required to prevent these positional respiratory function reductions [51,52]. Furthermore, since abnormal sagittal plane postures cause an increase in stress and strain on both neural and vascular tissues in the cervical spine [46,47], and it is known that neuronal tissues are highly oxygen-energy dependent [53], it is probable that increased neural strain coupled with reductions in respiratory efficiency may be a mechanism subtly impacting oxygenation to the spinal cord, nerve roots, and cerebral areas, leading to the alteration in the sensorimotor integration disturbances identified in our study. Supporting these assertions, there is evidence of an alteration in vertebral artery hemodynamics and cerebral blood flow intensity on MRA due to alterations in sagittal cervical alignment [54,55].

4.3. Clinical Implications

While the observed differences in our neurophysiological data in terms of actual numerical differences can be arbitrary and should not be construed as rigorous in isolation, relating Cohen's d between our two groups (as in Table 3) to other existing reports in the literature offers context to the meaning or implications of our findings. Of interest, the mean difference and effect sizes for central somatosensory conduction time (N13–N20), sensorimotor integration (N30 potential), and somatosensory processing potentials (spinal N13, brainstem P14, parietal N20 and P27) found in the current study are very similar to the mean differences and effect sizes reported in a previous experimental study [56]. In relation to clinical interpretation, it is thought that alterations in normal afferentation may influence the processing of neural networks located in cortical motor areas and, in turn, impact motor control [14,15]. In support of this concept, it has been identified that collegiate athletes with increased FHP exhibited altered sensorimotor processing, integration, and concomitantly. They were found to have less efficient athletic performance compared to athletes with normal sagittal head posture alignment [21]. Furthermore, a recent randomized trial demonstrated that structural rehabilitation (correction of abnormal alignment) of the sagittal cervical spine allowed for more efficient responses in several sensorimotor control outcome measurements (balance, oculomotor control, head repositioning error) [57]. Since it has been reported that central condition time (N13–N20) and the amplitude of sensorimotor integration (N30) are linearly related to the amount of improvement in FHP and cervical lordosis following an intervention [56], it seems probable that restoration of the sagittal cervical alignment is a primary mechanism for improving the somatosensory system and sensorimotor integration regions, yielding improved sensorimotor control and more efficient motor control output in general. Future studies, however, are needed to clarify this and identify precisely which, if any, specific motor control outcome variables are dependent on and influenced by improved sagittal cervical alignment.

4.4. Limitations

By using a matched design, we attempted to adjust for potential confounding characteristics, such as age, sex, BMI, smoking status, marital status, education, and weekly work hours. However, as with any observational study, residual confounding factors, such as the length of the participant's neck, may exist. N13 is measured from the back of the C6 spinous process and N20 from the scalp. Thus, the latency of the N20 versus the latency of the N13 may be influenced by the length of the neck and the size of the scalp/brain. However, our participant groups were matched for sex and size, so it seems unlikely that neck length would be a significant source of confounding in our populations. Further, any differences in the length of the neck in our two matched groups are likely due to the forward head posture effects on cervical spine kinematics, thus, strengthening our study results [17–19]. Still, we recommend that future studies adjust the interpeak latencies to each participant's neck length.

Additionally, we did not control for certain lifestyle factors, such as physical activity (exercise), and we did not assess the stress or anxiety level experienced by participants, which can affect neural function. Our investigation focused on an asymptomatic population of younger adults; therefore, participants of varying ages and with specific musculo-skeletal disorders should be included in future studies. A further limitation is our method of FHP measurement in that although the CVA is both a reliable and valid quantification method for external FHP [23], the CVA cannot describe the shape and magnitude of the cervical lordotic curve on spine radiographs [45]. Future investigations should use imaging (spine radiographs, MRI, CT) to identify the role that actual vertebral alignment plays in altering sensorimotor integration and somatosensory processing systems. Additionally, we recommend the assessment of patients before and after cervical spine surgical interventions for spine disorders to identify if reductions in FHP to the recommended surgical cutoff values (radiographic FHP < 40 mm) have an effect on improving central conduction time (N13–N20) [5]. Finally, there are several other measurements that represent the sagittal alignment of the head and neck, such as the sagittal head tilt (flexion/extension), sagittal shoulder-C7 angle (protraction/retraction) [58], and these may influence the neurophysiological measures of sensorimotor integration and somatosensory processing. Future investigations should look at more comprehensive measurements of sagittal cervical spine posture in order to confirm, add to, or refute the findings of the current investigation.

4.5. Conclusions

Using a matched case-control design in asymptomatic young adults, we identified that forward head posture is associated with differences in central conduction time, sensorimotor integration, and somatosensory processing amplitudes at different neural regions. Full-time work increased the odds of having a higher amplitude of neurophysiological potentials and slower N13–N20 conduction time. Additionally, increases in the CVA (less forward head posture) were found to decrease the amplitudes of somatosensory processing potentials and resulted in a faster N13–N20 conduction time.

Author Contributions: I.M.M., A.A.M.D. and D.E.H. conceived the research idea and participated in its design. I.M.M., A.A.M.D. and D.E.H. contributed to the statistical analysis. I.M.M. and A.A.M.D. participated in data collection and study supervision. I.M.M., A.A.M.D. and D.E.H. contributed to the interpretation of the results and wrote the drafts. All authors have read and agreed to the published version of the manuscript.

Funding: CBP Nonprofit (Eagle, ID, USA) approved the funding of this manuscript for publication fees in the JCM. Deed Harrison's role as a senior author and conflicts of interest are outlined below.

Institutional Review Board Statement: The research was conducted in accordance with the senior citizen's services department and approved by the Research Institute of Medical & Health Sciences of the University of Sharjah (reference number: REC-21-03-11-03-S).

Informed Consent Statement: All participant's pictures in the study were included after written informed consent was signed and obtained.

Data Availability Statement: The datasets analyzed in the current study are available from the corresponding author upon reasonable request.

Conflicts of Interest: DEH teaches rehabilitation methods and is the CEO of a company that distributes products to physicians in the U.S.A. used for the rehabilitation of postural abnormalities. All the other authors declare that they have no competing interests.

References

1. Machado, S.; Cunha, M.; Velasques, B.; Minc, D.; Teixeira, S.; Domingues, C.A.; Silva, J.G.; Bastos, V.H.; Budde, H.; Cagy, M.; et al. Sensorimotor integration: Basic concepts, abnormalities related to movement disorders and sensorimotor training-induced cortical reorganization. *Rev. Neurol.* **2010**, *51*, 427–436. [PubMed]
2. Machado, D.; Bastos, V.H.; Cunha, M.; Velasques, B.; Machado, S.; Basile, L.; Cagy, M.; Piedade, R.; Ribeiro, P. Efectos del bromacepam en el desarrollo de una actividad sensoriomotora: Un estudio electroencefalográfico. *Rev. Neurol.* **2009**, *49*, 295–299. [PubMed]
3. Krakauer, J.W.; Mazzoni, P.; Ghazizadeh, A.; Ravindran, R.; Shadmehr, R. Generalization of Motor Learning Depends on the History of Prior Action. *PLoS Biol.* **2006**, *4*, e316. [CrossRef] [PubMed]
4. Grosso, M.J.; Hwang, R.; Mroz, T.; Benzel, E.; Steinmetz, M.P. Relationship between degree of focal kyphosis correction and neurological outcomes for patients undergoing cervical deformity correction surgery. *J. Neurosurg. Spine* **2013**, *18*, 537–544. [CrossRef]
5. Smith, J.S.; Lafage, V.; Ryan, D.J.; Shaffrey, C.I.; Schwab, F.J.; Patel, A.A.; Brodke, D.S.; Arnold, P.M.; Riew, K.D.; Traynelis, V.C.; et al. Association of Myelopathy Scores With Cervical Sagittal Balance and Normalized Spinal Cord Volume. *Spine* **2013**, *38* (Suppl. 1), S161–S170. [CrossRef]
6. Flor, H. The modification of cortical reorganization and chronic pain by sensory feedback. *Appl. Psychophysiol. Biofeedback* **2002**, *27*, 215–227. [CrossRef]
7. Mercier, C.; Léonard, G. Interactions between Pain and the Motor Cortex: Insights from Research on Phantom Limb Pain and Complex Regional Pain Syndrome. *Physiother. Can.* **2011**, *63*, 305–314. [CrossRef]
8. Bank, P.J.M.; Peper, C.E.; Marinus, J.; Beek, P.J.; van Hilten, J.J. Motor consequences of experimentally induced limb pain: A systematic review. *Eur. J. Pain.* **2013**, *17*, 145–157. [CrossRef]
9. Bowering, K.J.; O'Connell, N.; Tabor, A.; Catley, M.; Leake, H.B.; Moseley, L.; Stanton, T. The Effects of Graded Motor Imagery and Its Components on Chronic Pain: A Systematic Review and Meta-Analysis. *J. Pain.* **2013**, *14*, 3–13. [CrossRef]
10. Moseley, L.G. Graded motor imagery is effective for long-standing complex regional pain syndrome: A randomised controlled trial. *Pain* **2004**, *108*, 192–198. [CrossRef]
11. Daligadu, J.; Haavik, H.; Yielder, P.C.; Baarbe, J.; Murphy, B. Alterations in Cortical and Cerebellar Motor Processing in Subclinical Neck Pain Patients Following Spinal Manipulation. *J. Manip. Physiol. Ther.* **2013**, *36*, 527–537. [CrossRef]
12. Haavik-Taylor, H.; Murphy, B. Cervical spine manipulation alters sensorimotor integration: A somatosensory evoked potential study. *Clin. Neurophysiol.* **2007**, *118*, 391–402. [CrossRef]
13. Taylor, H.H.; Murphy, B. Altered Sensorimotor Integration With Cervical Spine Manipulation. *J. Manip. Physiol. Ther.* **2008**, *31*, 115–126. [CrossRef]
14. Hishinuma, M.; Yamaguchi, T. Axonal projection of descending pathways responsible for eliciting forelimb stepping into the cat cervical spinal cord. *Exp. Brain Res.* **1990**, *82*, 597–605. [CrossRef]
15. Knight, R.T.; Staines, W.R.; Swick, D.; Chao, L.L. Prefrontal cortex regulates inhibition and excitation in distributed neural networks. *Acta Psychol.* **1999**, *101*, 159–178. [CrossRef]
16. Fernandez-de-las-Penas, C.; Alonso-Blanco, C.; Cuadrado, M.L.; Pareja, J.A. Forward head posture and neck mobility in chronic tension-type headache: A blinded, controlled study. *Cephalgia* **2006**, *26*, 314–319. [CrossRef]

17. Patwardhan AGKhayatzadeh, S.; Havey, R.M.; Voronov, L.I.; Smith, Z.A.; Kalmanson, O.; Ghanayem, A.J.; Sears, W. Cervical sagittal balance: A biomechanical perspecive can help clinical practice. *Eur. Spine J.* **2018**, *27* (Suppl. 1), 25–28. [CrossRef]
18. Khayatzadey, S.; Kalmanson, O.A.; Schuit, D.; Havey, R.M.; Voronov, L.I.; Ghanayem, A.J.; Patwardhan, A.G. Cervical Spine Muscle-Tendon Unit Length Differences between Neutral and Forward Head Postures: Biomechanical Study Using Human Cadaveric Specimens. *Phys. Ther.* **2017**, *97*, 756–766. [CrossRef]
19. Mousavi-Khatir, R.; Talebian, S.; Toosizadeh, N.; Olyaei, G.R.; Maroufi, N. Disturbance of neck proprioception and feed-forward motor control following static neck flexion in healthy young adults. *J. Electromyogr. Kinesiol.* **2018**, *41*, 160–167. [CrossRef]
20. Nese, G.Y.; Yasemin, E. Diagnostic value of the F-wave in loss of the cervical lordosis. *Neurophysiology* **2020**, *52*, 192–197. [CrossRef]
21. Moustafa, I.; Kim, M.; Harrison, D.E. Comparison of Sensorimotor Integration and Skill-Related Physical Fitness Components Between College Athletes with and Without Forward Head Posture. *J. Sport. Rehabil.* **2022**, *32*, 53–62. [CrossRef] [PubMed]
22. Moustafa, I.M.; Youssef, A.; Ahbouch, A.; Tamim, M.; Harrison, D.E. Is forward head posture relevant to autonomic nervous system function and cervical sensorimotor control? Cross sectional study. *Gait Posture* **2020**, *77*, 29–35. [CrossRef] [PubMed]
23. Yip, C.H.T.; Chiu, T.T.W.; Poon, A.T.K. The relationship between head posture and severity and disability of patients with neck pain. *Man. Ther.* **2008**, *13*, 148–154. [CrossRef] [PubMed]
24. Rossi, S.; della Volpe, R.; Ginanneschi, F.; Ulivelli, M.; Bartolini, S.; Spidalieri, R.; Rossi, A. Early somatosensory processing during tonic muscle pain in humans: Relation to loss of proprioception and motor 'defensive' strategies. *Clin. Neurophysiol.* **2003**, *114*, 1351–1358. [CrossRef] [PubMed]
25. Van Niekerk, S.M.; Louw, Q.; Vaughan, C.; Grimmer-Somers, K.; Schreve, K. Photographic measurement of upper-body sitting posture of high school students: A reliability and validity study. *BMC Musculoskelet. Disord.* **2008**, *9*, 113. [CrossRef] [PubMed]
26. Falla, D.; Jull, G.; Russell, T.; Vicenzino, B.; Hodges, P. Effect of Neck Exercise on Sitting Posture in Patients With Chronic Neck Pain. *Phys. Ther.* **2007**, *87*, 408–417. [CrossRef]
27. Mauguière, F.; Allison, T.; Babiloni, C.; Buchner, H.; Eisen, A.A.; Goodin, D.S.; Jones, S.J.; Kakigi, R.; Matsuoka, S.; Nuwer, M.; et al. Somatosensory evoked potentials. The International Federation of Clinical Neurophysiology. *Electroencephalogr. Clin. Neurophysiol. Suppl.* **1999**, *52*, 79–90.
28. Ulas, U.H.; Özdag, F.; Eroglu, E.; Odabasi, Z.; Kutukcu, Y.; Demirkaya, S.; Gökçil, Z.; Hamamcioglu, K.; Vural, O. Median Nerve Somatosensory Evoked Potentials Recorded with Cephalic and Noncephalic References in Central and Peripheral Nervous System Lesions. *Clin. EEG Neurosci.* **2001**, *32*, 191–196. [CrossRef]
29. Tinazzi, M.; Priori, A.; Bertolasi, L.; Frasson, E.; Mauguière, F.; Fiaschi, A. Abnormal central integration of a dual somatosensory input in dystonia. Evidence for sensory overflow. *Brain* **2000**, *123*, 42–50. [CrossRef]
30. Tinazzi, M.; Fiaschi, A.; Rosso, T.; Faccioli, F.; Grosslercher, J.; Aglioti, S.M. Neuroplastic Changes Related to Pain Occur at Multiple Levels of the Human Somatosensory System: A Somatosensory-Evoked Potentials Study in Patients with Cervical Radicular Pain. *J. Neurosci.* **2000**, *20*, 9277–9283. [CrossRef]
31. Desmedt, J.E.; Cheron, G. Prevertebral (oesophageal) recording of subcortical somatosensory evoked potentials in man: The spinal P13 component and the dual nature of the spinal generators. *Electroencephalogr. Clin. Neurophysiol.* **1981**, *52*, 257–275. [CrossRef]
32. Allison, T.; McCarthy, G.; Wood, C.C.; Jones, S.J. Potentials evoked in human and monkey cerebral cortex by stimulation of the median nerve. A review of scalp and intracranial recordings. *Brain* **1991**, *114*, 2465–2503. [CrossRef]
33. Mauguière, F.; Desmedt, J.E.; Courjon, J. Astereognosis and dissociated loss of frontal or parietal components of somatosensory evoked potentials in hemispheric lesions. Detailed correlations with clinical signs and computerized tomographic scanning. *Brain* **1983**, *106 Pt 2*, 271–311. [CrossRef]
34. Andrew, D.; Haavik, H.; Dancey, E.; Yielder, P.; Murphy, B. Somatosensory evoked potentials show plastic changes following a novel motor training task with the thumb. *Clin. Neurophysiol.* **2015**, *126*, 575–580. [CrossRef]
35. Cebolla, A.M.; Palmero-Soler, E.; Dan, B.; Cheron, G. Frontal phasic and oscillatory generators of the N30 somatosensory evoked potential. *Neuroimage* **2011**, *54*, 1297–1306. [CrossRef]
36. Zabihhosseinian, M.; Yielder, P.; Wise, M.; Holmes, M.; Murphy, B. Effect of Neck Muscle Fatigue on Hand Muscle Motor Performance and Early Somatosensory Evoked Potentials. *Brain Sci.* **2021**, *11*, 1481. [CrossRef]
37. Mochizuki, H.; Yagi, K.; Tsuruta, K.; Taniguchi, A.; Ishii, N.; Shiomi, K.; Nakazato, M. Prolonged central sensory conduction time in patients with chronic arsenic exposure. *J. Neurol. Sci.* **2016**, *361*, 39–42. [CrossRef]
38. Bouwes, A.; Doesborg, P.G.G.; Laman, D.M.; Koelman, J.H.T.M.; Imanse, J.G.; Tromp, S.C.; van Geel, B.M.; van der Kooi, E.L.; Zandbergen, E.G.J.; Horn, J. Hypothermia after CPR prolongs conduction times of somatosensory evoked potentials. *Neurocrit Care* **2013**, *19*, 25–30. [CrossRef]
39. Cohen, J. Some statistical issues in psychological research. In *Handbook of Clinical Psychology*; Wolman, B.B., Ed.; McGraw-Hill: New York, NY, USA, 1965; pp. 95–121.
40. Parker, J.L.; Dostrovsky, J.O. Cortical involvement in the induction, but not expression, of thalamic plasticity. *J. Neurosci.* **1999**, *19*, 8623–8629. [CrossRef]
41. Florence, S.L.; Hackett, T.A.; Strata, F. Thalamic and cortical contributions to neural plasticity after limb amputation. *J. Neurophysiol.* **2000**, *83*, 3154–3159. [CrossRef]
42. Taylor, H.H.; Murphy, B. Altered Central Integration of Dual Somatosensory Input After Cervical Spine Manipulation. *J. Manip. Physiol. Ther.* **2010**, *33*, 178–188. [CrossRef] [PubMed]

43. Harrison, D.E.; Jones, E.W.; Janik, T.J.; Harrison, D.D. Evaluation of axial and flexural stresses in the vertebral body cortex and trabecular bone in lordosis and two sagittal cervical translation configurations with an elliptical shell model. *J. Manip. Physiol. Ther.* **2002**, *25*, 391–401. [CrossRef] [PubMed]
44. Thoomes, E.J.; Scholten-Peeters, W.; Koes, B.; Falla, D.; Verhagen, A.P. The effectiveness of conservative treatment for patients with cervical radiculopathy: A systematic review. *Clin. J. Pain.* **2013**, *29*, 1073–1086. [CrossRef] [PubMed]
45. Sun, A.; Yeo, H.G.; Kim, T.U.; Hyun, J.K.; Kim, J.Y. Radiologic assessment of forward head posture and its relation to myofascial pain syndrome. *Ann. Rehabil. Med.* **2014**, *38*, 821–826. [CrossRef]
46. Harrison, D.D.E.; Cailliet, R.; Harrison, D.D.E.; Troyanovich, S.J.; Harrison, S.O. A review of biomechanics of the central nervous system–part II: Spinal cord strains from postural loads. *J. Manip. Physiol. Ther.* **1999**, *22*, 322–332. [CrossRef]
47. Breig, A. *Adverse Mechanical Tension in the Central Nervous System: An Analysis of Cause and Effect: Relief by Functional Neurosurgery*; Wiley: New York, NY, USA, 1978; 130p.
48. Moustafa, I.M.; Diab, A.A. The effect of adding forward head posture corrective exercises in the management of lumbosacral radiculopathy: A randomized controlled study. *J. Manip. Physiol. Ther.* **2015**, *38*, 167–178. [CrossRef]
49. Diab, A.A.; Moustafa, I.M. The efficacy of forward head correction on nerve root function and pain in cervical spondylotic radiculopathy: A randomized trial. *Clin. Rehab* **2012**, *26*, 351–361. [CrossRef]
50. Baker, P.F.; Ladds, M.; Rubinson, K.A. Measurement of the flow properties of isolated axoplasm in a defined chemical environment. *J. Physiol.* **1977**, *269*, 10P–11P.
51. Kim, M.S.; Cha, Y.J.; Choi, J.D. Correlation between forward head posture, respiratory functions, and respiratory accessory muscles in young adults. *J. Back. Musculoskelet. Rehabil.* **2017**, *30*, 711–715. [CrossRef]
52. Zafar, H.; Albarrati, A.; Alghadir, A.H.; Iqbal, Z.A. Effect of different head-nec postures on the respiratory function in healthy males. *Biomed. Res. Int.* **2018**, *2018*, 4518269. [CrossRef]
53. McCormick, P.C.; Stein, B.M. Functional anatomy of the spinal cord and related structures. *Neurosurg. Clin. N. Am.* **1990**, *1*, 469–489. [CrossRef]
54. Bulut, M.D.; Alpayci, M.; Şenköy, E.; Bora, A.; Yazmalar, L.; Yavuz, A.; Gülşen, I. Decreased Vertebral Artery Hemodynamics in Patients with Loss of Cervical Lordosis. *Med. Sci. Monit.* **2016**, *22*, 495–500. [CrossRef]
55. Katz, E.; Katz, S.; Fedorchuk, C.; Lightstone, D.; Banach, C.; Podoll, J. Increase in cerebral blood flow indicated by increased cerebral arterial area and pixel intensity on brain magnetic resonance angiogram following correction of cervical lordosis. *Brain Circ.* **2019**, *5*, 19. [CrossRef]
56. Moustafa, I.M.; Diab, A.A.; Hegazy, F.; Harrison, D.E. Demonstration of central conduction time and neuroplastic changes after cervical lordosis rehabilitation in asymptomatic subjects: A randomized, placebo-controlled trial. *Sci. Rep.* **2021**, *11*, 15379. [CrossRef]
57. Moustafa, I.; Youssef, A.S.A.; Ahbouch, A.; Harrison, D. Demonstration of Autonomic Nervous Function and Cervical Sensorimotor Control After Cervical Lordosis Rehabilitation: A Randomized Controlled Trial. *J. Athl. Train.* **2021**, *56*, 427–436. [CrossRef]
58. Singla, D.; Veqar, Z.; Hussain, M.E. Photogrammetric Assessment of Upper Body Posture Using Postural Angles: A Literature Review. *J. Chiropr. Med.* **2017**, *16*, 131–138. [CrossRef]

Disclaimer/Publisher's Note: The statements, opinions and data contained in all publications are solely those of the individual author(s) and contributor(s) and not of MDPI and/or the editor(s). MDPI and/or the editor(s) disclaim responsibility for any injury to people or property resulting from any ideas, methods, instructions or products referred to in the content.

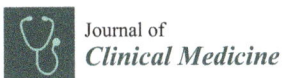

Article

Alterations in Cervical Nerve Root Function during Different Sitting Positions in Adults with and without Forward Head Posture: A Cross-Sectional Study

Maryam Kamel [1], Ibrahim M. Moustafa [1,2], Meeyoung Kim [1], Paul A. Oakley [3,4,5] and Deed E. Harrison [3,*]

1. Department of Physiotherapy, College of Health Sciences, University of Sharjah, Sharjah 27272, United Arab Emirates
2. Neuromusculoskeletal Rehabilitation Research Group, Research Institute of Medical and Health Sciences, University of Sharjah, Sharjah 27272, United Arab Emirates
3. CBP Nonprofit (A Spine Research Foundation), Eagle, ID 83616, USA
4. Independent Researcher, Newmarket, ON L3Y 8Y8, Canada
5. Kinesiology and Health Sciences, York University, Toronto, ON M3J 1P3, Canada
* Correspondence: drdeed@idealspine.com or drdeedharrison@gmail.com

Citation: Kamel, M.; Moustafa, I.M.; Kim, M.; Oakley, P.A.; Harrison, D.E. Alterations in Cervical Nerve Root Function during Different Sitting Positions in Adults with and without Forward Head Posture: A Cross-Sectional Study. *J. Clin. Med.* **2023**, *12*, 1780. https://doi.org/10.3390/jcm12051780

Academic Editor: Nada Andelic

Received: 21 January 2023
Revised: 12 February 2023
Accepted: 20 February 2023
Published: 23 February 2023

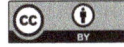

Copyright: © 2023 by the authors. Licensee MDPI, Basel, Switzerland. This article is an open access article distributed under the terms and conditions of the Creative Commons Attribution (CC BY) license (https:// creativecommons.org/licenses/by/ 4.0/).

Abstract: The current study aimed to determine whether participants with and without forward head posture (FHP) would respond differently in cervical nerve root function to various sitting positions. We measured peak-to-peak dermatomal somatosensory-evoked potentials (DSSEPs) in 30 participants with FHP and in 30 participants matched for age, sex, and body mass index (BMI) with normal head posture (NHP), defined as having a craniovertebral angle (CVA) >55°. Additional inclusion criteria for recruitment were individuals between the ages of 18 and 28 who were in good health and had no musculoskeletal pain. All 60 participants underwent C6, C7, and C8 DSSEPs evaluation. The measurements were taken in three positions: erect sitting, slouched sitting, and supine. We identified statistically significant differences in the cervical nerve root function in all postures between the NHP and FHP groups ($p < 0.001$), indicating that the FHP and NHP reacted differently in different positions. No significant differences between groups for the DSSEPs were identified for the supine position ($p > 0.05$), in contrast to the erect and slouched sitting positions, which showed a significant difference in nerve root function between the NHP and FHP ($p < 0.001$). The NHP group results were consistent with the prior literature and had the greatest DSSEP peaks when in the upright position. However, the participants in the FHP group demonstrated the largest peak-to-peak amplitude of DSSEPs while in the slouched position as opposed to an erect position. The optimal sitting posture for cervical nerve root function may be dependent upon the underlying CVA of a person, however, further research is needed to corroborate these findings.

Keywords: sitting; cervical spine; posture; evoked potentials; radiculopathy

1. Introduction

Sustained sitting postures and the related load on the cervical spine are important contributors to the high prevalence of neck pain [1]. Prolonged hours of sitting have shown a large incidence of pain in the head, neck, and shoulder region [2–5]. The optimum sitting position is generally accepted to be a maintained and erect upright spinal position [6]. As described by physiotherapists, an optimal sitting posture is the position with the least amount of muscle activation and the most relaxed and comfortable posture for the entire spine [7,8]. Presumptuously, any deviations away from this erect sitting posture is causative of pain and discomfort [9].

One issue regarding these mechanical ideologies, and popular clinical assumptions supporting the erect sitting posture, is that there is no evidence-based agreement on the optimal sitting posture, especially regarding the neck region [9–12]. Several studies support the erect sitting as an optimal posture for the head and neck region as mechanically, a more upright sitting posture reduces forward head translation and cervical flexion positions [11,13]. Reducing forward head posture (FHP) and cervical flexion posture by changes in sitting position modification has a direct influence on neck flexor and extensor muscles [14,15].

An issue that is not typically addressed when assessing sitting posture is the presence of pre-existing spinal misalignment or poor postures. FHP is a common poor posture that is associated with a greater load transmitted to the neck [16,17], greater muscle activation and fatigue [18], lower endurance of the deep neck extensors and flexors [19], as well as substantial effects on the biomechanics of the nervous system by causing unfavorable mechanical strain [20,21], which causes the blood vessels to constrict [22] and the nerve root sleeves to unfold and become taut, predisposing individuals to altered or inefficient neurophysiological symptoms [23,24]. Accordingly, we believe the combined effects of sitting with a pre-existing FHP may likely exacerbate any overstraining of the spine and soft tissues, including any neurophysiological effects.

Those with FHP have been demonstrated to exhibit abnormal sensorimotor control as well as autonomic nervous system dysfunction as compared to persons without FHP [23]. It has also been shown that the therapeutic correction of FHP and cervical lordosis aids in the improvement of sensorimotor control [24]. It is unknown, however, whether immediate changes in sitting posture have the potential to create alterations in neurophysiologic parameters and how these may differ between persons with and without pre-existing FHP. Consequently, the current study aimed to determine whether participants with and without FHP would respond differently in terms of dermatomal somatosensory-evoked potentials (DSSEPs) to variations in sitting positions versus a supine posture. In terms of neurophysiological outcomes, dermatomal somatosensory-evoked potentials (DSSEPs) are methods for recording cerebral-evoked reactions to the stimulation of specific regions innervated by single nerve roots, with the goal of supplying pure sensory input to the central nervous system through individual spinal segments to provide reliable information about segmental nerve root function [25].

2. Methods

Sixty (60) healthy participants voluntarily agreed to participate in this cross-sectional study. These two groups were parallel matched in age, body mass index (BMI), and sex. Ethics approval was obtained from University of Sharjah Research Ethics Committee in April 2021 REC-19-10-31-02-S. Following Ethics Committee approval, participant recruitment was from April 2021 to August 2022. Informed consent was obtained from all participants prior to the experiment according to relevant guidelines and regulations.

Participants in the NHP group were allocated as closely as possible to match those in the FHP group. Their age was accepted if it was within 2 years apart, the BMI was likewise matched if their BMI varied within 1–2 points. All participants were screened prior to enrollment into the study. The exclusion criteria were as follows: any inflammatory joint disease, systemic pathologies, previous history of musculoskeletal injuries or surgery, spinal disorders, extremity pathologies, or musculoskeletal pain 3 months prior to the study. Exclusion criteria information was obtained through each participant's medical records. Exclusions were further made of participants during the analysis of the peripheral nerve folly (N9), as detailed below in the neurophysiological assessment section. Participants with an abnormal N9 were excluded. DSSEP peaks follow a normal known structure, and any abnormalities appear clearly. The N9 DSSEP peak represents the afferent signals coming from the brachial plexus. Therefore, any participants with an abnormal N9 were excluded, to remove any possibility of unrelated peripheral factors.

The study inclusion criteria for recruitment were any individual between the ages of 18 and 28 who was in good health and had no musculoskeletal pain. The specific allocation of participants to either the FHP or the NHP group was determined by the photogrammetric craniovertebral angle (CVA) of each person [26]. Participants having a

CVA below 50° were assigned to the FHP group while participants having a CVA greater than 55° (considered as the cut-off for non-FHP) were assigned to the normal head posture (NHP) group. The CVA measurement method is shown in Figure 1.

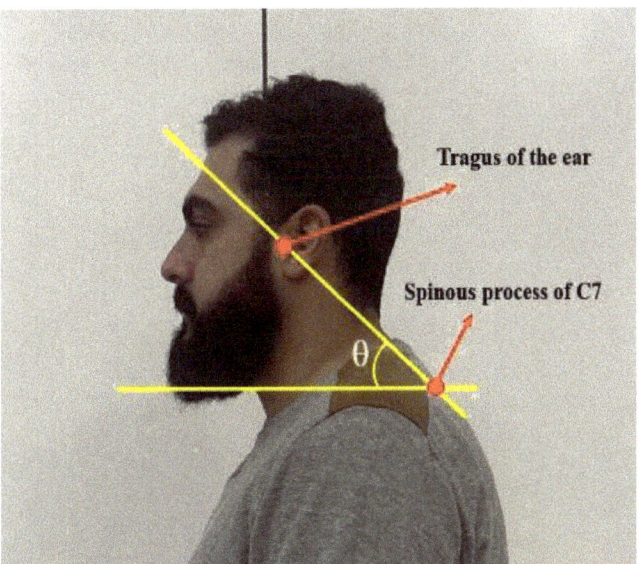

Figure 1. Measurement of the cranio-vertebral angle (CVA). The CVA is represented as the angle above. It is formed by the line connecting two adhesive markers placed at the tragus of the ear and the C7 spinous process; then, this line is assessed relative to a horizontal line drawn through the C7 marker. The angle θ represents the CVA.

2.1. Procedures

2.1.1. Evaluation of CVA

The CVA has a high inter-rater and intra-rater reliability in the assessment of FHP [27]. CVA is defined by the angle measured between the horizontal line bisecting the spinous process of C7 and the diagonal line going from the C7 spinous process to the tragus of the ear. As mentioned, we considered a CVA less than 50° to be the threshold for our FHP as this is related to an increased FHP, and FHP is related to increased disability [27].

We followed the published protocol of Falla et al. for the CVA assessment [28]: neutral lateral photos of every participant were taken. Each participant was instructed to sit up in a neutral and comfortable position on a chair and look forward. The photograph was then assessed for the CVA. A digital single-lens reflex camera was placed on a tripod 0.8 m away from the participant. The camera was perpendicular to the sagittal plane of the individuals' seated position at a height that corresponded with the seventh cervical vertebra of each seated participant. Florescent adhesive markers were used to identify the tragus and the C7 spinous process for the photos. All participants assumed and were assessed in the following three positions for the experiment.

2.1.2. Positions

All 60 participants in their respective group underwent C6, C7 and C8 dermatomal somatosensory-evoked potentials (DSSEPs). For each of the cervical nerves (C6, C7 and C8), measurements were taken in three positions for each participant:

- Supine position (which acted as a reference for DSSEPs measurement);
- After assuming the erect sitting posture for 30 min;
- After assuming the slouched sitting posture for 30 min.

Erect Sitting Position

As shown in Figure 2, the participants sat on a chair supporting their back. Their hips and knees were positioned at a 90° angle, where the base of support was perpendicular to the chair. The arms were rested on the armrest and the spine was assumed in a 'neutral upright position' (i.e., neutral kyphosis and lordosis angles); therefore, achieving a slight anterior rotation of the pelvis. Participants were instructed to look forward at a stationary point straight ahead of them.

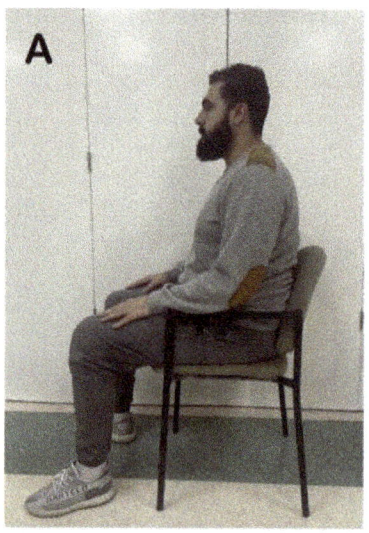 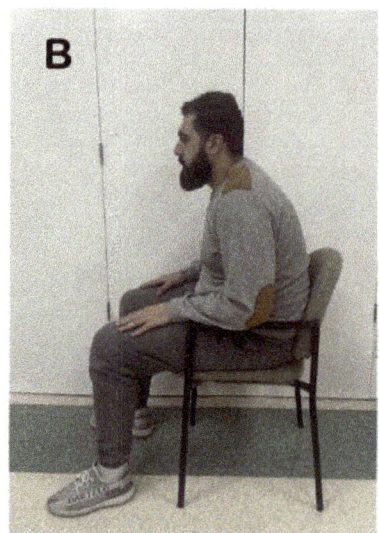

Figure 2. Sitting Positions. (**A**): Erect sitting, (**B**): Slouched sitting.

Slouched Sitting Position

Participants sat on the same chair with their back supported and were instructed to relax their thoracolumbar spine to produce a hyperkyphotic angle at the thorax and a straightened lordotic curve at the lumbar region, as shown in Figure 2. This causes a posterior tilt of the pelvis, hyper-kyphosis of the thoracic spine, and a pronounced forward head posture.

Supine Position

Participants were instructed to lay back on a flat plinth with the arms in an extended anatomical position. The hip angle was at 180 degrees [29]. The head was supported by a pillow to prevent interference or movement of the electrode placements [30].

2.2. Neurophysiological Outcome Measures
DSSEPs

Neurophysiological findings for C6, C7, and C8 were measured in this study as the peak-to-peak amplitude of DSSEPs. An electromyography device (Neuropack S1 MEB-9400K, Nihon Koden, Tokyo, Japan) was used for these neurophysiological assessments. DSSEPs were stimulated with a continuous electrical pulse wave (0.5 ms) at 3 Hz, delivered by three standard surface gel electrodes (20 mm) placed over the respective cervical dermatome; a reference electrode, a recording electrode, and a grounding electrode were used. The stimulation intensity used was above each participant's perception threshold. All participants initially assumed a relaxed supine position where they were instructed to lay quietly and with eyes closed during the procedure. After parting the hair and using alcohol to prepare the skin, Nuprep gel and Ag–AgCl disc recording electrodes (10 mm with 60 inch lead wires) were fixed with Elefix paste to the scalp (Nihon Kohden, Tokyo, Japan) (Figure 3 shows the electrode placement). The grounding electrode was attached to a strap, which was secured around the forearm. The impedance of all three electrodes was kept below 5 kΩ for an even reading. Three recordings were done for each of the dermatomes stimulated (C6, C7, and C8). The stimulation points were radial forearm 1 inch above the wrist, the middle of the palm right below the middle finger, and the ulnar side of the palm, respectively.

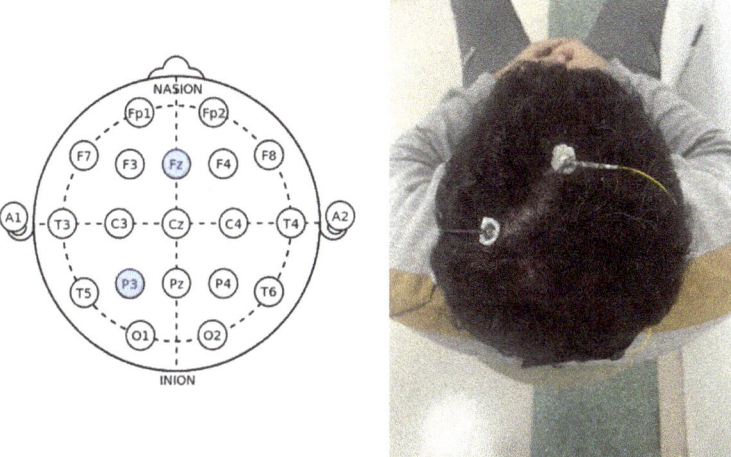

Figure 3. Left: Electrode placement following the 10–20 international EEG system; **Right**: Reference and recording electrode placements.

2.3. Statistical Analysis

2.3.1. Sample Size

Estimates of mean and standard deviations (SD) from a pilot study of 10 individuals who received the same program were collected to determine the required number of participants in this study. The mean differences and SD of the peak-to-peak amplitude of DSSEPs for different levels C6, 7, and 8 for the different sitting postures: supine, erect and slouched, were: C6: −0.1 (SD 0.3), −0.17 (SD 01.2), −0.86 (SD 0.6); C7: −0.07 (SD 0.9), −0.6 (SD 0.9), −1.6 (SD 1.00); and C8: −0.1 (SD 0.4), −0.9 (SD 0.8), −1.6 (SD 0.9), respectively. The sample size was calculated independently for each of the key outcomes using a Bonferroni correction to adjust the significance level. The greatest sample size value was then used as the trial's final sample size. Given a statistical power of 80%, the current investigation required at least 25 individuals in each group. To accommodate for probable dropouts, the sample size was increased by 20%.

2.3.2. Data Analysis

Levene's test of equality of error variances was used to determine the normality distribution of the dataset at 95% confidence interval and p-value < 0.05. The dataset had a 2 × 3 factorial design. Descriptive statistics (mean ± SD) were summarized for each position and cervical nerve root. The unpaired t-test for continuous variables was used to compare the means and determine the significance of the interaction between the nerve roots in the different sitting positions. A two-way analysis of variance (ANOVA) was then used to test the relationships between the head posture (NHP vs. FHP) and sitting position (supine, slouched, and erect) on the cervical nerve roots (C6, C7, and C8). A p-value of 0.05 or less was considered a statistically significant difference in the dataset. Following that, the Tukey honestly significant difference (HSD) post hoc tests were used. SPSS version 29.0 software was used for analyzing data (SPSS Inc., Chicago, IL, USA).

3. Results

Ninety-five potential participants were initially screened. Thirty participants with FHP and thirty age-, BMI-, and sex-matched controls without FHP were recruited for the NHP group. Figure 4 shows the participant flow chart with numbers excluded and reasons why. Descriptive data for the baseline participant demographics are presented in Table 1. No statistically significant differences between the NHP and the FHP group were found at baseline for their demographic variables. Table 1 shows the mean and distribution of CVA for both groups.

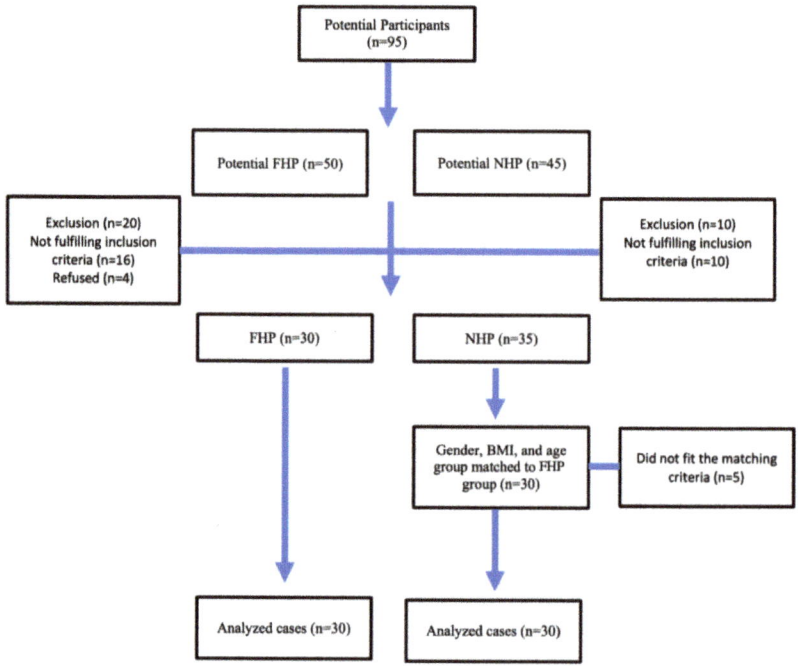

Figure 4. Participant flowchart.

Table 1. Participant demographic variables listed as means and standard deviations. There were no statistically significant differences between the NHP and FHP groups; $p > 0.05$ for all variables, using the independent t-test for continuous data and chi-squared test of independence for categorical data.

Characteristic	Forward Head Group (n = 30)	Normal Head Group (n = 30)	Significance
Age (years)	20.5 ± 2	20 ± 3	0.4
Weight (kg)	61.2 ± 4	62.2 ± 5	0.3
BMI	18.4 ± 1.2	18.3 ± 1.4	0.7
Smoking			
Nonsmoker	15	14	
Light Smoker	10	12	0.6
Heavy smoker	5	4	
Sex			
Male	11	11	-
Female	19	19	
CVA	41.7 ± 2	66.9 ± 4.6	<0.001

While the number of females in both groups was nearly double that of males, adding sex as a fixed variable to our statistical models in this study did not produce any difference in the outcome findings. A two-way analysis of variance (two-way ANOVA) identified significant head posture × sitting position effects on the outcome of peak-to-peak amplitudes of the cervical nerve roots C6, C7 and C8. Results showed a statistically significant interaction between the head posture and sitting position (F = 32.867) ($p < 0.001$), (F = 38.926) ($p < 0.001$), (F = 40.348) ($p < 0.001$) for C6, C7 and C8, respectively. Tables 2–4 presents these data.

Table 2. Two-way analysis of variance results. FHP = forward head posture group, NHP = neutral head posture group, Erect = neutral upright sitting posture, Slouched = slouched or slumped sitting posture, Supine = lying supine analysis, C6, C7, C8 = the respective nerve roots tested, C.I. = confidence interval.

		Erect	Slouched	Supine
C6	FHP	1.84 ± 0.33	2.30 ± 0.38	2.50 ± 0.37
	NHP	2.51 ± 0.36	1.92 ± 0.30	2.60 ± 0.42
p-value		$p < 0.001$	$p < 0.001$	$p = 0.09$
C.I.		[−0.80, −0.44]	[0.27, 0.62]	[−0.38, 0.03]
C7	FHP	1.71 ± 0.23	2.24 ± 0.15	2.22 ± 0.20
	NHP	2.11 ± 0.38	1.60 ± 0.25	2.22 ± 0.42
p-value		$p = 0.001$	$p < 0.001$	$p = 0.72$
C.I.		[−0.50, −0.17]	[0.49, 0.70]	[−0.14, 0.20]
C8	FHP	1.71 ± 0.41	2.61 ± 0.56	2.73 ± 0.55
	NHP	2.21 ± 0.40	1.70 ± 0.31	2.34 ± 0.46
p-value		$p < 0.001$	$p < 0.001$	$p = 0.01$
C.I.		[−0.80, −0.38]	[0.66, 1.13]	[0.08, 0.61]

Table 3. Two-way analysis of variance results.

Tests of Between-Subjects Effects						
	Type III Sum of Squares	df	Mean Square	F	Sig.	Partial Eta Squared
C6 amplitude						
Corrected Model	17.272	5	3.454	26.294	<0.001	0.430
Intercept	917.742	1	917.742	6985.400	<0.001	0.976
Head Posture	0.629	1	0.629	4.787	0.030	0.027
Sitting	8.007	2	4.004	30.474	<0.001	0.259
Head Posture * Sitting	8.636	2	4.318	32.867	<0.001	0.274
Error	22.860	174	0.131			
C7 amplitude						
Corrected Model	11.095	5	2.219	26.217	<0.001	0.430
Intercept	726.374	1	726.374	8581.961	<0.001	0.980
Head Posture	0.431	1	0.431	5.095	0.025	0.028
Sitting	4.075	2	2.037	24.070	<0.001	0.217
Head Posture * Sitting	6.589	2	3.295	38.926	<0.001	0.309
Error	14.727	174	0.085			
C8 amplitude						
Corrected Model	28.892	5	5.778	27.731	<0.001	0.443
Intercept	885.470	1	885.470	4249.485	<0.001	0.961
Head Posture	2.185	1	2.185	10.484	0.001	0.057
Sitting	9.892	2	4.946	23.737	<0.001	0.214
Head Posture * Sitting	16.815	2	8.407	40.348	<0.001	0.317
Error	36.257	174	0.208			

Table 4. Pairwise comparisons.

(I) Sitting	(J) Sitting	Mean Difference (I−J)	Std. Error	Sig. b	95% Confidence Interval for Difference b	
					Lower Bound	Upper Bound
Dependent Variable: C6 Amplitude						
Erect	Slouched	0.051	0.066	1	−0.109	0.211
	Supine	−0.420 *	0.066	<0.001	−0.580	−0.260
Dependent Variable: C7 Amplitude						
Erect	Slouched	−0.237 *	0.083	0.015	−0.439	−0.036
	Supine	−0.572 *	0.083	<0.001	−0.773	−0.370
Dependent Variable: C8 Amplitude						
Erect	Slouched	−0.012	0.053	1	−0.140	0.117
	Supine	−0.325 *	0.053	<0.001	−0.453	−0.196

* The mean difference is significant at the 0.05 level. b. Adjustment for multiple comparisons: Bonferroni.

Following the prolonged sitting position of 30 min, the between-group statistical analysis was significantly different, showing a more favorable nerve root function in the slouched sitting position for the FHP group compared to the NHP group, while the erect sitting position demonstrated a significant favorability to the NHP group, as shown in Table 2. Figures 5 and 6 show short latency DSSEPs for C6, C7 and C8 pre and post 30 min of sitting in a participant from the NHP group.

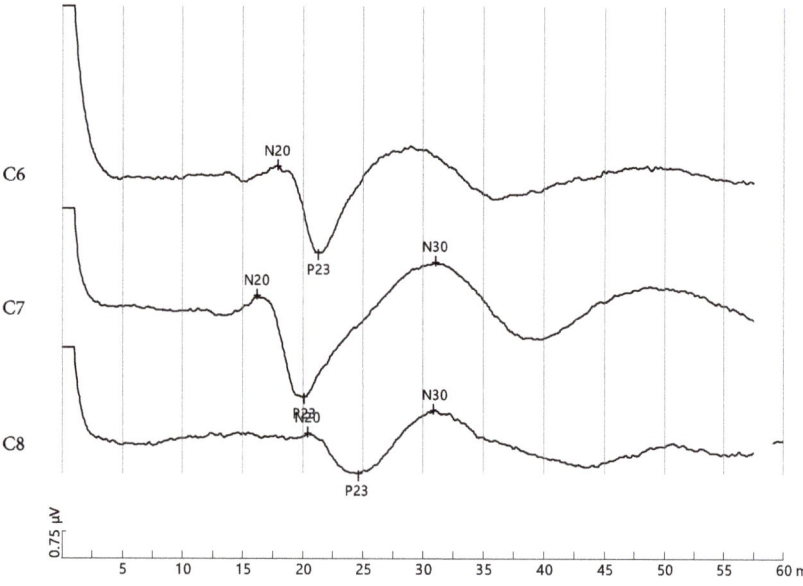

Figure 5. Short latency somatosensory-evoked potential of a normal head posture (NHP) participant before prolonged slouched sitting for C6, C7 and C8. The amplitudes measured between N20 and P23 are: 2.45 µV, 2.8 µV, and 1.14 µV, respectively.

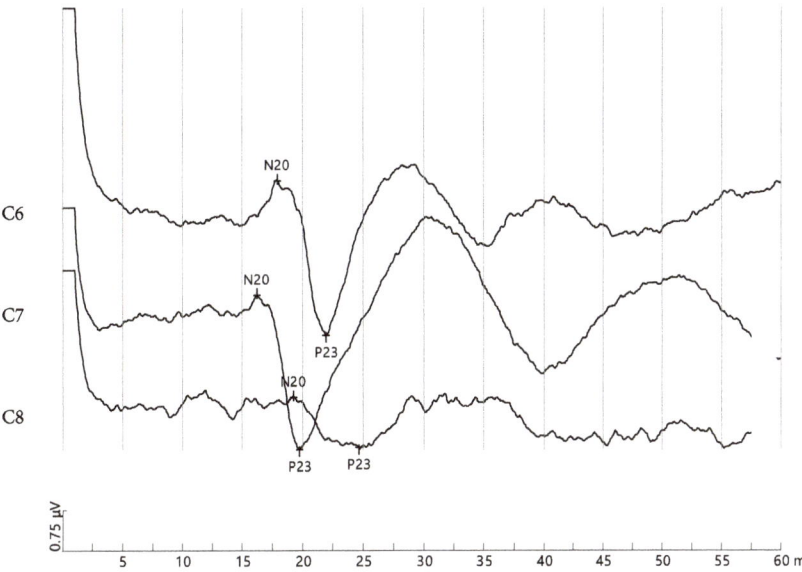

Figure 6. Short latency somatosensory-evoked potential of normal head posture (NHP) participant after prolonged slouched sitting for C6, C7, and C8. The amplitudes measured between N20 and P23 are: 2.81 µV, 2.81 µV, and 0.945 µV, respectively.

The scatterplots in Figures 7–9 show that for all three cervical nerve roots (C6, C7, C8), their amplitudes increased in the slouched position for the FHP group compared to the erect position. Contrarily, the NHP group displayed a higher amplitude in the erect position than the slouched position. Both groups showed similarity in the nerve root functions in the prolonged supine position.

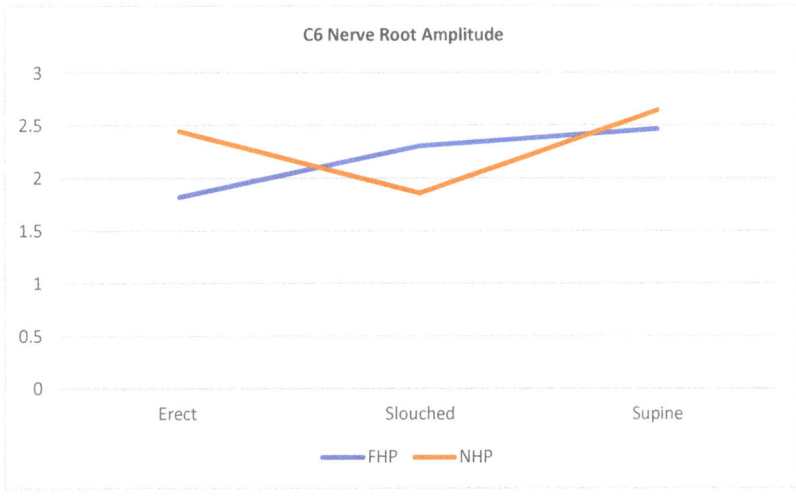

Figure 7. Scatterplot line of cervical nerve C6 amplitude relationship with the different sitting positions for participants with forward head posture (FHP) and normal head posture (NHP). The graph highlights that the FHP group has shown an increased amplitude during slouched sitting compared to erect sitting. The supine position shows the highest nerve peak from all three positions.

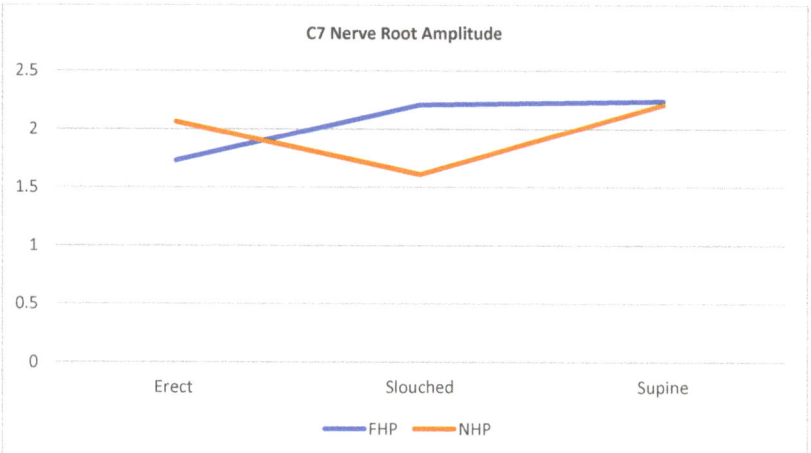

Figure 8. Scatterplot line of cervical nerve C7 amplitude relationship with the different sitting positions for participants with forward head posture (FHP) and normal head posture (NHP). The graph highlights that the FHP group has shown an increased amplitude during slouched sitting compared to erect sitting. The supine position shows the highest nerve peak from all three positions.

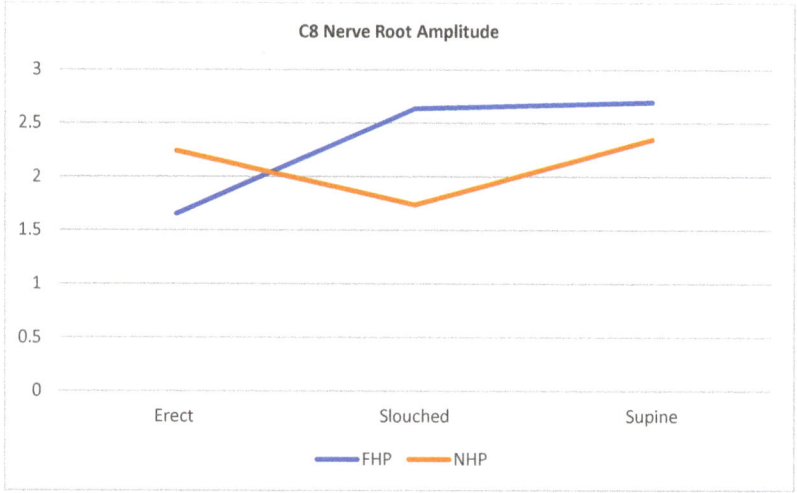

Figure 9. Scatterplot line of cervical nerve C8 amplitude relationship with the different sitting positions for participants with forward head posture (FHP) and normal head posture (NHP). The graph highlights that the FHP group has shown an increased amplitude during slouched sitting compared to erect sitting. The supine position shows the highest nerve peak from all three positions.

Simple main effects analysis showed that the head posture had a statistically significant effect on the cervical nerve root functions of C6 ($p = 0.030$), C7 ($p = 0.025$), and C8 ($p < 0.001$). As for the sitting posture, a statistical significance was also detected on the cervical nerve roots C6 ($p < 0.001$), C7 ($p = 0.025$), and C8 ($p < 0.001$). Analysis with Levene's test of equality of error variances showed that the homogeneity of variances in our data can be assumed for C6 ($p = 0.235$), for C7 ($p = 0.02$), and for C8 ($p = 0.068$).

4. Discussion

As we had initially hypothesized, the cervical nerve root DSSEPs were identified to have significant differences between each of the positions tested: erect sitting, slouched sitting, and lying supine. Interestingly, our intergroup results (NHP vs. FHP groups) showed a pattern contrary to popular belief. The NHP group displayed the greatest peaks for DSSEPs while in the erect sitting position, and this is generally consistent with the previous literature on ideal sitting posture; namely, that altered cervical posture has damaging effects. In contrast, the individuals in the FHP group had the greatest peak-to-peak amplitude of DSSEPs while in the slouched position as opposed to the erect position. While the erect position is deemed the most correct and healthy position for the spine, our results show otherwise relative to the initial posture of the participant. Thus, our findings indicate the importance of considering the initial presenting cervical sagittal alignment of the individual as a significant factor when determining the ideal sitting posture. To our knowledge, this is the first research investigation that considers the cervical sagittal alignment as a contributing factor when assessing different sitting postures. These findings give new insights into an essential consensus of sitting that seem to suggest the uniqueness of the individual's alignment. In other words, what works well for one person may create discomfort for another. Our main findings are in agreement with that of Dunk et al. who reported that individuals may respond differently to various sitting postures and the variables that influence sitting posture are still not fully understood [31]. Similarly, Adams suggested that sustained postures, including the erect posture if maintained for a prolonged period, can lead to discomfort and even injury [32].

One of the most important findings in this study was that for participants who already had FHP, adopting the erect sitting position negatively affected their nerve root function, as manifested by significant reductions in the peak-to-peak amplitude of the DSSEPs for the nerve roots tested. Some authors have noted that an erect sitting posture [14,15] may lead to increased levels of fatigue resulting from increased muscle activation compared with the habitual sitting posture of an individual. In contrast, Nishikawa et al. [18] identified that FHP compared to NHP was associated with a greater cervical spine muscle activity and subjective fatigue using high density surface EMG. These seemingly contradictory findings are challenging to explain and likely involve complex interactions between an individual's perception of their natural posture, specific spine geometric alignments of the sagittal plane curvatures, muscle length tension relationships, and yet-undetermined variables.

It has been reported that FHP is associated with the weakening of isometric strength and endurance of the deep neck flexors [33]. The endurance of the deep neck flexor muscles directly affects the function of the cervical spine, and the strength of these muscles are important in maintaining the posture and stability of the neck [33–35]. Along with the shoulder girdle muscles, the deep neck flexors are crucial for the control and support of the neck, supporting the weight of the head against gravity and stabilizing the head [36]. Accordingly, it is expected that assuming the erect posture for people with FHP will induce more fatigue. Due to this, it is believed that FHP participants will be more comfortable if they adopt a slouched posture while relying on passive structures of the spine (ligaments and bone). During a slouched or slumped posture, it is proposed that this posture relies mainly on the passive (e.g., spinal ligaments) structures to maintain a resting sitting position. This results in a diminished requirement for muscle activity [37,38].

Related research has shown that muscle fatigue occurs when erect postures (such as upright sitting) are sustained for as little as 30 min, even if contractions are as low as 2% to 5% of the maximum voluntary contraction [39]. This offers a possible explanation as to why participants might prefer a slumped sitting posture—because it is perceived as less physically demanding [37,38]. Still, it is necessary to note that the decline in stabilizing potential of the paraspinal muscles, the associated compensatory antagonistic coactivation, and the related increase in spinal load are associated with muscle fatigue. As documented in many studies, fatigue-related changes in muscle stiffness may reduce the capacity of the paraspinal muscles to stabilize the spine. If fatigue is not severe (as expected in our study), then the compensatory recruitment of antagonistic co-contraction may restore stability, but this will contribute to increased spinal load and an associated risk of overload injury [40–42]. This aberrant spinal load caused by muscular fatigue might be a possible explanation for the decrease in the peak-to-peak amplitude of DSSEPs.

A final explanation for the reduced amplitude of the DSSEPs being different in the NHP vs. FHP groups during different sitting positions could be the amount and distribution of the cervical lordotic curve in the participants. It is known that abnormal cervical sagittal alignment (kyphosis, s-curves, etc.) creates changes in loading on the vertebrae and soft tissues [43]. Gong et al. [33] reported that reduced and kyphotic cervical curves coupled with FHP reduced the endurance of the deep neck flexors. Since it is known that increased FHP causes flexion of the lower cervical spine and extension of the upper cervical spine [44], it could be that slumped sitting in already FHP individuals causes a more dramatic increase in the lower cervical spine due to the increased thoracic kyphosis that also occurs in this posture. The increased cervical lordosis in this specific 'exaggerated' postural position might reduce the net tension on the lower cervical spinal cord and nerve roots, leading to an increased amplitude of the DSSEPs [20,45]. Though speculative, this seems like a plausible explanation that needs to be confirmed in future investigations using spine imaging.

Study Limitations and Suggestions for Future Research

The following limitations should be considered when interpreting the current study's findings. We only examined the lower cervical spine nerve roots C5, C6 and C7, without looking at other cervical levels. Additionally, participants in this study were young adults, and as result, the findings might not be applicable to other age groups. Given the limitations of the current study, future research is needed to analyze the other cervical nerve roots, to shed more light on the upper cervical region related to different sitting postures. Investigating the effects of different sitting postures in different age groups may also help researchers in understanding the function of age as a contributing factor. Lastly, we did not specifically investigate the smoking status of a participant as an independent variable herein. However, the fact that there were almost an equal number of smokers in the two groups eliminated the possibility that smoking could have an impact on the outcome measure as a confounding variable between our two groups, as was shown. Still, we suggest that future research should take smoking status into consideration. Finally, our investigation did not formally investigate the true ideal geometric sitting posture of the thoracic and thoraco-lumbar pelvic region, nor did it investigate mechanisms for attaining or improving altered posture positions in participants, as has been performed in previous investigations [46,47]. Future work could incorporate the key findings herein of how the CVA of an individual affects nerve root function in different sitting positions and how variations in ideal sitting postures and its training or re-training are affected.

5. Conclusions

We identified statistically significant differences in the cervical nerve root function in all postures between the NHP and FHP groups ($p < 0.001$), indicating that the FHP and NHP reacted differently in different positions. For the supine reference position, we found no significant differences between the FHP and NHP groups for the DSSEPs of nerve roots C6–C8. In contrast, both the erect and slouched sitting positions were found to have significant differences in nerve root amplitudes between the NHP and FHP groups. Specifically, the NHP group was found to have the greatest peaks for nerve root DSSEPs while in the erect sitting position and this is generally consistent with the previous literature on ideal sitting posture; namely, that altered cervical posture has damaging effects in sitting posture. However, the participants in the FHP group demonstrated the largest peak-to-peak amplitude of DSSEPs for nerve roots C6–C8 while in the slouched position as opposed to an erect position. The ideal sitting posture and its influence on cervical nerve root function may be dependent upon the underlying initial forward head posture presentation of a person, however, further research is needed to corroborate these findings in patients with and without cervical spine disorders.

Author Contributions: M.K. (Maryam Kamel), I.M.M. and M.K. (Meeyoung Kim) conceived the research idea. M.K. (Maryam Kamel), I.M.M., M.K. (Meeyoung Kim), P.A.O. and D.E.H. all contributed to the statistical analysis. M.K. (Maryam Kamel), I.M.M. and M.K. (Meeyoung Kim) participated in the data collection and study supervision. M.K. (Maryam Kamel), I.M.M., M.K. (Meeyoung Kim), P.A.O. and D.E.H. all contributed to the interpretation of the results and wrote the drafts. All authors have read and agreed to the published version of the manuscript.

Funding: Funding for the publication fee was provided by CBP Nonprofit, Inc. Deed E. Harrison is President of CBP Nonprofit and is a member of a 13 member board that approves funding of clinical trials. Deed Harrison's role as a senior author and conflicts of interest are outlined above lines 489–497.

Institutional Review Board Statement: The research was conducted in accordance with ethics committee of the College of Health Sciences, University of Sharjah and approved by the Research Institute of Medical and Health Sciences of the University of Sharjah (reference number: REC-19-10-31-02-S.). Consent forms were signed by participants prior to data collection and we also followed the CONSORT guidelines.

Informed Consent Statement: All participant's pictured in the study were after written informed consent was signed and obtained.

Data Availability Statement: The datasets analyzed in the current study are available from the corresponding author on reasonable request.

Conflicts of Interest: P.A.O. is a paid consultant for CBP NonProfit, Inc. D.E.H. teaches continuing education conferences to health care providers, is the CEO of Chiropractic BioPhysics, teaches rehabilitation methods, and sells products for patient rehabilitation to physicians in the USA. All the other authors declare that they have no competing interests.

References

1. Kallings, L.V.; Blom, V.; Ekblom, B.; Holmlund, T.; Eriksson, J.S.; Andersson, G.; Wallin, P.; Ekblom-Bak, E. Workplace Sitting Is Associated with Self-Reported General Health and Back/Neck Pain: A Cross-Sectional Analysis in 44,978 Employees. *BMC Public Health* **2021**, *21*, 875. [CrossRef]
2. Waongenngarm, P.; van der Beek, A.J.; Akkarakittichoke, N.; Janwantanakul, P. Perceived Musculoskeletal Discomfort and Its Association with Postural Shifts during 4-h Prolonged Sitting in Office Workers. *Appl. Ergon.* **2020**, *89*, 103225. [CrossRef]
3. Pattath, P.; Webb, L. Computer-usage and associated musculoskeletal discomfort in college students. *Work* **2022**, *73*, 327–334. [CrossRef]
4. Yang, F.; Di, N.; Guo, W.W.; Ding, W.B.; Jia, N.; Zhang, H.; Li, D.; Wang, D.; Wang, R.; Zhang, D.; et al. The prevalence and risk factors of work related musculoskeletal disorders among electronics manufacturing workers: A cross-sectional analytical study in China. *BMC Public Health* **2023**, *23*, 10. [CrossRef] [PubMed]
5. De Carvalho, D.E. *Spine Biomechanics of Prolonged Sitting: Exploring the Effect Chair Features, Walking Breaks and Spine Manipulation Have on Posture and Perceived Pain in Men and Women*; UWSpace, University of Waterloo: Waterloo, ON, Canada, 2015.
6. Harrison, D.D.; Harrison, S.O.; Croft, A.C.; Harrison, D.E.; Troyanovich, S.J. Sitting biomechanics part I: Review of the literature. *J. Manip. Physiol. Ther.* **1999**, *2*, 594–609. [CrossRef] [PubMed]
7. Hey, H.W.D.; Wong, C.G.; Lau, E.T.C.; Tan, K.A.; Lau, L.L.; Liu, K.P.G.; Wong, H.K. Differences in Erect Sitting and Natural Sitting Spinal Alignment—Insights into a New Paradigm and Implications in Deformity Correction. *Spine J.* **2017**, *17*, 183–189. [CrossRef] [PubMed]
8. O'Sullivan, K.; O'Sullivan, P.; O'Sullivan, L.; Dankaerts, W. What Do Physiotherapists Consider to Be the Best Sitting Spinal Posture? *Man. Ther.* **2012**, *17*, 432–437. [CrossRef]
9. Ye, J.; Jiang, Z.; Chen, S.; Cheng, R.; Xu, L.; Tsai, T.-Y. Rehabilitation Practitioners' Perceptions of Optimal Sitting and Standing Posture in Men with Normal Weight and Obesity. *Bioengineering* **2023**, *10*, 210. [CrossRef]
10. Czaprowski, D.; Leszczewska, J.; Sitarski, D.; Rehabilitacji, K.; Rehabilitacji, W.; Fizycznego, W.; Piłsudskiego, J.; Warszawie, A.; Wychowania Fizycznego, W.; Fizjoterapii, W.; et al. Czy Istnieje "Idealna" Pozycja Siedząca? Does "Ideal" Sitting Position Exist? *Postęp. Rehabil.* **2014**, *28*, 47–54. [CrossRef]
11. Harrison, D.D.; Harrison, S.O.; Croft, A.C.; Harrison, D.E.; Troyanovich, S.J. Sitting biomechanics, part II: Optimal car driver's seat and optimal driver's spinal model. *J. Manip. Physiol. Ther.* **2000**, *23*, 37–47. [CrossRef]
12. Claus, A.P.; Hides, J.A.; Moseley, G.L.; Hodges, P.W. Is "ideal" Sitting Posture Real: Measurement of Spinal Curves in Four Sitting Postures. *Man. Ther.* **2009**, *14*, 404–408. [CrossRef] [PubMed]

13. Douglas, E.C.; Gallagher, K.M. The Influence of a Semi-Reclined Seated Posture on Head and Neck Kinematics and Muscle Activity While Reading a Tablet Computer. *Appl. Ergon.* **2017**, *60*, 342–347. [CrossRef] [PubMed]
14. Kwon, J.W.; Son, S.M.; Lee, K. Changes in Upper-Extremity Muscle Activities Due to Head Position in Subjects with a Forward Head Posture and Rounded Shoulders. *J. Phys. Ther. Sci.* **2015**, *27*, 1739–1742. [CrossRef] [PubMed]
15. Falla, D.; O'Leary, S.; Fagan, A.; Jull, G. Recruitment of the Deep Cervical Flexor Muscles during a Postural-Correction Exercise Performed in Sitting. *Man. Ther.* **2007**, *12*, 139–143. [CrossRef] [PubMed]
16. Choi, H. Quantitative Assessment of Co-Contraction in Cervical Musculature. *Med. Eng. Phys.* **2003**, *25*, 133–140. [CrossRef]
17. Eitivipart, A.C.; Viriyarojanakul, S.; Redhead, L. Musculoskeletal disorder and pain associated with smartphone use: A systematic review of biomechanical evidence. *Hong Kong Physiother. J.* **2018**, *38*, 77–90. [CrossRef]
18. Nishikawa, Y.; Watanabe, K.; Chihara, T.; Sakamoto, J.; Komatsuzaki, T.; Kawano, K.; Kobayashi, A.; Inoue, K.; Maeda, N.; Tanaka, S.; et al. Influence of Forward Head Posture on Muscle Activation Pattern of the Trapezius Pars Descendens Muscle in Young Adults. *Sci. Rep.* **2022**, *12*, 19484. [CrossRef]
19. Oliveira, A.C.; Silva, A.G. Neck Muscle Endurance and Head Posture: A Comparison between Adolescents with and without Neck Pain. *Man. Ther.* **2016**, *22*, 62–67. [CrossRef]
20. Harrison, D.E.; Cailliet, R.; Harrison, D.D.; Troyanovich, S.J.; Harrison, S.O. A Review of Biomechanics of the Central Nervous System—Part II: Spinal Cord Strains from Postural Loads. *J. Manip. Physiol. Ther.* **1999**, *22*, 322–332. [CrossRef]
21. Diab, A.A.; Moustafa, I.M. The Efficacy of Forward Head Correction on Nerve Root Function and Pain in Cervical Spondylotic Radiculopathy: A Randomized Trial. *Clin. Rehabil.* **2012**, *26*, 351–361. [CrossRef]
22. Thosar, S.S.; Bielko, S.L.; Wiggins, C.C.; Wallace, J.P. Differences in Brachial and Femoral Artery Responses to Prolonged Sitting. *Cardiovasc. Ultrasound* **2014**, *12*, 1–7. [CrossRef] [PubMed]
23. Moustafa, I.M.; Youssef, A.; Ahbouch, A.; Tamim, M.; Harrison, D.E. Is Forward Head Posture Relevant to Autonomic Nervous System Function and Cervical Sensorimotor Control? Cross Sectional Study. *Gait Posture* **2020**, *77*, 29–35. [CrossRef] [PubMed]
24. Moustafa, I.; Youssef, A.S.A.; Ahbouch, A.; Harrison, D. Demonstration of Autonomic Nervous Function and Cervical Sensorimotor Control after Cervical Lordosis Rehabilitation: A Randomized Controlled Trial. *J. Athl. Train.* **2021**, *56*, 427–436. [CrossRef] [PubMed]
25. Muzyka, I.M.; Estephan, B. Somatosensory Evoked Potentials. *Handb. Clin. Neurol.* **2019**, *160*, 523–540. [CrossRef]
26. Yip, C.H.T.; Chiu, T.T.W.; Poon, A.T.K. The relationship between head posture and severity and disability of patients with neck pain. *Man. Ther.* **2008**, *13*, 148–154. [CrossRef]
27. Singla, D.; Veqar, Z.; Hussain, M.E. Photogrammetric Assessment of Upper Body Posture Using Postural Angles: A Literature Review. *J. Chiropr. Med.* **2017**, *16*, 131–138. [CrossRef]
28. Falla, D.; Jull, G.; Russell, T.; Vicenzino, B.; Hodges, P. Effect of neck exercise on sitting posture in patients with chronic neck pain. *Phys. Ther.* **2007**, *87*, 408–417. [CrossRef]
29. Acharya, J.N.; Hani, A.J.; Cheek, J.; Thirumala, P.; Tsuchida, T.N. American Clinical Neurophysiology Society Guideline 2: Guidelines for Standard Electrode Position Nomenclature. *Neurodiagn. J.* **2016**, *56*, 245–252. [CrossRef]
30. Morley, A.; Hill, L.; Kaditis, A.G. *10-20 System EEG Placement*; European Respiratory Society: Lausanne, Switzerland, 2016.
31. Dunk, N.M.; Callaghan, J.P. Gender-Based Differences in Postural Responses to Seated Exposures. *Clin. Biomech. (Bristol. Avon)* **2005**, *20*, 1101–1110. [CrossRef] [PubMed]
32. Adams, M.A. Biomechanics of Back Pain. *Acupunct. Med.* **2004**, *22*, 178–188. [CrossRef] [PubMed]
33. Gong, W.; Kim, C.; Lee, Y. Correlations between Cervical Lordosis, Forward Head Posture, Cervical ROM and the Strength and Endurance of the Deep Neck Flexor Muscles in College Students. *J. Phys. Ther. Sci.* **2012**, *24*, 275–277. [CrossRef]
34. Ha, S.Y.; Sung, Y.H. Vojta Approach Affects Neck Stability and Static Balance in Sitting Position of Children With Hypotonia. *Int. Neurourol. J.* **2021**, *25*, S90–S95, Erratum in *Int. Neurourol. J.* **2022**, *26*, 258. [CrossRef] [PubMed]
35. Iqbal, Z.A.; Alghadir, A.H.; Anwer, S. Efficacy of Deep Cervical Flexor Muscle Training on Neck Pain, Functional Disability, and Muscle Endurance in School Teachers: A Clinical Trial. *BioMed Res. Int.* **2021**, *2021*, 7190808. [CrossRef] [PubMed]
36. Lin, G.; Wang, W.; Wilkinson, T. Changes in deep neck muscle length from the neutral to forward head posture. A cadaveric study using Thiel cadavers. *Clin. Anat.* **2022**, *35*, 332–339. [CrossRef] [PubMed]
37. Larson, B.A.; Nicolaides, E.; Al Zu'bi, B.; Sukkar, N.; Laraki, K.; Matoussi, M.S.; Zaim, K.; Chouchani, C. Examination of the Flexion Relaxation Phenomenon in Erector Spinae Muscles during Short Duration Slumped Sitting. *Clin. Biomech.* **2002**, *17*, 353–360. [CrossRef]
38. Claus, A.P.; Hides, J.A.; Moseley, G.L.; Hodges, P.W. Different Ways to Balance the Spine: Subtle Changes in Sagittal Spinal Curves Affect Regional Muscle Activity. *Spine (Phila. Pa. 1976)* **2009**, *34*, E208–E214. [CrossRef] [PubMed]
39. van Dieën, J.H.; Westebring-van der Putten, E.P.; Kingma, I.; de Looze, M.P. Low-Level Activity of the Trunk Extensor Muscles Causes Electromyographic Manifestations of Fatigue in Absence of Decreased Oxygenation. *J. Electromyogr. Kinesiol.* **2009**, *19*, 398–406. [CrossRef] [PubMed]
40. Granata, K.P.; Slota, G.P.; Wilson, S.E. Influence of Fatigue in Neuromuscular Control of Spinal Stability. *Hum. Factors* **2004**, *46*, 81–91. [CrossRef] [PubMed]
41. Marras, W.S.; Granata, K.P. Changes in Trunk Dynamics and Spine Loading during Repeated Trunk Exertions. *Spine (Phila. Pa. 1976)* **1997**, *22*, 2564–2570. [CrossRef]

42. Kirsch, R.F.; Rymer, W.Z. Neural compensation for fatigue-induced changes in muscle stiffness during perturbations of elbow angle in human. *J. Neurophysiol.* **1992**, *68*, 449–470. [CrossRef]
43. Harrison, D.E.; Jones, E.W.; Janik, T.J.; Harrison, D.D. Evaluation of axial and flexural stresses in the vertebral body cortex and trabecular bone in lordosis and two sagittal cervical translation configurations with an elliptical shell model. *J. Manip. Physiol Ther.* **2002**, *25*, 391–401. [CrossRef] [PubMed]
44. Patwardhan, A.G.; Khayatzadeh, S.; Havey, R.M.; Voronov, L.I.; Smith, Z.A.; Kalmanson, O.; Sears, W. Cervical sagittal balance: A biomechanical perspective can help clinical practice. *Eur. Spine J.* **2018**, *27*, 25–38. [CrossRef] [PubMed]
45. Moustafa, I.M.; Diab, A.A.; Harrison, D.E. The Efficacy of Cervical Lordosis Rehabilitation for Nerve Root Function and Pain in Cervical Spondylotic Radiculopathy: A Randomized Trial with 2-Year Follow-Up. *J. Clin. Med.* **2022**, *11*, 6515. [CrossRef] [PubMed]
46. Kiebzak, W.P.; Żurawski, A.Ł.; Kosztołowicz, M. Alignment of the Sternum and Sacrum as a Marker of Sitting Body Posture in Children. *Int. J. Environ. Res. Public Health* **2022**, *19*, 16287. [CrossRef] [PubMed]
47. Kiebzak, W.P. Application of Euclidean geometry in the assessment of body posture in a sitting position. *Pol. Ann. Med.* **2022**, *29*, 167–171. [CrossRef]

Disclaimer/Publisher's Note: The statements, opinions and data contained in all publications are solely those of the individual author(s) and contributor(s) and not of MDPI and/or the editor(s). MDPI and/or the editor(s) disclaim responsibility for any injury to people or property resulting from any ideas, methods, instructions or products referred to in the content.

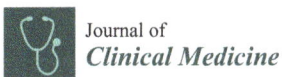

Article

A Comparison of Two Forward Head Posture Corrective Approaches in Elderly with Chronic Non-Specific Neck Pain: A Randomized Controlled Study

Aisha Salim Al Suwaidi [1], Ibrahim M. Moustafa [1,2], Meeyoung Kim [1], Paul A. Oakley [3,4,5] and Deed E. Harrison [3,*]

1. Department of Physiotherapy, College of Health Sciences, University of Sharjah, Sharjah 27272, United Arab Emirates
2. Neuromusculoskeletal Rehabilitation Research Group, Research Institute of Medical and Health Sciences, University of Sharjah, Sharjah 27272, United Arab Emirates
3. CBP Nonprofit (A Spine Research Foundation), Eagle, ID 83616, USA
4. Private Practice, Newmarket, ON L3Y 8Y8, Canada
5. Kinesiology and Health Sciences, York University, Toronto, ON M3J 1P3, Canada
* Correspondence: drdeed@idealspine.com

Abstract: Forward head posture (FHP) is a common postural displacement that is significantly associated with neck pain, with higher risks of having neck pain in female and older populations. This study investigated the effect of two different forward head posture (FHP) interventions in elderly participants with poor posture and non-specific neck pain. Sixty-six elderly participants with a craniovertebral angle (CVA) < 50° were randomized into either a Chiropractic Biophyics® (CBP®) or a standardized exercise based FHP correction group (Standard Group). Both groups were treated for 18 sessions over a 6-week period. A 3-month post-treatment follow-up was also assessed with no further interventions. The CBP group received a mirror image® exercise and a Denneroll™ cervical traction orthotic (DCTO); the standard group performed a protocol of commonly used stretching and strengthening exercises for the neck. Both groups received 30 min of their respective interventions per session. The primary outcome was the CVA, with secondary outcomes including pain intensity, Berg balance score (BBS), head repositioning accuracy (HRA), and cervical range of motion (CROM). After 18 sessions (6 weeks later), the CBP group had statistically significant improvement in the CVA ($p < 0.001$), whereas the standard group did not. In contrast, both groups showed improved functional measurements on the BBS and HRA as well as improved pain intensity. However, at the 3-month follow-up (with no further treatment), there were statistically significant differences favoring the CBP group for all outcomes ($p < 0.001$). The differences in the between group outcomes at the 3-month follow-up indicated that the improved outcomes were maintained in the CBP group, while the standard group experienced regression of the initially improved outcomes at 6 weeks. It is suggested that the improvement in the postural CVA (in the CBP group but not in the standard group) is the driver of superior and maintained pain and functional outcomes.

Keywords: neck pain; craniovertebral angle; forward head posture; exercise; orthotic

Citation: Suwaidi, A.S.A.; Moustafa, I.M.; Kim, M.; Oakley, P.A.; Harrison, D.E. A Comparison of Two Forward Head Posture Corrective Approaches in Elderly with Chronic Non-Specific Neck Pain: A Randomized Controlled Study. *J. Clin. Med.* **2023**, *12*, 542. https://doi.org/10.3390/jcm12020542

Academic Editor: Hideaki Nakajima

Received: 16 November 2022
Revised: 18 December 2022
Accepted: 7 January 2023
Published: 9 January 2023

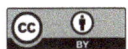

Copyright: © 2023 by the authors. Licensee MDPI, Basel, Switzerland. This article is an open access article distributed under the terms and conditions of the Creative Commons Attribution (CC BY) license (https:// creativecommons.org/licenses/by/ 4.0/).

1. Introduction

Forward head posture (FHP) has been shown to be a common postural displacement, with a conservative estimate of 66% of the patient population [1–3]. Studies have found that there is a significant association between neck pain and forward head posture, with higher risks of having neck pain in female and older populations [4]. It is generally believed that this abnormal posture is associated with the development and persistence of many types of spine pain and various biomechanically driven disorders [5–7]. For example, researchers have identified that FHP posture alters cervical range of motion (ROM) [5], contributes to abnormal balance [6], and alters respiratory efficiency [7]. Many studies indicate that biomechanical dysfunction of the spinal column, as seen with altered sagittal plane alignment, results in the degeneration of the muscles, ligaments, bony structures, and neural elements [8,9].

Therefore, there is an increased interest regarding the understanding and rehabilitation of the sagittal configuration of the cervical spine as a clinical outcome and goal of patient care. Despite the high prevalence of this condition, the available treatment approaches that are directed toward FHP correction are highly variable. The methods vary, from muscle therapy, cervical traction devices, adjustments and/or manipulations of the spinal vertebra, postural re-education, ergonomic modifications, to corrective pillows [5,10–12]. Of interest, while the relationship between FHP and health outcomes has been extensively studied, the literature does not provide specific evidence on whether different methods of FHP correction affect health outcomes differently.

In this regard, Chiropractic BioPhysics® (CBP®) rehabilitation and traditional exercise programs are two of the most well-known corrective techniques, while having different mechanisms to restore proper cervical alignment [11–14]. The CBP technique is a posture-correcting method that depends on stretching the viscous and plastic elements of the longitudinal ligament and intervertebral discs, in addition to effectively stretching the soft tissue through the entire neck area in the direction of normal head and neck postures [11,13]. The technique utilizes both mirror image® adjusting/manipulation, exercises, and the unique extension traction procedures [11–13]. Meanwhile, the mirror image refers to the reversal of the spine and posture in the opposite direction of the present malalignment during the performance of rehabilitative procedures; the unique extension traction methods are for restoring normal lordosis and reducing forward head posture [11,14–17].

A recent systematic review located nine controlled trials featuring Chiropractic BioPhysics (CBP) methods used in the rehabilitation of cervical lordosis (i.e., some form of cervical extension traction) [14]. It was determined that there were "several high-quality controlled clinical trials substantiating that increasing cervical lordosis by extension traction as part of a spinal rehabilitation program reduces pain and disability and improves functional measures and that these improvements are maintained long-term" [14]. Since this review (Oct., 2021), additional trials have emerged, further supporting the clinical importance of increasing the cervical curve and reducing forward head posture using the CBP cervical extension traction methods, but none of these trials have specifically investigated an elderly population [15,16].

On the other hand, exercise programs that aim to correct the FHP misalignment towards an ideal posture using a combination of strengthening and stretching exercises are commonplace for physical interventions provided to correct FHP. Several studies have shown that corrective exercise regimes can improve FHP and potentially related symptoms [10,17–25]. For example, exercise training protocols have resulted in improvements in the craniovertebral angle (CVA) [8,18,24,25], head tilt [17], cranial or cervical range of motion [24], neck disability [24], and pain [8,24]. A systematic review with pooled meta-analysis is necessary to clarify the strength of the effect of such exercises on FHP.

Despite both techniques (CBP vs. conventional physical exercise programs) being frequently used, to our knowledge, no research has been conducted comparing the two FHP rehabilitative techniques in terms of the magnitude of improved head posture and the impact of these different techniques on balance, cervical ROM, cervicocephalic kinesthetic sensibility, and pain. Furthermore, the majority of previous studies that explored the effectiveness of various posture correction procedures were conducted on young individuals [20,23,24] and these results might not be applicable to all age groups, particularly the elderly, due to age-related musculoskeletal and physiological changes [26]. Thus, there remains a gap in the body of knowledge on the effectiveness of the two approaches for treating elderly patients.

Therefore, the goal of this study was to ascertain if two different FHP correction techniques may have different effects on the CVA, balance, cervical range of motion, cervicocephalic kinesthetic sensitivity, and pain in a senior population. The study hypothesis is that the two FHP correction procedures will have different effects on CVA and other management outcomes such as balance, cervical ROM, cervical kinesthetic sensitivity, and pain in the short and intermediate terms.

2. Materials and Methods

A prospective, investigator-blinded, parallel-group, randomized clinical trial was conducted at a senior citizen service center in Sharjah, UAE. Recruitment began after approval was obtained from our University Research *Ethics Committee* (reference number: REC-18-02-27-02-S). A consent form was signed by participants before data collection. The study was registered at ClinicalTrials.gov with registration number: NCT05533853. The study's starting and ending dates were 10 July 2022, through 1 November 2022, respectively.

2.1. Participants

We recruited a sample of 66 elders (>60 years) who reported chronic, non-specific neck discomfort that had persisted for more than three months and was worse than a 3/10 on the visual analogue scale (VAS). Chronic non-specific neck pain was defined as neck pain provoked by neck postures, movements, or pressure for at least 3 months without a known pathology (neurological, trauma-induced, etc.) as the cause of the complaints. Patients were recruited from an outpatient facility at the senior citizen service center, Sharjah. Participants were screened prior to inclusion by measuring their CVA using a photographic method by a physiotherapist. After being screened, all potential participants were invited to undergo a comprehensive assessment by an orthopedist, where any known pathology (neurological, trauma-induced, etc.) as the cause of the complaints was excluded. Participants were included if their CVA was less than 50 degrees [8,27]. Exclusion criteria included neck pain associated with inflammatory, hormonal, and neurological disorders, neck pain related to previous surgery, positive radicular signs consistent with nerve root compression, severe referred pain, severe psychological disorders, and a history of spinal column fracture, spinal tumors and related malignancies, congenital spinal anomalies, or rheumatoid arthritis.

2.2. Randomization

The patients were randomly assigned to the CBP group ($n = 33$) or the standardized exercise-based FHP correction group (standard group) ($n = 33$) by an independent person who selected numbers from sealed envelopes containing numbers chosen by a random number generator. The randomization was restricted to permuted blocks of different sizes to ensure that equal numbers were allocated to each group. Each random permuted block was transferred to a sequence of consecutively numbered, sealed, opaque envelopes that were stored in a locked drawer until required. As each participant formally entered the trial, the researcher opened the next envelope in sequence in the presence of the patient. Participants in the CBP group completed a 6-week-long, 3x per week, total of 18 sessions of the CBP technique, consisting of Denneroll cervical extension traction and mirror image exercises. Participants in the standard group completed a 6-week long, 3x per week, total of 18 sessions of a standardized protocol of stretching and strengthening exercises according to the randomized trial protocol of Harman et al. [1].

2.3. Interventions

Denneroll™ Cervical Traction Orthotic (DCTO)

The CBP group received DCTO (Denneroll Industries (www.denneroll.com, accessed on 1 October 2022) of Sydney, Australia). The patient lies flat on their back (supine) on the ground with their legs extended and arms by their sides. The patient is encouraged to relax while lying on the Denneroll [15,16]. The denneroll was placed on the ground and positioned in the posterior aspect of the neck depending on the area to be addressed, as shown in Figure 1. Participants were screened and tested for tolerance to the slightly extended and posterior head translation position on the device to ensure they were capable of performing this position; while the Denneroll takes the segments of the cervical spine near the apex of the curve to their end range of extension motion, it does not create hyperextension of the skull relative to the torso. The apex of the DCTO was placed in one of three regions based on lateral cervical radiographic displacements of the cervical curve and forward head posture:

(1) In the upper cervical area (C2-C4). This position allows for upper cervical segment extension bending while providing minor anterior head translation (AHT). This placement site was assigned to two participants.
(2) In the mid-cervical area (C4-C6). This position allows for mid-upper cervical extension bending while causing a significant posterior head translation. This placement location was assigned to 8 participants.
(3) Upper thoracic/lower cervical (C6-T1) area. This position allows for lower to intermediate cervical segment extension bending while causing substantial posterior head translation. This placement location was assigned to 23 participants.

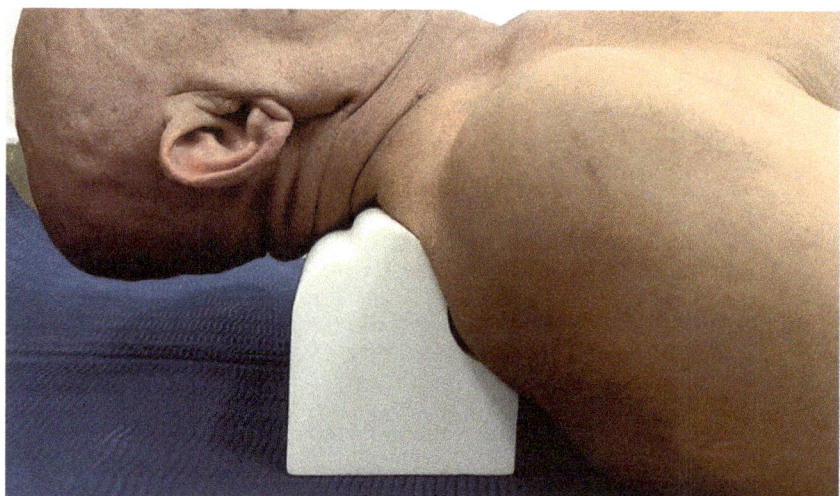

Figure 1. Cervical Denneroll™ traction.

All participants began with 3-min sessions of the DCTO application and were encouraged to extend the duration by 2–3 min each visit until they reached the goal of 15–20 min each session. Mirror image® traction allows for viscoelastic plastic deformation of spinal ligaments as well as correcting the patient's incorrect posture by initiating muscle and ligament creep, resulting in long-term restorative improvement [11].

2.4. Mirror Image Exercises

The patient performed a sequence of mirror image exercises in the sagittal plane to add to the correction of FHP and the cervical curvature. This sequence of maneuvers was first proposed by Fedorchuk [28,29] and included the following steps using a right-handed cartesian coordinate system describing rotations and translations of the head in three dimensions [12]:

(1) Maximum anterior head translation ($+T_zH$) Anterior head translation generates a cervical spine coupling pattern that results in lordosis of the upper cervical spine and kyphosis (curve reversal) of the lower cervical spine.
(2) While maintaining $+T_zH$, maximum head extension ($-R_xH$). Maintaining anterior head translation permits the upper cervical spine to keep its lordosis, while maximal head extension allows the lower cervical spine to progress toward a healthy lordotic curvature.

(3) While maintaining the −RxH, a posterior head translation (−TzH) with a slight inferior compression down the long axis of the spine (−TyH) is initiated. The posterior head translation with compression from this position allows for the head to return to a normal postural position while maintaining the induced cervical lordosis from the previous movements.

The patient held the final position for 10 s before relaxing and repeating it for 20 repetitions. Mirror Image® exercises strengthen weak musculature and lengthen tight musculatures that have adapted to unhealthy posture to correct and maintain corrections in spinal alignment and postural abnormalities [11–13]. Figure 2 depicts a simple bike chain analogy of this sequence of movements and its proposed effect on the sagittal cervical spine alignment. Figure 3 depicts a patient's lateral cervical x-rays showing the change in alignment from neutral with this sequence of movements. A motion x-ray video analysis of a patient performing this procedure is shown in the Supplemental Video attachment.

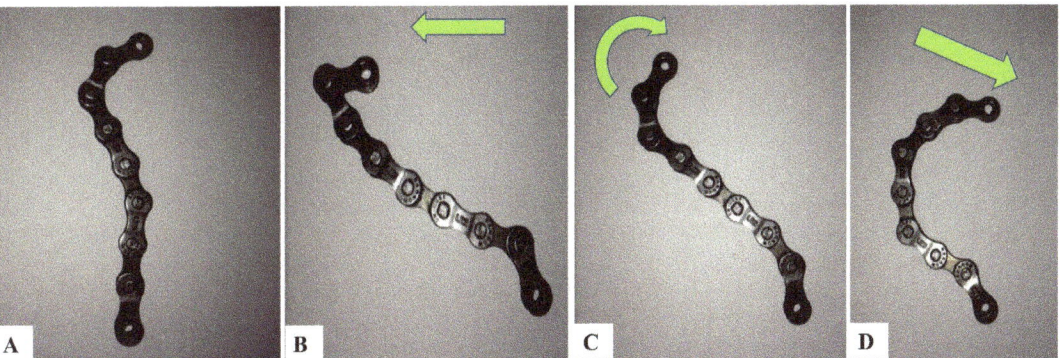

Figure 2. A simple bike chain analogy of the sequence of movements for the CBP group's mirror image exercise and its proposed effect on the sagittal cervical spine alignment. (**A**) depicts neutral alignment with an altered curve; (**B**) depicts forward head posture (+TzH); (**C**) depicts upper neck/head extension (-RxH); and (**D**) depicts the effects of posterior head translation (-TzH) with slight inferior compression (-TyH). Images courtesy of Curtis Fedorchuk, reprinted with permission [28,29].

Video Supplement File S1. A motion x-ray of a patient's lateral cervical spine demonstrating the mirror image exercise in the following sequence: first, forward head posture (+TzH); second, upper neck/head extension (−RxH); and third, posterior head translation (−TzH) with slight inferior compression (−TyH).

2.5. The Standardized Exercise Based FHP Correction Group (Standard Group)

Patients in the standard group were given a posture correction exercise program that included two strengthening exercises (deep cervical flexors and shoulder retractors) and two stretching exercises (cervical extensors and pectoral muscles). The exercise program was conducted according to Harman et al.'s [1] protocol and based on Kendall et al. [2] approach. The rationale for using the exercise protocol and exercise types herein is that it is a known standardized protocol used in randomized trials and clinical settings for the treatment and improvement of FHP in patient populations [1,2,20]. Further, this FHP exercise protocol is the accepted protocol in the senior citizen care center in Sharjah, UAE, where our trial was conducted. The protocol involved the following:

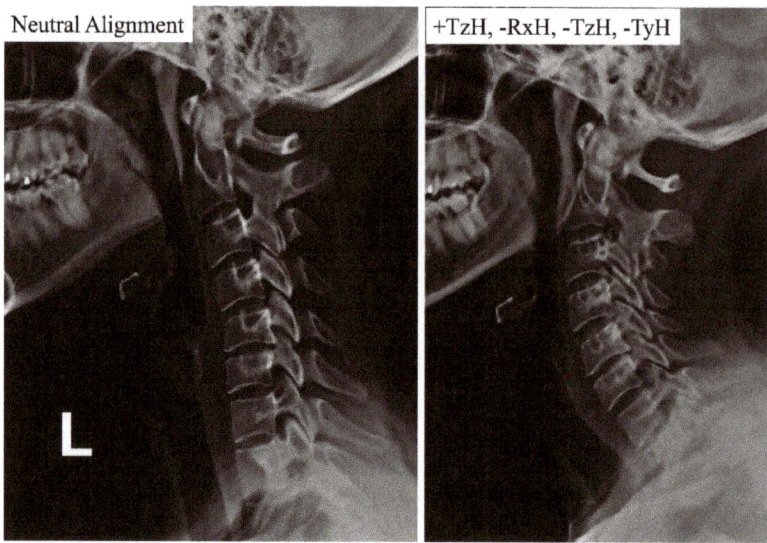

Figure 3. A patient's lateral cervical x-rays are shown in neutral and after the mirror image exercise sequence (+TzH, −RxH, −TzH, −TyH) demonstrating the change in alignment from neutral with this sequence of movements: forward head posture (+TzH), upper neck/head extension (−RxH), followed by posterior head translation (−TzH) with an inferior compression component (−TyH). Images courtesy of Curtis Fedorchuk, reprinted with permission [28,29].

1. Chin tucks were performed while lying supine with the head in touch with the floor, which progressed to lifting the head off the floor in a tucked posture and holding it for varied periods of time (this was to progress by two-second holds starting at two seconds, i.e., 2, 4, 6, and 8 s. During the session, patients completed five chin tuck repetitions and five to seven sets of five chin tucks with a 1-min rest between each set. Figure 4 presents this exercise.
2. Chin drop while sitting to stretch cervical extensors (the progression of this exercise was to drop the chin with hand assistance). The patients were instructed to flex the neck until a good stretch was felt at the base of the head and top of the neck. The patient held the final position for 5 s. This chin drop exercise was repeated a total of 10 times, or as tolerated. A modification of the chin tuck that further emphasizes strengthening of the deep neck flexor muscles is to apply resistance with a hand placed under the tucked chin and apply light downward pressure into the hand, or by adding manual resistance to the forehead using the 5-s hold time approach. Figure 5 demonstrates this exercise maneuver.
3. Pulling the shoulders back using a theraband while standing to strengthen the shoulder retractors. The patient was instructed to squeeze their scapulae together tightly for at least 6 s without elevating or extending their shoulder. The initial progression step was to use weights to do shoulder retraction from a prone posture. The second stage involved the use of elastic resistance and weights. Each progression was carried out by the participants for two weeks. At the consultation, they were moved to the second progression if they could complete three sets of 12 repetitions, with 2 min of rest in between, accurately for appropriate strengthening. Figure 6 demonstrates this exercise maneuver.
4. Every two weeks, participants alternated between unilateral and bilateral pectoralis stretches. The patient was seated comfortably with their hand behind their head for bilateral pectoralis stretching. From this posture, the patient's elbow was pushed up and out to the limit of its possible range. The arm at the affected location was shifted

into abduction and external rotation for unilateral stretching. The end position was maintained for 20–30 s and repeated 3–5 times. For unilateral stretching, the patients were directed to bring their hands up such that their forearms and elbows rested on the side of the doorway. The elbow and shoulder should be at a 90-degree angle. The patient was encouraged to move his or her body toward the opposite side away from the doorway until a stretch was felt anteriorly between the chest and shoulder. Each stretch was performed with slow, steady movements without any bouncing. The same process was repeated on the opposite side. This posture was maintained for 20–30 s and repeated 3–5 times. Two sets of 3–5 repetitions of unilateral self-stretching with a 1-min rest were performed for each patient. Figure 7 shows this exercise maneuver.

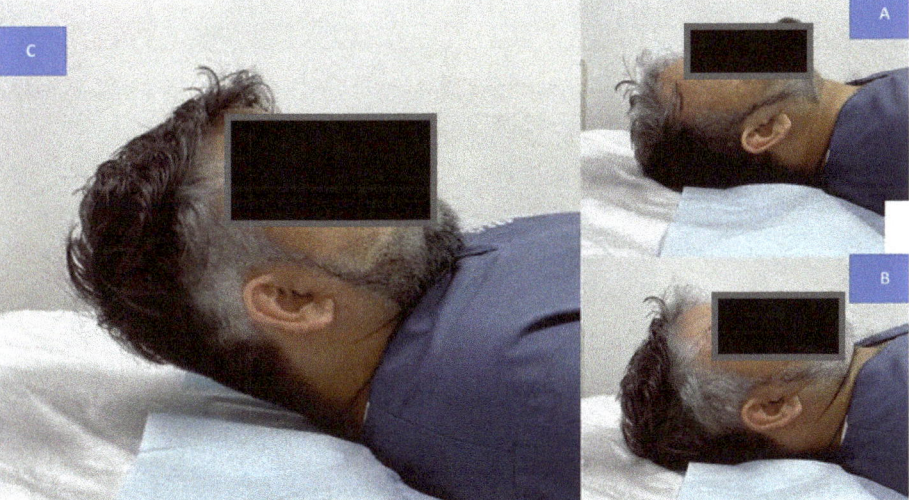

Figure 4. The chin tuck exercise: (**A**) starting position; (**B**) chin tucks performed while lying supine with the posterior aspect of the skull in contact with the floor; (**C**) the head is then lifted off the floor in a tucked posture.

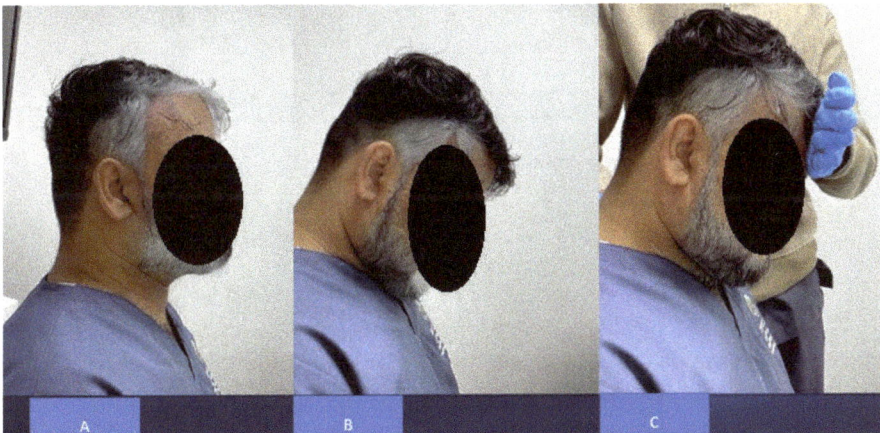

Figure 5. The chin drop exercise: (**A**) the starting position; (**B**) the end stretching position; (**C**) a modification of the chin tuck that further emphasizes strengthening of the deep neck flexor muscles.

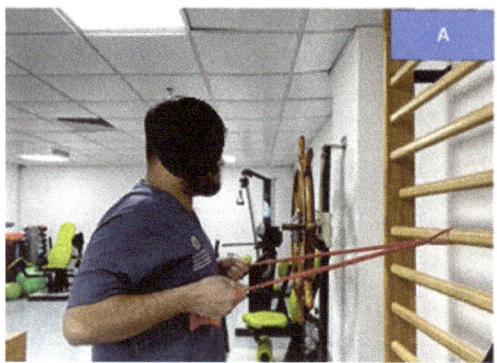
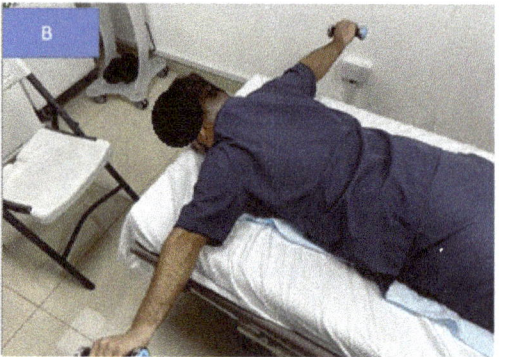

Figure 6. Scapular retractors strengthening exercise: (**A**) pulling the shoulders back using a theraband for resistance while standing to strengthen the shoulder retractors; (**B**) the initial progression step was to use weights to do shoulder retraction from a prone posture.

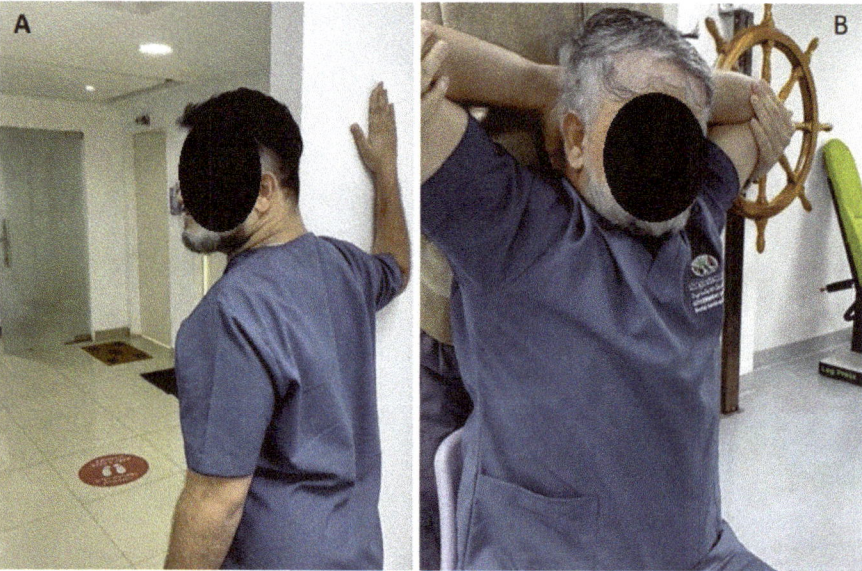

Figure 7. In (**A**) a unilateral pectoralis stretch is shown. In (**B**) a bilateral pectoralis stretch position is shown.

While the CBP group seemingly received an extra intervention (the DCTO plus mirror image exercises), the standard group received more exercise types and number of repetitions. Thus, both groups were exposed to and received similar treatment durations, which were approximately 30 min per session.

2.6. Outcome Measures

A series of outcome measures were obtained at three intervals: (1) baseline, (2) one day following the completion of 18 visits after 6 weeks of treatment, and (3) three months after the participants' 18-session re-evaluation. The sequence of measurements was identical for all participants. The primary outcome measure was the cranio-vertebral angle (*CVA*). Whereas secondary outcomes included (1) neck pain, (2) Berg balance scale (BBS), (3) head repositioning accuracy (HRA), and (4) cervical ROM. All outcome assessments were carried out with the same data collectors, who were blinded to group allocation to prevent potential recorder and ascertainment bias. Participants were blinded to their measurement scores to address potential expectation bias and were instructed not to inform the assessors of their intervention status.

2.6.1. Craniovertebral Angle

The assessment of forward head posture (FHP) was conducted by measuring the craniovertebral angle. If the angle was less than 50 degrees, it was considered to be FHP, as guided by Yip et al.'s study, where the normal range is between 55 and 86 [27]. The CVA as an assessment measurement for FHP has good reliability and excellent validity [30,31]. The measurement technique was duplicated, as in the study by Diab and Moustafa [8], as follows: adhesive markers (8 mm in diameter) were placed on the participant's C7 spinous process and tragus of the ear. The physical therapist observed the participant from the lateral side while standing and then took a picture of the participant from a fixed distance (75 cm) and height (150 cm), then with the help of an application sealed by a password, the angle was measured by placing each vector as following a line from the tragus of the ear to the C7 spinous process and another horizontal line through the C7 spinous process [8]. Figure 8 demonstrates the CVA as used.

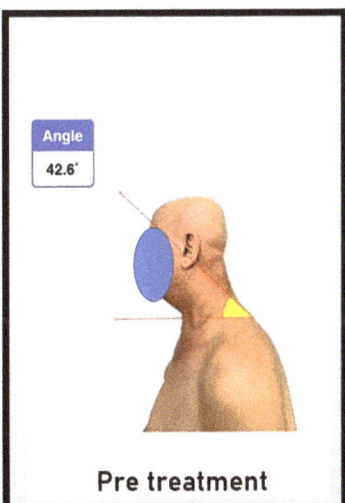 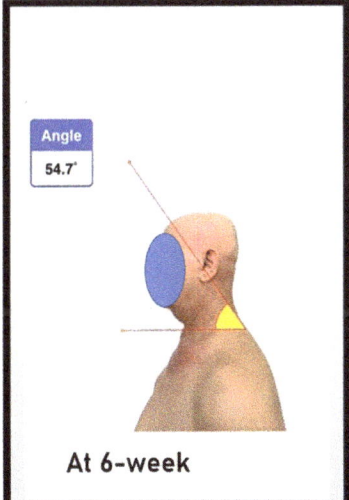 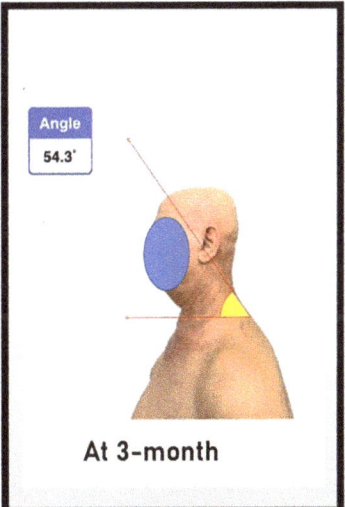

Figure 8. CVA at three intervals: (1) baseline, (2) one day following the completion of 18 visits after 6 weeks of treatment, and (3) three months after the participants' 18-session re-evaluation.

2.6.2. Berg Balance Scale

Balance was measured by the Berg balance scale with a total score of 56; if the score was less than 45, this predicted the risk of falling. The scale has excellent reliability and concurrent validity [32].

2.6.3. Numeric Pain Rating Scale

The numeric pain rating scale (NPRS), where 10 is the worst pain and 0 is no pain, was used to assess pain. It is valid and has moderate reliability in assessing cervical pain [33].

2.6.4. Cervicocephalic Kinesthetic Sensibility

Cervicocephalic kinesthetic sensibility was used to detect alterations in cervical proprioception. The blindfolded subject must be able to accurately relocate the head into a straight-head position after being actively moved to the new maximum position, either in the horizontal or vertical plane. The deep suboccipital muscle is the main contributor to proprioception signaling when vision is occluded. Muscular and articular pain will lead to functional deficits that will affect the kinesthetic findings [34]. The reliability of cervicocephalic kinesthetic sensibility ranges from fair to excellent; however, it is acceptable [35]. The assessment procedure was the same as Ravi et al.'s, and the cervical range of motion instrument (CROM) was used [36]. CROM has good reliability and validity for use in cervicocephalic kinesthetic sensibility measurement [35,36].

2.7. Sample Size Determination

Sample size estimates of mean and standard deviations were collected from previous studies that utilized a similar protocol to our study. The mean differences and standard deviation of the CVA were estimated to be 14° and 12°, respectively, from these studies [14,37–39]. Accordingly, 25 participants for each treatment arm, given a significance level of 5% and statistical power of 80%, were needed in the current study. To compensate for potential participant withdrawal, a 10% increase in sample size was implemented.

2.8. Data Analysis

The statistical procedure depended on the principle of intention-to-treat for between group comparisons. Significance was set to P-values less than 0.05. In order to manage any missing data, multiple imputations were used. Parametric methods for significance testing were determined with Levene's test for equality of variances and the Kolmogorov–Smirnov test, expressing continuous data as means with standard deviation (SD) in text and tables.

In order to follow-up and compare the effects of the two alternative treatments, the results were examined through a two-way analysis of covariance (ANCOVA). The model was working as follows: a group and time were used as a single independent factor, and group × time as an interaction factor. The level of significance used for the study was set at $\alpha = 0.05$. The Pearson correlation coefficient (r) was used to investigate the correlation between FHP and outcome variables. To impute the missing values for both groups, multiple regression models were constructed, including the potentially related variables from the missing data that correlated with that outcome. SPSS version 20.0 software was used for analyzing data (SPSS Inc., Chicago, IL, USA), with normality and equal variance assumptions ensured prior to the analysis.

3. Results

A diagram of patients' retention and randomization throughout the study is shown in Figure 9. One hundred and twenty patients were initially screened. After the screening process, 66 patients were eligible to participate in the study, and 66 (100%) completed the first follow-up at 6 weeks, while 62 of them completed the entire study, including the 3-month follow-up. Three participants in the standard group tested positive for COVID and were unable to make the 3-month follow-up, while one participant in the CBP group had travel conflicts and was unable to complete the 3-month follow-up. See Figure 9. The study design did not include a pre-determined adverse event protocol. However, participants were formally asked during their treatment sessions if they were experiencing any unusual adverse events or increased pain due to the interventions. No adverse events were documented by the treating therapist aside from minimal and transient discomfort in the neck as the patient acclimatized to using the DCTO at the point of cervical spine contact over the apex of the device.

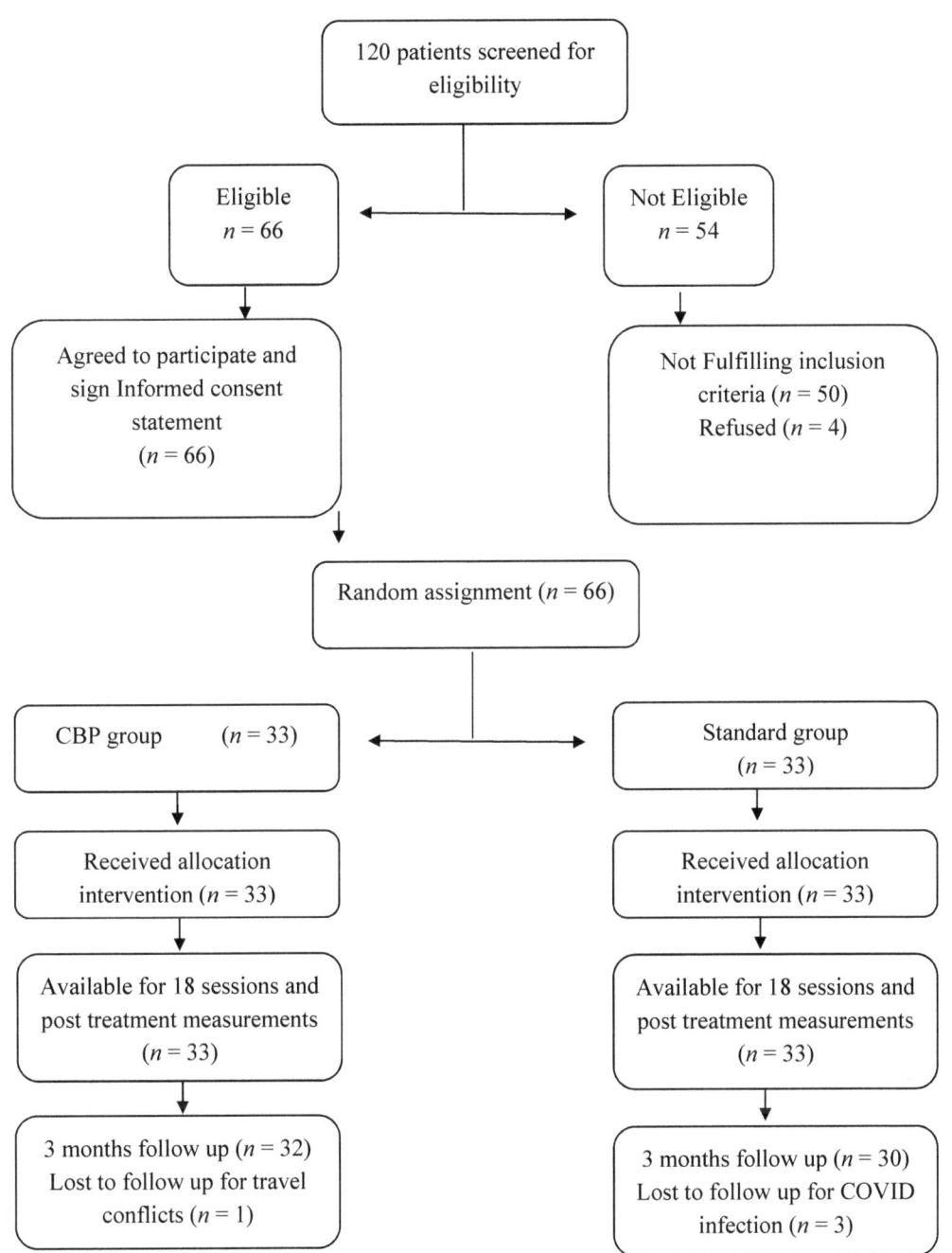

Figure 9. Flow chart of study participants.

The demographic characteristics of the patients are shown in Table 1.

Table 1. Baseline participant demographics. CBP is the group receiving mirror image exercise plus the Denneroll™ cervical traction orthotic (DCTO). The standard group is the group receiving standardized strengthening and stretching exercises to correct FHP. Values are expressed as means ± standard deviation (SD) where indicated.

Demographic Information		CBP Group (n = 33)	Standard Group (n = 33)	p Value
Age (y)		63.5 ± 3	65 ± 4.2	0.09
Weight (kg)		66 ± 10	60 ± 19	0.1
Sex, Marital status				
Male		22 (67%)	20 (60%)	
Female		11 (33%)	13 (40%)	
Single		1 (3%)	2 (7%)	0.3
Married		22 (67%)	20 (60%)	
Separated, divorced, or widowed		10 (30%)	11 (33%)	
Pain duration (%) [Mean ± SD]				
< 1 y		1 (3%)	3 (10%)	
1–2 y		21 (67%)	20 (60%)	0.1
>2 y		10 (30%)	10 (30%)	
Smoking history				
Light smoker		8 (24%)	7 (21%)	
Heavy smoker		0	1	0.2
Non-Smoker		25 (76%)	26 (79%)	

Group Outcomes

The general linear model with repeated measures identified significant group * time effects in favor of the CBP group for the following management outcomes: CVA ($F_{(3.114)} = 131$, $p < 0.001$); pain intensity ($F_{(3.114)} = 54$, $p < 0.001$); HRA right ($F_{(3.114)} = 183$, $p < 0.001$); HRA left ($F_{(3.114)} = 208$, $p < 0.001$); Berg balance score ($F_{(3.114)} = 29.2$, $p < 0.001$); and cervical ROM, $p < 0.001$. However, subsequent analyses indicated that, after 6 weeks of treatment, both treatments were similarly improved in some management outcomes. At 6 weeks, the unpaired *t*-test analyses found insignificant differences between groups for the following parameters: Berg balance score ($p = 0.48$), HRA Right ($p = 0.6$), and HRA left ($p = 0.3$). Tables 2–4 show these details for each variable.

Table 2. The changes in pain and CVA in both groups vs. time. CBP = CBP group; standard = standard exercise groups; CVA = craniovertebral angle; pain intensity is 0–10 where 0 is no pain and 10 is incapacitated; G = group; T = time; G vs. T = group vs. time; all values are expressed as means ± standard deviation; [] = 95% confidence interval; *p*-Value = statistical significance; * = statistically significant difference.

		Baseline	6-Weeks	3-Month Follow-Up	p-Value		
					G	T	G vs. T
CVA	CBP G	41.4 ± 2.6	54.9 ± 3.2	54 ± 2.6	<0.001 * F = 76 Partial Eta squared = 0.5	<0.001 * F = 248 Partial Eta squared = 0.8	<0.001 * F = 131 Partial Eta squared = 0.7
	Standard G	42.7 ± 3.2	45 ± 2.4	45.6 ± 5.9			
	p-Value 95% C.I.	0.08 [−2.7, 0.2]	<0.001 * [8.7, 11.1]	<0.001 * [6.1, 10.7]			
Pain intensity	CBP G	4.7 ± 0.8	1.1 ± 0.7	0.5 ± 0.8	<0.001 * F = 209 Partial Eta squared = 0.7	<0.001 * F = 244 Partial Eta squared = 0.8	<0.001 * F = 54 Partial Eta squared = 0.6
	Standard G	5.3 ± 1.5	2.9 ± 1.2	4.3 ± 1			
	p-Value 95% C.I.	0.08 [−1.19, 0.008]	<0.001 * [−2.2, −1.2]	<0.001 * [−4.2, −3.2]			

Table 3. The changes in the Berg balance score for balance assessment and HRA in both groups vs. time. CBP = CBP group; standard: standard exercise group; HRA = head repositioning accuracy; G = group; T = time; G vs. T = group vs. time; all values are expressed as means ± standard deviation; C.I. [] = 95% confidence interval; p-Value = statistical significance; * = statistically significant difference.

		Baseline	6-Weeks	3-Month Follow-Up	p-Value G	p-Value T	p-Value G vs. T
Berg Balance Score	CBP G	43 ± 2.1	48.1 ± 3	48.2 ± 3.2	<0.001 * F = 28.3 Partial Eta squared = 0.3	<0.001 * F = 91.3 Partial Eta squared = 0.6	<0.001 * F = 29.2 Partial Eta squared = 0.7
	Standard G	42.3 ± 2.2	44.6 ± 1.7	43.8 ± 2.1			
p-Value C.I.		0.2 [−0.49, 1.7]	0.48 [2.2, 4.7]	<0.001 * [2.9, 5.5]			
HRA Right	CBP G	3.4 ± 0.6	2.1 ± 0.9	0.3 ± 0.5	<0.001 * F = 43 Partial Eta squared = 0.5	<0.001 * F = 193 Partial Eta squared = 0.8	<0.001 * F = 183 Partial Eta squared = 0.8
	Standard G	3 ± 0.9	2.2 ± 1.1	2.7 ± 1			
p-Value C.I.		0.06 [0.023, −0.77]	0.6 [−0.3, 0.2]	<0.001 * [−2.5, −2.1]			
HRA Left	CBP G	3.8 ± 1.4	2.2 ± 1.4	.4 ± 1.1	<0.001 * F = 20.3 Partial Eta squared = 0.2	<0.001 * F = 184 Partial Eta squared = 0.8	<0.001 * F = 208 Partial Eta squared = 0.8
	Standard G	3.2 ± 0.9	2.5 ± 1.6	2.9 ± 1.2			
p-Value C.I.		0.07 [0.02, −1.1]	0.3 [−0.6, 0.07]	<0.001 * [−2.8, −2.1]			

Table 4. The changes in ROM outcomes in both groups vs. time. The values are mean ± standard deviation. CBP = CBP group; standard: standard exercise group; G = group, T = time, C.I. [] = 95% confidence interval, p-Value = statistical significance; * = statistically significant difference.

		Baseline	6-Weeks	3-Month Follow-Up	p-Value G	p-Value T	p-Value G vs. T
CROM lateral flexion right	CBP G	36.9 ± 2.8	42.4 ± 2	42.1 ± 2.2	<0.001 * F = 44.2 Partial Eta squared = 0.5	<0.001 * F = 132 Partial Eta squared = 0.6	<0.001 * F = 44.9 Partial Eta squared = 0.5
	Standard G	37.2 ± 2	40.6 ± 3	37.4 ± 3.8			
p-Value C.I.		0.5 [−0.9, 1.3]	<0.008 * [0.5, 3.1]	<0.001 * [3.6, 5.7]			
CROM lateral flexion left	CBP G	37.5 ± 2.3	42.6 ± 1.8	42.2 ± 2.6	<0.001 * F = 23 Partial Eta squared = 0.3	<0.001 * F = 104 Partial ETA squared = 0.7	<0.001 * F = 40 Partial Eta squared = 0.5
	Standard G	37.1 ± 2.7	40.1 ± 2.6	37.8 ± 2.5			
p-Value C.I.		0.4 [−0.6, 1.4]	<0.001 * [0.8, 3.1]	<0.001 * [3.3, 5.4]			
CROM rotation right	CBP G	61.1 ± 5.3	71.40 ± 2.3	70.8 ± 4	<0.001 * F = 24 Partial Eta squared = 0.2	<0.001 * F = 150 Partial Eta squared = 0.8	<0.001 * F = 72 Partial Eta squared = 0.7
	Standard G	62.3 ± 5.6	63.6 ± 4.8	62 ± 6.1			
p-Value C.I.		0.1 [−2.8, 2.5]	<0.001 * [5.8, 9.6]	<0.001 * [6.4, 11.2]			
CROM rotation left	CBP G	62.15 ± 4.5	70.7 ± 3.9	70 ± 5.7	<0.001 * F = 24.6 Partial Eta squared = 0.3	F = 73 Partial Eta squared = 0.7	F = 46 Partial Eta squared = 0.6
	Standard G	60.9 ± 6.4	63.4 ± 4.5	61.2 ± 6.7			
p-Value C.I.		0.3 [−1.4, 4.2]	<0.001 * [5.2, 9.1]	<0.001 * [6, 11.4]			

In contrast to the 6-week outcomes, the between-group analyses at the 3-month follow-up revealed statistically significant between-group differences for all the management variables. Tables 2–4 show these details for each variable.

Correlations (Pearson's r) between the amount of change in CVA angle and the amount of change in all measured outcomes at 3-month follow up compared to the initial scores are shown in Table 5. All measured variable change scores in both groups were moderately to strongly negatively correlated (pain intensity and HRA left and right) and positively correlated (all other variables) to the amount of change in the CVA, indicating that as FHP decreased, the various outcome variables were found to be improved. Specially, a negative correlation between CVA and pain and HRA indicates that as CVA increases (FHP decreases) pain intensity and HRA decrease. See Table 5 for details.

Table 5. Correlations (Pearson's r) between the amount of change in CVA angle and the amount of change of all measured outcomes (3-month follow-up scores and initial scores).

Correlation between Variables	Δ CVA CBP Group r (p Value) n = 33	Δ CVA Standard Group r (p Value) n = 33
ΔPain intensity	−0.7 (<0.001)	−0.67 (<0.001)
ΔBerg Balance Score	0.64 (<0.001)	0.49 (<0.001)
Δ Head repositioning accuracy (Right)	−0.69 (<0.001)	−0.71 (<0.001)
Δ Head repositioning accuracy (Left)	−0.72 (<0.001)	−0.72 (<0.001)
Δ CROM lateral flexion Right	0.49 (<0.001)	0.61 (<0.001)
Δ CROM lateral flexion Left	0.57 (<0.001)	0.52 (<0.001)
Δ CROM rotation right	0.49 (<0.001)	0.61 (<0.001)
Δ CROM rotation left	0.57 (<0.001)	0.52 (<0.001)

CVA = craniovertebral angle; Δ = change.

4. Discussion

Unexpectedly, there was a significant difference between the groups regarding the CVA, favoring the CBP group. However, the patient perceptive outcomes of neck pain and the functional outcome measures (berg balance, HRA, and cervical ROM) showed fewer differences between the groups at 6 weeks of treatment. In contrast, after 3 months of follow-up with no further interventions, the standard exercise group's improvements regressed back to baseline values, while the CBP group showed sustained improved management outcomes for all variables. Thus, these contrasting trends of changes in outcomes at 3 months after the treatment between our two groups may indicate that our hypothesis is supported, namely, that using different FHP correction techniques will differently affect the amount of CVA and other related outcomes.

4.1. Sagittal Cervical Alignment

The improvement in FHP and cervical lordotic curve recorded by the CBP group was anticipated in as much as previous investigations have identified that this DCTO does indeed improve cervical lordosis and reduce anterior head translation [37–39]. Sustained extension loading on devices like the Denneroll causes stretching of the visco-elastic tissues (discs, ligaments, and muscles) of the cervical spine in the direction of the neutral head and neck posture and increased lordosis; this is the likely explanation and rationale for sustained extension loading restoring the cervical lordosis and improving anterior head translation [37–41].

There was considerable improvement in the CBP group in comparison with the standard group, and our study identified a similar mean improvement in the CVA compared to a previous investigation using the DCTO [37]. Interestingly, the similar improvement in the CVA in the current study compared to the previous investigation seems contradictory in as much as only 18 sessions were used herein on the Denneroll, while the previous investigation used 30 sessions [37]. The fact that 60% of the treatments yielded similar postural changes may be attributed to the elderly age range and decreased elastic recovery in comparison to younger age groups. Previously, Oliver and Twomey [42] identified that elderly cadaveric spines obtained more viscoelastic creep deformation and less elastic recovery compared to younger aged specimens under the same extension loading scenario. It is important to understand the role of collagen and how age-related changes to collagen matrices are linked to the declining mechanical properties of aging bones and joints [43,44]. Physical and biochemical changes occur in collagen with increasing age, resulting in decreased extensibility. These changes include an increased formation of intramolecular and intermolecular cross-links that restrict the ability of the collagen fibers to move past each other as tissue length changes [45]. Another possible explanation for the same magnitude of improvement in the CVA in 40% fewer treatment sessions could be the effectiveness of the new mirror image exercise sequence as performed herein. Problematically, we did not have a group that compared this exercise alone, so it remains unknown which intervention created the most improvement in the CVA.

Regardless of which intervention improved the CVA more significantly in the CBP group, we suggest it is likely that the improvement of cervical sagittal alignment is the main modulator for the enhanced and maintained changes in the pain and functional outcome measures in our CBP group, as supported by the strong correlation between the amount of change in the CVA in both groups and measurement outcomes at the two intervals of re-assessment. It is likely that the continuous asymmetrical loading from altered posture (forward head posture) may be the possible explanation for the decline in functional status for the control group at 3 months follow-up, as supported by predictions from experimental and biomechanical spine-posture modeling studies [46,47], surgical outcomes [48,49], and large cohort investigations [50]. Abnormal posture is considered a predisposing factor for pain because it elicits abnormal stresses and strains in many structures, including bone, intervertebral discs, facet joints, musculotendinous tissues, and neural elements [46–52].

The participants in our standard exercise group completed a 6-week-long, 3 x per week, 18-session protocol of standardized stretching and strengthening exercises according to the randomized trial protocol of Harman et al. [1]. We followed this methodology because it built on the known protocols from Kendall et al. [2], and it has been documented that these types of standardized stretching and strengthening exercises are effective at reducing FHP and improving patient cervical spine conditions in clinical trials [1,2,20]. Thus, this standard treatment of exercises provided an established evidence-based protocol to compare and contrast the CBP group's treatment to. There are several other exercise systems in the literature designed to improve FHP abnormalities (Pilates [24], McKenzie [23], biofeedback methods [22], and Feldenkrais techniques [53]) that we could have used to compare the CBP group outcomes to. However, we elected to use the standard exercises herein, as they are commonly used in clinical settings, have documented results in clinical trials, and this is the accepted protocol that is actively used in our university's senior care center. However, to our knowledge, none of these protocols have been uniquely investigated in an elderly population with defined FHP and neck pain such as in our investigation, making our trial and results unique.

4.2. Balance, Pain, Cervicocephalic Kinesthetic Sensibility and ROM

Importantly, after restoring the proper cervical sagittal alignment, there were recorded improvements in a wide range of main complaints that were not just related to neck pain; balance, ROM, and repositioning accuracy were all reported to have improved. According to the most recent research, neck pain relief following cervical spine therapy, including better radiographic sagittal plane alignment, shows a clear causal relationship. For instance, Harrison et al. statistically differentiate symptomatic neck pain patients from asymptomatic volunteers based on discriminant analysis based on the cervical sagittal alignment [54]. According to McAviney et al. [55], individuals with neck curves (C2-7 posterior tangents) less than 20° had a two-fold increased risk of suffering neck discomfort, and those with curves less than 0° (straight and kyphotic curves) had an 18-fold increased risk. Neck pain is also linked to a forward head posture, which can happen with lordosis loss [49].

A growing body of research suggests that the FHP and balance are directly related. For instance, Moustafa et al. found a significant association between the CVA and the postural stability index as a measure of balance and posture stability [56]. In terms of ROM improvements, our findings are in line with the findings of Darnel's research [57], which stated that "correct mechanical alignment is crucial for cervical joint performance". These results are generally consistent with those of White and Panjabi [58], who claimed that coupled motions in the cervical spine rely on a variety of variables, including the posture of the spine, the geometry of the individual vertebrae, and the orientation of the facet joints. Additionally, Miyazaki et al. [59] performed a retrospective study employing kinetic magnetic resonance imaging looking at the connection between disc degeneration and changes in the sagittal alignments of the cervical spine. According to them, when the alignment changed from normal to a cervical lordotic curvature that was smaller, the segmental translational motion and angular displacements tended to decrease at all levels [59].

4.3. Limitations

As with all investigations, our study has some limitations, each of which lends itself to a future investigation. A primary limitation was that our sample was a convenient sample rather than a random sample of the entire aging population. Second, we did not include a natural history group, and we did not assess the effects of different numbers of treatment interventions to identify the optimum frequency and duration of treatment in seniors with FHP and neck pain. Thus, it remains to be seen what effect a greater frequency and number of traction sessions will produce and what effect the Denneroll would have on improvement of altered posture alignment in disorders other than chronic neck pain in the elderly population. Third, we used a combined treatment approach of Denneroll extension traction with a new sagittal plane mirror image exercise sequence, and we were not able to discern the effects on the CVA and outcome measures from each individual therapeutic intervention. Additionally, despite better outcomes in the CBP group, clinically they remained at an average CVA value that is on the cusp of normal [27]. Therefore, in practice, many of these patients would require continued treatment to correct the CVA to below the normative threshold. It is yet to be determined if this would translate into continued outcome improvements. Likewise, this investigation used a relatively short duration of follow-up at 3 months; it is therefore not known how long the improvements in the CBP group would remain. Lastly, the results of the current RCT do not indicate the superiority of the CBP technique for postural correction in comparison to other FHP corrective methodological systems. There are several other postural corrective techniques used in conservative care of patients (Pilates [24], McKenzie [23], Biofeedback [22], and Feldenkrais [53] techniques for examples), and these techniques should be looked at in future randomized trials to identify their effects on the CVA, pain, balance, and cervical spine mobility in elderly populations in an effort to identify the optimum course of treatment for seniors presenting with neck pain, disability, and abnormal FHP.

4.4. Conclusions

This study demonstrated that although both the CBP and standardized exercise-based FHP correction groups demonstrated initial immediate (post-intervention) improved outcomes, the CBP group that included use of the DCTO resulted in greater immediate improved outcomes and also a maintenance of improved outcomes at the 3-month follow-up. The standard FHP exercise group experienced regression of the improved outcomes at the 3-month follow-up. It is suggested that the improvement in the postural CVA (in the CBP group but not in the standard exercise group) is the driver of superior and maintained pain and functional outcomes at final follow-up. Therefore, clinical treatments that are known to improve forward head posture should be added to the clinical armamentarium for the rehabilitation of properly selected seniors with chronic neck pain and forward head posture.

Supplementary Materials: The following supporting information can be downloaded at: https://www.mdpi.com/article/10.3390/jcm12020542/s1, Video S1: Mirror image sagittal plane exercise.

Author Contributions: A.S.A.S., I.M.M., M.K. and A.S.A.S. conceived the research idea and participated in its design; A.S.A.S., I.M.M., M.K., A.S.A.S., P.A.O. and D.E.H. All contributed to the statistical analysis; A.S.A.S., I.M.M., M.K. and A.S.A.S. participated in the data collection and study supervision; I.M.M., P.A.O. and D.E.H. All contributed to the interpretation of the results and wrote the drafts. All authors have read and approved the final version of the manuscript and agree with the order of presentation of the authors. All authors have read and agreed to the published version of the manuscript.

Funding: Cervical Dennerolls for use in this trial were supplied by CBP Nonprofit, Inc. Deed E. Harrison is President of CBP Nonprofit and is a member of a 13-member board that approves funding of clinical trials. Deed Harrison's role as a senior author and conflicts of interest are outlined below in the conflicts of interest section.

Institutional Review Board Statement: The research was conducted in accordance with the Senior Citizens Services Department and approved by the Research Institute of Medical & Health Sciences of the University of Sharjah (reference number: REC-18-02-27-02-S). The consent form was signed by participants prior to data collection, we also followed the CONSORT guidelines. The study was registered at ClinicalTrials.gov with registration number: NCT05533853.

Informed Consent Statement: All participant's pictures in the study were after written informed consent was signed and obtained.

Data Availability Statement: The datasets analyzed in the current study are available from the corresponding author on reasonable request.

Conflicts of Interest: PAO is a paid consultant for CBP NonProfit, Inc. DEH teaches is the CEO of Chiropractic BioPhysics, owns the registered trademark, teaches rehabilitation methods, and sells products used in this manuscript for patient rehabilitation to physicians in the USA. All the other authors declare that they have no competing interests.

References

1. Harman, K.; Hubley-Kozey, C.L.; Butler, H. Effectiveness of an Exercise Program to Improve Forward Head Posture in Normal Adults: A Randomized, Controlled 10-Week Trial. *J. Man. Manip. Ther.* **2005**, *13*, 163–176. [CrossRef]
2. Kendall, F.P.; McCreary, E.K.; Provance, P.G.; Rodgers, M.M.I.; Romani, W.A. *Muscles: Testing and Function, with Posture and Pain*; LWW: Baltimore, MD, USA, 2014.
3. Griegel-Morris, P.; Larson, K.; Mueller-Klaus, K.; Oatis, C.A. Incidence of Common Postural Abnormalities in the Cervical, Shoulder, and Thoracic Regions and Their Association with Pain in Two Age Groups of Healthy Subjects. *Phys. Ther.* **1992**, *72*, 425–431. [CrossRef] [PubMed]
4. Mahmoud, N.F.; Hassan, K.A.; Abdelmajeed, S.F.; Moustafa, I.M.; Silva, A.G. The Relationship Between Forward Head Posture and Neck Pain: A Systematic Review and Meta-Analysis. *Curr. Rev. Musculoskelet. Med.* **2019**, *12*, 562–577. [CrossRef]
5. Quek, J.; Pua, Y.H.; Clark, R.A.; Bryant, A.L. Effects of Thoracic Kyphosis and Forward Head Posture on Cervical Range of Motion in Older Adults. *Man. Ther.* **2013**, *18*, 65–71. [CrossRef]
6. Lee, J.H. Effects of Forward Head Posture on Static and Dynamic Balance Control. *J. Phys. Ther. Sci.* **2016**, *28*, 274–277. [CrossRef]

7. Koseki, T.; Kakizaki, F.; Hayashi, S.; Nishida, N.; Itoh, M. Effect of Forward Head Posture on Thoracic Shape and Respiratory Function. *J. Phys. Ther. Sci.* **2019**, *31*, 63–68. [CrossRef] [PubMed]
8. Diab, A.A.; Moustafa, I.M. The Efficacy of Forward Head Correction on Nerve Root Function and Pain in Cervical Spondylotic Radiculopathy: A Randomized Trial. *Clin. Rehabil.* **2012**, *26*, 351–361. [CrossRef]
9. Ling, F.P.; Chevillotte, T.; Leglise, A.; Thompson, W.; Bouthors, C.; Le Huec, J.C. Which parameters are relevant in sagittal balance analysis of the cervical spine? A literature review. *Eur. Spine J.* **2018**, *27* (Suppl. S1), 8–15. [CrossRef]
10. Ruivo, R.M.; Pezarat-Correia, P.; Carita, A.I. Effects of a Resistance and Stretching Training Program on Forward Head and Protracted Shoulder Posture in Adolescents. *J. Manip. Physiol. Ther.* **2017**, *40*, 1–10. [CrossRef]
11. Oakley, P.A.; Moustafa, I.M.; Harrison, D.E. Restoration of Cervical and Lumbar Lordosis: CBP® Methods Overview. In *Spinal Deformities in Adolescents, Adults and Older Adults*; IntechOpen: London, UK, 2021.
12. Harrison, D.D.; Janik, T.J.; Harrison, G.R.; Troyanovich, S.; Harrison, D.E.; Harrison, S.O. Chiropractic biophysics technique: A linear algebra approach to posture in chiropractic. *J. Manip. Physiol. Ther.* **1996**, *19*, 525–535.
13. Oakley, P.A.; Harrison, D.D.; Harrison, D.E.; Haas, J.W. Evidence-Based Protocol for Structural Rehabilitation of the Spine and Posture: Review of Clinical Biomechanics of Posture (CBP) Publications. *J. Can. Chiropr. Assoc.* **2005**, *49*, 270–296. [PubMed]
14. Oakley, P.A.; Ehsani, N.N.; Moustafa, I.M.; Harrison, D.E. Restoring Cervical Lordosis by Cervical Extension Traction Methods in the Treatment of Cervical Spine Disorders: A Systematic Review of Controlled Trials. *J. Phys. Ther. Sci.* **2021**, *33*, 784–794. [CrossRef] [PubMed]
15. Moustafa, I.M.; Diab, A.A.; Harrison, D.E. The Efficacy of Cervical Lordosis Rehabilitation for Nerve Root Function and Pain in Cervical Spondylotic Radiculopathy: A Randomized Trial with 2-Year Follow-Up. *J. Clin. Med.* **2022**, *11*, 6515. [CrossRef] [PubMed]
16. Moustafa, I.M.; Diab, A.A.M.; Harrison, D.E. Does Improvement towards a Normal Cervical Sagittal Configuration Aid in the Management of Lumbosacral Radiculopathy: A Randomized Controlled Trial. *J. Clin. Med.* **2022**, *11*, 5768. [CrossRef]
17. Ruivo, R.M.; Carita, A.I.; Pezarat-Correia, P. The Effects of Training and Detraining after an 8 Month Resistance and Stretching Training Program on Forward Head and Protracted Shoulder Postures in Adolescents: Randomised Controlled Study. *Man. Ther.* **2016**, *21*, 76–82. [CrossRef]
18. Diab, A.A. The Role of Forward Head Correction in Management of Adolescent Idiopathic Scoliotic Patients: A Randomized Controlled Trial. *Clin. Rehabil.* **2012**, *26*, 1123–1132. [CrossRef]
19. Mulet, M.; Decker, K.L.; Look, J.O.; Lenton, P.A.; Schiffman, E.L. A Randomized Clinical Trial Assessing the Efficacy of Adding 6 x 6 Exercises to Self-Care for the Treatment of Masticatory Myofascial Pain. *J. Orofac. Pain* **2007**, *21*, 318–328.
20. Im, B.; Kim, Y.; Chung, Y.; Hwang, S. Effects of Scapular Stabilization Exercise on Neck Posture and Muscle Activation in Individuals with Neck Pain and Forward Head Posture. *J. Physical. Ther. Sci.* **2015**, *28*, 951–955. [CrossRef]
21. Jang, H.J.; Kim, M.J.; Kim, S.Y. Effect of Thorax Correction Exercises on Flexed Posture and Chest Function in Older Women with Age-Related Hyperkyphosis. *J. Phys. Ther. Sci.* **2015**, *27*, 1161–1164. [CrossRef]
22. Kang, D.Y. Deep Cervical Flexor Training with a Pressure Biofeedback Unit Is an Effective Method for Maintaining Neck Mobility and Muscular Endurance in College Students with Forward Head Posture. *J. Phys. Ther. Sci.* **2015**, *27*, 3207–3210. [CrossRef]
23. Kang, J.-I.; Jeong, D.-K.; Choi, H. The Effect of Feedback Respiratory Exercise on Muscle Activity, Craniovertebral Angle, and Neck Disability Index of the Neck Flexors of Patients with Forward Head Posture. *J. Phys. Ther. Sci.* **2016**, *28*, 2477–2481. [CrossRef] [PubMed]
24. Lee, S.M.; Lee, C.H.; O'Sullivan, D.; Jung, J.H.; Park, J.J. Clinical Effectiveness of a Pilates Treatment for Forward Head Posture. *J. Phys. Ther. Sci.* **2016**, *28*, 2009–2013. [CrossRef] [PubMed]
25. Seidi, F.; Rajabi, R.; Ebrahimi, I.; Alizadeh, M.H.; Minoonejad, H. The Efficiency of Corrective Exercise Interventions on Thoracic Hyper-Kyphosis Angle. *J. Back Musculoskelet. Rehabil.* **2014**, *27*, 7–16. [CrossRef] [PubMed]
26. Ikegami, S.; Uehara, M.; Tokida, R.; Nishimura, H.; Sakai, N.; Horiuchi, H.; Kato, H.; Takahashi, J. Cervical Spinal Alignment Change Accompanying Spondylosis Exposes Harmonization Failure with Total Spinal Balance: A Japanese Cohort Survey Randomly Sampled from a Basic Resident Registry. *J. Clin. Med.* **2021**, *10*, 5797. [CrossRef]
27. Yip, C.H.T.; Chiu, T.T.W.; Poon, A.T.K. The relationship between head posture and severity and disability of patients with neck pain. *Man. Ther.* **2008**, *13*, 148–154. [CrossRef]
28. Fedorchuk, C. Cervical Coupling Patterns following head retraction with compression to neutral: A Prospective Study. In Proceedings of the 39th CBP Annual Convention, Scottsdale, AZ, USA, 13–15 October 2017.
29. Fedorchuk, C.; Lightstone, D.; Comer, R. Radiographic stress analysis to determine the proper coupling patterns of the cervical spine prior to intervention. In Proceedings of the 2nd International Conference on Medical Imaging and Case Reports (MICR) 2019, Newton, Boston, MA, USA, 20–22 November 2019.
30. SolakoÄa&lu, Ö.; Yalçın, P.; Dinçer, G. The Effects of Forward Head Posture on Expiratory Muscle Strength in Chronic Neck Pain Patients: A Cross-Sectional Study. *Turk. J. Phys. Med. Rehabil.* **2020**, *66*, 161–168. [CrossRef]
31. Subbarayalu, A.V. Measurement of Craniovertebral Angle by the Modified Head Posture Spinal Curvature Instrument: A Reliability and Validity Study. *Physiother. Theory Pract.* **2016**, *32*, 144–152. [CrossRef]
32. Pickenbrock, H.M.; Diel, A.; Zapf, A. A Comparison between the Static Balance Test and the Berg Balance Scale: Validity, Reliability, and Comparative Resource Use. *Clin. Rehabil.* **2016**, *30*, 288–293. [CrossRef]

33. Young, I.A.; Dunning, J.; Butts, R.; Mourad, F.; Cleland, J.A. Reliability, Construct Validity, and Responsiveness of the Neck Disability Index and Numeric Pain Rating Scale in Patients with Mechanical Neck Pain without Upper Extremity Symptoms. *Physiother. Theory Pract.* **2019**, *35*, 1328–1335. [CrossRef]
34. Rix, G.D.; Bagust, J. Cervicocephalic Kinesthetic Sensibility in Patients with Chronic, Nontraumatic Cervical Spine Pain. *Arch. Phys. Med. Rehabil.* **2001**, *82*, 911–919. [CrossRef]
35. Lee, H.Y.; Teng, C.C.; Chai, H.M.; Wang, S.F. Test-Retest Reliability of Cervicocephalic Kinesthetic Sensibility in Three Cardinal Planes. *Man. Ther.* **2006**, *11*, 61–68. [CrossRef] [PubMed]
36. Reddy, R.S.Y.; Maiya, A.G.; Rao, S.K. Effect of age on cervicocephalic kinesthetic sensibiity. *Int. J. Curr. Res. Rev.* **2011**, *3*, 42–48.
37. Moustafa, I.M.; Diab, A.A.; Hegazy, F.; Harrison, D.E. Does Improvement towards a Normal Cervical Sagittal Configuration Aid in the Management of Cervical Myofascial Pain Syndrome: A 1- Year Randomized Controlled Trial. *BMC Musculoskelet. Disord.* **2018**, *19*, 396. [CrossRef] [PubMed]
38. Moustafa, I.M.; Diab, A.A.; Harrison, D.E. The Effect of Normalizing the Sagittal Cervical Configuration on Dizziness, Neck Pain, and Cervicocephalic Kinesthetic Sensibility: A 1-Year Randomized Controlled Study. *Eur. J. Phys. Rehabil. Med.* **2017**, *53*, 57–71. [CrossRef] [PubMed]
39. Moustafa, I.M.; Diab, A.A.; Taha, S.; Harrison, D.E. Addition of a Sagittal Cervical Posture Corrective Orthotic Device to a Multimodal Rehabilitation Program Improves Short- and Long-Term Outcomes in Patients With Discogenic Cervical Radiculopathy. *Arch. Phys. Med. Rehabil.* **2016**, *97*, 2034–2044. [CrossRef] [PubMed]
40. Harrison, D.E.; Harrison, D.D.; Betz, J.J.; Janik, T.J.; Holland, B.; Colloca, C.J.; Haas, J.W. Increasing the Cervical Lordosis with Chiropractic Biophysics Seated Combined Extension-Compression and Transverse Load Cervical Traction with Cervical Manipulation: Nonrandomized Clinical Control Trial. *J. Manip. Physiol. Ther.* **2003**, *26*, 139–151, Erratum in *J. Manip. Physiol. Ther.* **2005**, *28*, 214. [CrossRef]
41. Harrison, D.E.; Cailliet, R.; Harrison, D.D.; Janik, T.J.; Holland, B. A New 3-Point Bending Traction Method for Restoring Cervical Lordosis and Cervical Manipulation: A Nonrandomized Clinical Controlled Trial. *Arch. Phys. Med. Rehabil.* **2002**, *83*, 447–453. [CrossRef]
42. Oliver, M.J.; Twomey, L.T. Extension creep in the lumbar spine. *Clin. Biomech.* **1995**, *10*, 363–368. [CrossRef]
43. Jackson, A.; Gu, W. Transport Properties of Cartilaginous Tissues. *Curr. Rheumatol. Rev.* **2009**, *5*, 40–50. [CrossRef]
44. Zioupos, P.; Currey, J.D.; Hamer, A.J. The Role of Collagen in the Declining Mechanical Properties of Aging Human Cortical Bone. *J. Biomed. Mater. Res.* **1999**, *45*, 108–116. [CrossRef]
45. Wallmann, H.W. Stretching and Flexibility in the Aging Adult. *Home Health Care Manag. Pract.* **2009**, *21*, 355–357. [CrossRef]
46. Harrison, D.E.; Colloca, C.J.; Harrison, D.D.; Janik, T.J.; Haas, J.W.; Keller, T.S. Anterior Thoracic Posture Increases Thoracolumbar Disc Loading. *Eur. Spine J.* **2005**, *14*, 234–242. [CrossRef] [PubMed]
47. Keller, T.S.; Colloca, C.J.; Harrison, D.E.; Harrison, D.D.; Janik, T.J. Influence of Spine Morphology on Intervertebral Disc Loads and Stresses in Asymptomatic Adults: Implications for the Ideal Spine. *Spine J.* **2005**, *5*, 297–309. [CrossRef] [PubMed]
48. Protopsaltis, T.S.; Scheer, J.K.; Terran, J.S.; Smith, J.S.; Hamilton, D.K.; Kim, H.J.; Mundis, G.M.; Hart, R.A.; McCarthy, I.M.; Klineberg, E.; et al. How the Neck Affects the Back: Changes in Regional Cervical Sagittal Alignment Correlate to HRQOL Improvement in Adult Thoracolumbar Deformity Patients at 2-Year Follow-Up. *J. Neurosurg. Spine* **2015**, *23*, 153–158. [CrossRef] [PubMed]
49. Scheer, J.K.; Passias, P.G.; Sorocean, A.M.; Boniello, A.J.; Mundis, G.M.; Klineberg, E.; Kim, H.J.; Protopsaltis, T.S.; Gupta, M.; Bess, S.; et al. Association between Preoperative Cervical Sagittal Deformity and Inferior Outcomes at 2-Year Follow-up in Patients with Adult Thoracolumbar Deformity: Analysis of 182 Patients. *J. Neurosurg. Spine* **2016**, *24*, 108–115. [CrossRef] [PubMed]
50. Glassman, S.D.; Bridwell, K.; Dimar, J.R.; Horton, W.; Berven, S.; Schwab, F. The Impact of Positive Sagittal Balance in Adult Spinal Deformity. *Spine* **2005**, *30*, 2024–2029. [CrossRef] [PubMed]
51. Harrison, D.E.; Cailliet, R.; Harrison, D.D.; Troyanovich, S.J.; Harrison, S.O. A Review of Biomechanics of the Central Nervous System—Part II: Spinal Cord Strains from Postural Loads. *J. Manip. Physiol. Ther.* **1999**, *22*, 322–332. [CrossRef]
52. Breig, A.; Marions, O. Biomechanics of the Lumbosacral Nerve Roots. *Acta Radiol.* **1963**, *1*, 1141–1160. [CrossRef]
53. Berland, R.; Marques-Sule, E.; Marín-Mateo, J.L.; Moreno-Segura, N.; López-Ridaura, A.; Sentandreu-Mañó, T. Effects of the Feldenkrais Method as a Physiotherapy Tool: A Systematic Review and Meta-Analysis of Randomized Controlled Trials. *Int. J. Environ. Res. Public Health* **2022**, *19*, 13734. [CrossRef]
54. Harrison, D.D.; Harrison, D.E.; Janik, T.J.; Cailliet, R.; Ferrantelli, J.R.; Haas, J.W.; Holland, B. Modeling of the Sagittal Cervical Spine as a Method to Discriminate Hypolordosis: Results of Elliptical and Circular Modeling in 72 Asymptomatic Subjects, 52 Acute Neck Pain Subjects, and 70 Chronic Neck Pain Subjects. *Spine* **2004**, *29*, 2485–2492. [CrossRef]
55. McAviney, J.; Schulz, D.; Bock, R.; Harrison, D.E.; Holland, B. Determining the Relationship between Cervical Lordosis and Neck Complaints. *J. Manip. Physiol. Ther.* **2005**, *28*, 187–193. [CrossRef]
56. Moustafa, I.M.; Youssef, A.; Ahbouch, A.; Tamim, M.; Harrison, D.E. Is Forward Head Posture Relevant to Autonomic Nervous System Function and Cervical Sensorimotor Control? Cross Sectional Study. *Gait Posture* **2020**, *77*, 29–35. [CrossRef] [PubMed]
57. Darnell, M.W. A Proposed Chronology of Events for Forward Head Posture. *J. Craniomandib. Pract.* **1983**, *1*, 49–54. [CrossRef] [PubMed]

58. White, M.; Panjabi, A.A. *Clinical Biomechanics of the Spine*, 2nd ed.; Lippincott Williams and Wilkins: Philadelphia, PA, USA, 1990; Volume 2.
59. Miyazaki, M.; Hymanson, H.J.; Morishita, Y.; He, W.; Zhang, H.; Wu, G.; Kong, M.H.; Tsumura, H.; Wang, J.C. Kinematic Analysis of the Relationship between Sagittal Alignment and Disc Degeneration in the Cervical Spine. *Spine* **2008**, *33*, E870–E876. [CrossRef] [PubMed]

Disclaimer/Publisher's Note: The statements, opinions and data contained in all publications are solely those of the individual author(s) and contributor(s) and not of MDPI and/or the editor(s). MDPI and/or the editor(s) disclaim responsibility for any injury to people or property resulting from any ideas, methods, instructions or products referred to in the content.

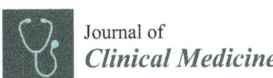

Article

The Efficacy of Cervical Lordosis Rehabilitation for Nerve Root Function and Pain in Cervical Spondylotic Radiculopathy: A Randomized Trial with 2-Year Follow-Up

Ibrahim M. Moustafa [1,2], Aliaa A. Diab [2] and Deed E. Harrison [3,*]

1. Department of Physiotherapy, College of Health Sciences, University of Sharjah, Sharjah P.O. Box 27272, United Arab Emirates
2. Basic Science Department, Faculty of Physical Therapy, Cairo University, Giza 12613, Egypt
3. CBP Nonprofit—A Spine Research Foundation, Eagle, ID 83616, USA
* Correspondence: drdeed@idealspine.com; Tel.: +1-775-340-4734

Abstract: Sagittal cervical alignment is a clinically related feature in patients suffering from chronic cervical spondylotic radiculopathy (CSR). We designed this randomized trial to explore the effects of cervical lordosis (CL) correction in thirty chronic lower CSR patients with CL < 20°. Patients were assigned randomly into two equal groups, study (SG) and control (CG). Both groups received neck stretching and exercises and infrared radiation; additionally, the SG received cervical extension traction. Treatments were applied 3× per week for 10 weeks after which groups were followed for 3 months and 2 years. The amplitude of dermatomal somatosensory evoked potentials (DSSEPS), CL C2–C7, and pain scales (NRS) were measured. The SG had an increase in CL post-treatment ($p < 0.0001$), this was maintained at 3 months and 2 years. No statistical improvement in CL was found for the CG. A significant reduction in NRS for SG after 10 weeks of treatment with non-significant loss of change at 3 months and continued improvement at 2 years was found. CG had less significant improvement in post-treatment NRS; the 3-month and 2-year measures revealed significant worsening in NRS. An inverse linear correlation between increased CL and NRS was found ($r = -0.49$; $p = 0.005$) for both groups initially and maintained in SG at the final 2-year follow-up ($r = -0.6$; $p = 0.01$). At 10 weeks, we found significant improvements in DSSEPS for both groups ($p < 0.0001$). We identified a linear correlation between initial DSSEPs and CL for both groups ($p < 0.0001$), maintained only in the SG at the final follow-up for all levels ($p < 0.0001$). Improved CL in the SG correlated with significant improvements in nerve root function and pain rating in patients with CSR at short and long-term follow-up. These observed effects indicate that clinicians involved in the treatment of patients with symptoms of cervical degenerative disorders should add sagittal curve correction to their armamentarium of rehabilitation procedures for relevant patient populations.

Keywords: cervical spine; dermatomal somatosensory evoked potential; lordosis; randomized trial; spondylotic radiculopathy; traction

Citation: Moustafa, I.M.; Diab, A.A.; Harrison, D.E. The Efficacy of Cervical Lordosis Rehabilitation for Nerve Root Function and Pain in Cervical Spondylotic Radiculopathy: A Randomized Trial with 2-Year Follow-Up. *J. Clin. Med.* **2022**, *11*, 6515. https://doi.org/10.3390/jcm11216515

Academic Editors: Panagiotis Korovessis and Hiroshi Horiuchi

Received: 21 September 2022
Accepted: 1 November 2022
Published: 2 November 2022

Publisher's Note: MDPI stays neutral with regard to jurisdictional claims in published maps and institutional affiliations.

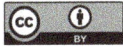

Copyright: © 2022 by the authors. Licensee MDPI, Basel, Switzerland. This article is an open access article distributed under the terms and conditions of the Creative Commons Attribution (CC BY) license (https://creativecommons.org/licenses/by/4.0/).

1. Introduction

Cervical spondylotic radiculopathy (CSR) is one of the most common causes of cervical radiculopathy [1,2]. It has been documented that the incidence of cervical degenerative abnormalities increases with age having the greatest frequency in the fifth to sixth decade of life [3]. Spondylotic degenerative findings appear to be the most common followed by disc damage and these are most common in the lower cervical spine discs (C5–C6) [3,4]. The degenerative state of the intervertebral disc, vertebral body and adjacent structures, occurs as a result of several factors including segmental injury/trauma and alterations in the sagittal alignment of the cervical spine; including reductions in the segmental and total angle of cervical curvature [4–7].

Causation of CSR involves multiple factors but the mechanical compression and shear loads acting on the nerve roots result in inflammation and this is the primary driver of the pain, decreased cervical movement, and consequent neurological disturbances. CSR incidence increases with age and has an estimated frequency of 0.35% in the fifth to sixth decade of life [2]. Recently, multiple systematic literature reviews have been published seeking to understand the complexities of CSM and its natural history, conservative management strategies, and the need for surgical interventions [2,8–13]. For patients with intractable pain and with motor loss of less than three out of five, surgical intervention is warranted [2]. However, in comparison between conservative and surgical management trials, the long-term outcomes at 1–2 years generally show conservative care to be equally effective for less severe CSM patients [2,8–12].

Although there is general agreement regarding the need for conservative treatment for CSR, the precise treatment protocols for the best results and when to use them for CSR disorders still remain an enigma [2,8–13]. Conservative treatments for CSM include rehabilitative exercise therapy, mechanical cervical traction, transcutaneous electrical nerve stimulation, pain management, education, cervical collars, and spinal manipulative therapy [2,8–13]. Problematically, the primary outcomes in CSR populations depend on pain measurements, which are subjective in nature, and it is rare that investigations include measurements of neurophysiological outcomes to demonstrate improvement in nerve root function concomitant with pain improvements [8]. One exception to this is the trial by Moustafa and Diab [14] where they used three different cervical traction setups in an attempt to identify the optimum angle of combined distraction with flexion, neutral, or extension angles. The authors identified that distraction combined with slight head extension was found to be associated with the best improvement in neurophysiological measures in patients with cervical radiculopathy.

Regarding the development of signs and symptoms of CSR, the patho-anatomy of the vertebra and disc is not the only cause of a given patient's pain; it is likely that the patho-anatomy, inflammatory mediators, functional disturbances, and altered spine alignment all interact to produce clinical symptoms [15]. In this regard, various studies point to the fact that biomechanical dysfunction of the spinal column, as seen with altered cervical sagittal plane alignment, results in degenerative changes in the muscles, ligaments, and bony structures [4–7]; altered spine alignment coupled with degenerative spine changes will increase the stress and strain on the neural elements potentially leading to and increasing the magnitude of neurologic dysfunctions in CSR [16–21]. Clinically, the goals of CSR patient care include sagittal plane alignment improvement in surgical [19–22] and conservative [13–17] settings. Regarding the conservative care setting, it is rare that investigations seek to address the radiographic alignment of the sagittal cervical spine as an outcome measure or predictive variable in CSR patients; [14,16] this may be due to the fact that the vast majority of conservative care techniques do not have the capability to significantly improve the shape and magnitude of the cervical lordotic curve [23–25]. The exception to this rule is three-point bending extension traction devices which are known to increase cervical curvature following a program of consistent care over the course of 8–12 weeks [25].

In an original collection of case studies, Pope [23] first incorporated a counter-stressing strap system (front pull pulling posterior-anterior in the posterior aspect of the cervical spine) to cervical extension traction with slight distraction on the skull, drawing attention to the possibility of cervical sagittal curve correction by a 'so-called 2 way' cervical extension traction. Later, in a non-randomized clinical trial, Harrison et al. [24] evaluated the effect of this three-point bending (two-way) cervical traction on restoring the sagittal curve in a chronic neck pain population without radiculopathy; they reported a significant increase in cervical lordosis and reduction in pain intensity.

In a pilot randomized trial looking at cervical spine disco-genic radiculopathy without spondylotic changes, Moustafa et al. [16], documented that cervical extension traction, using a novel cervical orthotic, improves the cervical lordosis and improves pain, disability, and neurophysiology. Regarding conservative care for CSM, cervical spine traction in flexion and distraction is one of the most commonly performed and investigated procedures, but this technique is not conducive to improving the abnormal cervical lordotic curve [2,8–13]. Furthermore, previous trials, [14,23–25] testing the effects of three-point bending types of cervical extension traction, have not clarified the relationship of cervical spine correction and its influence or effect on nerve root function and pain responses associated with improving an abnormal cervical lordosis in CSR patients. In terms of neurophysiological outcomes, dermatomal somatosensory evoked potentials (DSSEPs) can provide reliable information about segmental nerve root function and DSSEPs have been identified to correspond to clinical symptoms more closely than other electrophysiological examinations [26,27].

While it is known that the conservative management of cervical spondylotic radiculopathy is beneficial and multiple therapies (multi-modal) should be used simultaneously, a recent systematic literature review concluded that neck and arm pain improvements were 'trivial' at best and that further research into the best methods for specific patient populations is needed [8]. Accordingly, in properly selected patients, cervical curve restoration interventions might offer unknown benefits. Thus, the present randomized controlled trial was undertaken to investigate the neurophysiological and pain response outcomes of three-point bending (two-way) traction compared to standard care in patient cases with lower cervical spine CSR, chronic pain, and with a verified hypo-lordosis of the cervical spine. The primary hypothesis of this study was that cervical lordosis restoration will have short and long-term effects on DSSEPs and pain outcomes in CSR patients.

2. Materials and Methods

A prospective, investigator-blinded, parallel-group, randomized clinical trial was conducted at a research laboratory in our university and was retrospectively registered with ClinicalTrials.gov (NCT05547997) accessed on 20 September 2022. The reason for retrospective trial registration was that legislation in Egypt only required local registration for clinical trials at the time of study design and this is what was conducted initially by prospectively registration in a non-WHO-approved registry. Recruitment began after approval was obtained from the Ethics Committee of the Faculty of Physical Therapy, Cairo University with the ethical approval No Cairo23-987-12 M.S. All participants signed informed consent prior to data collection.

2.1. Patients

Thirty patients with lower cervical spine CSR participated in this study. There were nineteen females and eleven males ranging from 40 to 50 years of age. We randomly assigned the participants into a study group and a comparative control group. The study group, receiving three-point bending cervical traction, included nine females and six males. The comparative treatment (control) group consisted of five males and 10 females.

2.2. Inclusion and Exclusion Criteria

Patients were included if they had unilateral radiculopathy due to spondylotic changes of the lower cervical spine (C5–C6 and/or C6–C7). Participants were screened prior to inclusion by measuring their lateral cervical radiographs for a cervical absolute rotation angle (ARA) formed by two lines intersecting from the posterior body margins of C2–C7. If the ARA angle was less than 20°, then participants were included in the study and determined to have hypolordois of the cervical curve [28,29]. In addition to cervical lordosis $\geq 20°$, exclusion criteria included: (1) central spinal canal stenosis; (2) rheumatoid arthritis; (3) vestibulobasilar insufficiency; (4) osteoporosis; (5) any disorder that might affect the DSSEPs such as thoracic outlet syndrome, carpal tunnel syndrome, cubital tunnel syndrome, etc.; (6) patients who had received surgical treatment for CSR or neck injury; (7) patients with cervical spinal instability; (8) patients with comorbid severe primary diseases such as cardiovascular disease, cerebrovascular disease, diseases of the liver, kidneys, or hematopoietic system; (9) patients who were suffering from any malignant disease as well as those unable to tolerate the cervical extension position with increased axial pain and/or radiculopathy.

The diagnostic criteria of CSR in the current study included: pain and numbness in the distribution of spinal nerve roots C6, and/or C7; additionally, the brachial plexus tension test or foraminal compression test had to be positive. In all participants, the location of symptoms (e.g., dermatomal pain or neurological deficit) matched the evaluated nerve root. Moreover, the clinical manifestations and imaging findings were consistent with their clinical syndromes. Both plain cervical spine radiographs and MRI were used to assist in CSR diagnosis and rule out other diseases, such as disc herniation, infection, and tumor. Lastly, participants had to have side-to-side amplitude differences of 50% or more in their DSSEPs measurement, a duration of symptoms of more than 3 months, and a "present" pain score of 4 or higher on a scale of from 0 to 10. Included participants were randomly assigned to an intervention group (n = 15) or control group (n = 15) using a random number generator and were restricted to permuted blocks of different sizes, with the researcher blinded to the sequence designated for each person.

2.3. Treatment Procedures

Both groups (study and control) were provided standard comparative care to improve pain intensity and reduce muscle tension that might be responsible for a reduction in cervical lordosis; this standard care included stretching exercises and infrared radiation (IR). Additionally, the study group was treated with three-point bending cervical extension traction. All participants received their respective interventions, in a controlled environment, for three days per week for ten weeks for a total of 30 sessions. Participants were followed for 3 months and 2 years at which times re-assessments were performed.

Cervical traction procedure: The study group received three-point bending cervical extension traction following the protocol of Harrison et al. [24]. The head halter was fixed posteriorly to cause slight distraction, retraction, and slight extension and at the same time a front anterior strap had weight applied over a pulley that allows transverse traction load to be applied to the apex of the participants' cervical curve alteration. Following the findings of Moustafa et al. [14], the angle of the posterior head harness pull was positioned, relative to vertical, 5–30° backward in order to cause slight extension and distraction as this position was found to be associated with the best improvement in DSSEP's in patients with radiculopathy. Weights started at 15 lbs. (6.8 kg) on the anterior strap and increased over consecutive visits to patient tolerance or a maximum of 35 lbs. (15.9 kg). The duration of each session started at approximately three minutes and increased to one minute per session until reaching the goal of 20 min per session. Figure 1 represents the cervical 2-way traction method.

Stretching exercises: Exercises were performed in the following order: (1) stretching towards lateral flexion for the upper part of the trapezius; (2) ipsilateral flexion and rotation for the scalene, and (3) flexion for the extensor muscles. Each maneuver was held for 30 s as this is an optimum time to not create an alteration in the evoked potentials [30]. Each stretch was repeated three times. Patients performed the stretching program three times a week for 10 weeks and this treatment took approximately 10 min per session [31].

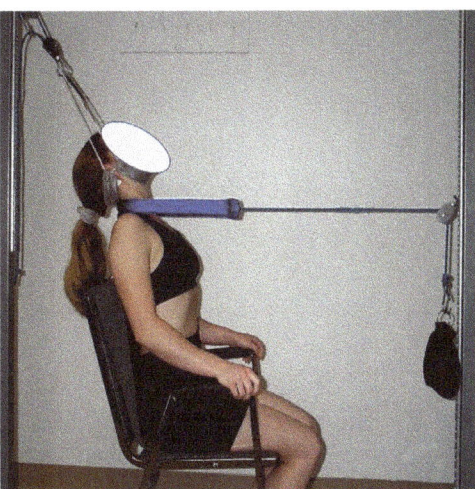

Figure 1. Three-point bending cervical traction. Photo reprinted with permission.

2.4. Outcome Measures

A series of outcome measures were obtained at three intervals: (1) baseline; (2) one day following the completion of 30 visits after 10 weeks of treatment; (3) at the 3-month follow-up after the 10-weeks of treatment re-evaluation; (4) at two years follow-up after the 10-weeks of treatment re-evaluation (1-year and 9-months after the 3-month follow-up). The sequence of measurements was identical for all participants. Radiographic cervical sagittal alignment of lordosis (ARA C2–C7) and neurophysiological findings were the primary treatment outcomes, whereas, the numerical pain rating scale (NPRS) variable was the secondary measure.

2.5. DSSEPs

The main outcome measure used to assess the nerve root function was the peak-to-peak amplitude of dermatomal somatosensory evoked potentials (DSSEPs). An electromyogram device (Tonneis neuroscreen plus version 1.59, Erich Jaeger, Inc., Rheda-Wiedenbrück, Germany) was used to measure this variable for all patients before starting the treatment, at the end of 10 weeks, at a follow-up of three months, and the long-term follow-up period of two years. All testing procedures for DSSEPs were conducted following the protocol of Liguori et al. [32] The patient was lying supine on a softly padded table with a pillow under their head and knees. After the skin was abraded and cleaned with alcohol, the stimulating electrodes were placed overlying dermatomes of C6 (about 7 cm above the styloid process of the radius) and C7 between the second and the third metacarpal bones and at C8 (medial side of the hand). Figure 2 demonstrates this procedure. A bipolar electrode was used for stimulation with an inter-electrode distance of 2.5 cm with the stimulation cathode placed proximally. The sensory threshold for the electrical stimulation was determined by increasing the intensity of the electrical current until the patient reported its sensation, tolerable and painless stimulus intensity was set at 2.5 times above this level. The recording was made with 9 mm diameter tin/lead electrodes affixed with electrolyte paste to the abraded skin. The recording electrodes were placed at C3 and C4 (between C3 and P3 and C4 and P4 of the international EEG 10–20 system), while the reference electrode was placed at Fz and the ground electrode at Fpz. See Figure 3. The cortical responses were amplified, averaged and displayed using an analysis time of 50 ms and a filter setting of 2 Hz to 1 kHz was used in this study. After the stimulation was performed and traces were superimposed to ensure reproducibility, negative near-field potentials were detected to measure the peak-to-peak amplitude.

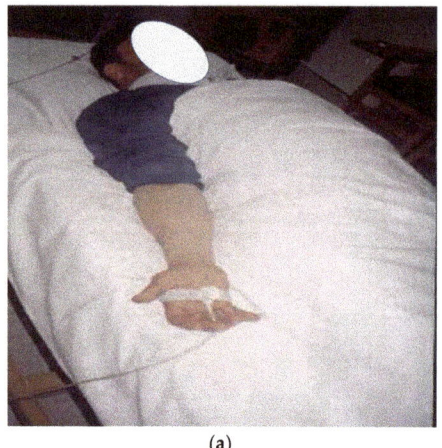 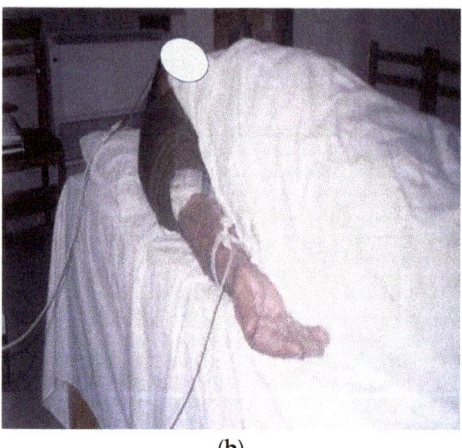

Figure 2. Location of stimulation sites indicated by arrow (**a**) for the C7 dermatome and (**b**) for the C6 dermatome.

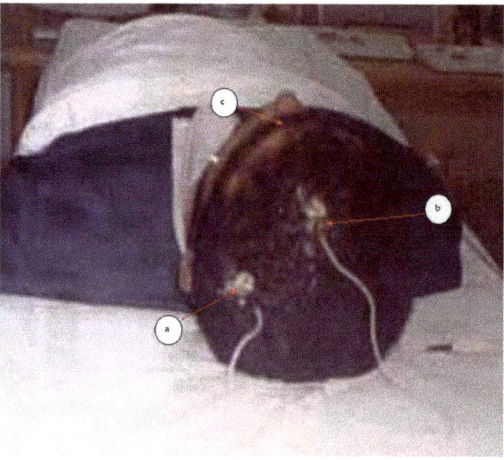

Figure 3. Sites of Recording: (**a**) active recording electrode at c3′, (**b**) reference electrode at Fz, and (**c**) grounding electrode at Fbz.

Cervical Lordosis: Cervical spine, standing, and lateral X-rays were obtained for each participant at four time periods: at baseline, following 10-weeks or 30 treatment sessions, at the 3-month follow-up, and at final follow-up of 2 years. The participants were asked to adopt a relaxed neutral posture and look straight forward as if staring into their own eyes in a mirror; this procedure has been investigated and has good to excellent examiner reliability [24]. The cervical lordosis was measured using the posterior body tangent method where a line is drawn along the posterior aspect of the C7 vertebral body and the angle of the curve is measured with an intersecting line drawn along the posterior vertebral body margin of C2; this is termed the absolute rotation angle or ARA of C2–C7. The ARA C2–C7 lordosis was measured using a standard protractor and sharp X-ray pencil; this measurement method has excellent examiner reliability [33].

Pain intensity: Neck and arm pain intensity were measured using the numerical pain rating scale (NPRS), which is considered a valid and reliable scale [34]. The patients were asked to place a mark along the line to denote their pain level; 0 reflecting "no pain" and 10 reflecting the "worst pain".

2.6. Sample Size Estimation

To determine the required number of participants needed in this study, estimates of mean and standard deviations (SD) were collected from a pilot study consisting of 10 participants who received the same program. The mean differences and SD of the ARA C2–C7 and peak-to-peak amplitude of DSSEPS for different levels C6, 7, and 8, were: ARA, −7 (SD 1.2); C6: −0.6 (SD 0.1); C7: −0.7 (SD 0.2); C8: −0.6 (SD 0.3), respectively. These values were used to calculate the sample size separately for each of the primary outcomes by applying a Bonferroni correction to adjust the significance level. The largest value of the sample size was then considered the final sample size for the trial. Accordingly, at least 14 participants in each group, given a statistical power of 80%, were needed in the current study. The sample size was enlarged by 10% to account for potential dropouts.

2.7. Data Analysis

Descriptive statistics were calculated including mean ± standard deviation (SD) for age, height and weight. For between-group repeated measures an analysis of covariance was used: Our model used the group as an independent variable, time as the repeated measurement, and group × time as the interactive variable. In order to assess between-group differences, participants' baseline variable outcomes were used as covariates; where each participant's value was subtracted from the population mean. The Bonferroni correction was used if we identified group × time interactions, ($p < 0.05$). In order to assess any possible linear correlation fits between variables, Pearson correlations between ARA C2–C7 and peak-to-peak amplitude values of DSSEPs, and ARA C2–C7 and pain scores were determined. The correlation findings were compiled into a pre-study set and a post-study set. The level of significance was set at $p < 0.05$.

3. Results

The study group, consisting of fifteen patients receiving the new extension traction, was compared with the fifteen control participants who received standard care only (IR and stretching exercises). Patient demographics are shown in Table 1 where it is shown that the two groups were statistically matched for age, weight and height. Patient retention throughout the study is shown in Figure 4.

Table 1. Baseline participant demographics.

	Study Group (n = 15)	Control Group (n = 15)	p ‡
Age (years)	46.3 ± 2.05	45.9 ± 2.1	0.5
Weight (kg)	73.3 ± 8.9	77.5 ± 9	0.2
Height (cm)	171.6 ± 5	168.3 ± 7.9	0.18
Male	6	5	0.7
Female	9	10	
Smoker	5	4	0.69
Non smoker	10	11	

‡ Two-sided two-sample *t*-test; SD: standard deviation, the values are mean (± SD) for age, height, weight and as the number for the term 'other'.

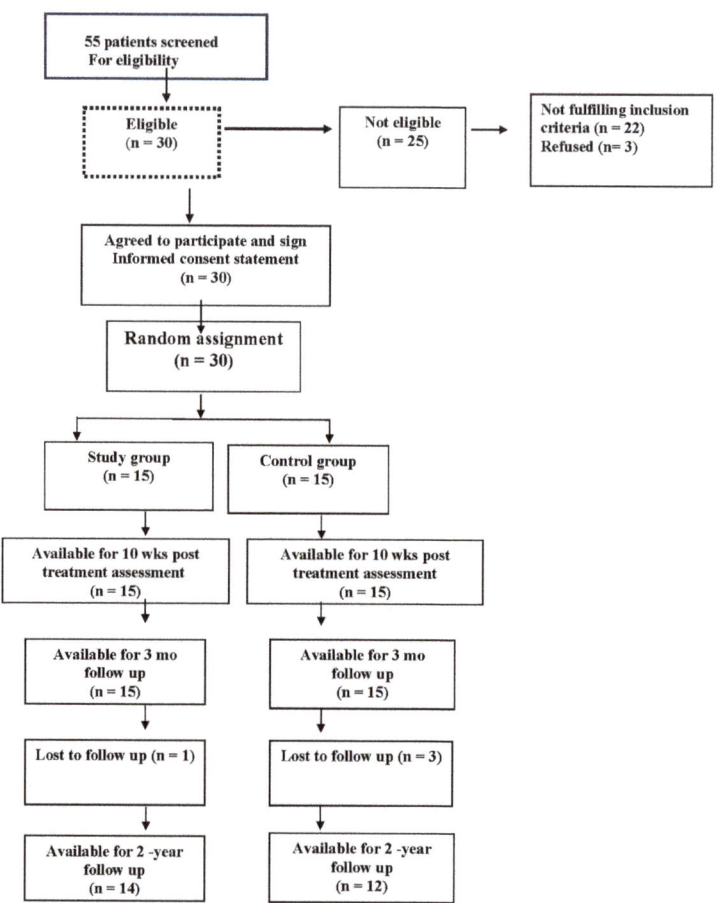

Figure 4. A diagram of patients' retention and randomization throughout the study is shown.

3.1. Pain Outcomes

At 10 weeks of treatment, pain intensity was significantly improved ($p < 0.0001$) for both the study and control groups; indicating a reduction in pain due to interventions in both groups. Using Tukey's Multiple Comparison Test, we identified that the study group's pain was unchanged at the 3-month follow-up compared to the 10-week values; $p > 0.05$. While at the 2-year follow-up the study group's pain continued to improve with a statistically significant decrease in pain at 2 years compared to 3 months, mean difference of 1.1 and $p < 0.05$. In contrast, the control group revealed a significant increase (worsening) in the mean pain at 3 months and 2 years compared to their 10 weeks of treatment evaluation; $p < 0.05$ at 3 months. The between-group analysis identified that the study group had statistically significant reductions in pain compared to the control group at each of the three follow-up measurements; $p < 0.0001$. See Table 2 and Figure 5.

Table 2. The results for the repeated measures one-way analysis of variance (ANOVA) for the absolute rotation angle (ARA) cervical lordosis and pain intensity in both groups.

Measures		Pretreatment	At 10 Weeks	At 3 Months	At 2 Years	p G	p T	p G × T	Post Hoc Test (MD)	
ARA	S	14.3 ± 4.1	20.87 ± 3	19.5 ± 3.2	18.8 ± 2.1	<0.001	<0.001	<0.001	1 vs. 2	−3.26 *
	C	14.6 ± 3.5	14.7± 3.3	14.1 ± 3.1	12.3 ± 2.7				1 vs. 3	−2.33 *
		0.8 [−3.1–2.5]	<0.001 [3.8–8.5]	<0.001 [3.02–7.7]	<0.001 [3.7–8.2]				1 vs. 4	−1.16 *
Pain	S	5.26 ± 0.96	3.2 ± 1.26	2.8 ± 1.27	1.71 ± 1.2	<0.001	<0.001	<0.001	1 vs. 2	1.7 *
	C	5.47 ± 1.18	3.9 ± 1.43	4.6 ± 1.49	4.3 ± 1.2				1 vs. 3	1.5 *
		0.7 [−0.8–0.9]	<0.001 [−1.7–0.29]	<0.001 [−2.9–−0.79]	<0.001 [−3.5–−1.8]				1 vs. 4	2.3 *

Study group: SG; Control group: CG; * Statistically significant difference: p-value; MD: mean difference.

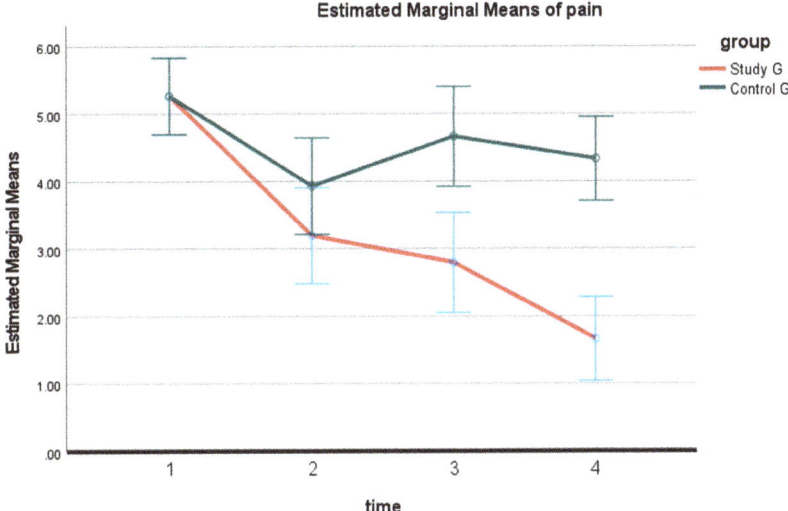

Figure 5. Differences in pain on the numerical rating scale (NRPS) during the study reported as mean ± SD for study and control groups at four time periods: baseline or pretreatment, after completion of the 10-week program, the 3-month follow-up, and the 2-year follow-up data. 1: pretreatment; 2: 10 weeks post-treatment; 3: at 3 months; 4: at 2-year follow-up.

3.2. ARA C2-C7 Cervical Lordosis

Regarding the cervical lordosis (ARA C2–C7), in the study group the one-way ANOVA (baseline versus 10 weeks), identified an increased cervical lordosis ARA C2–C7, $p < 0.0001$ and F = 49.8. In contrast, the control group was identified to have no statistical change in cervical lordosis; ($p > 0.05$). For the study group, using Tukey's Multiple Comparison Test, the ARA C2–C7 was unchanged at 3 months and 2 years in comparison to the 10-week data (mean difference of 1.333 at 10-weeks; $p > 0.05$). In contrast, for the control group, the post-test was not calculated due to insignificant differences; $p > 0.05$. The between-group analysis identified that the study group had statistically significant increases in ARA C2–C7 cervical lordosis compared to the control group at each of the three follow-up measurements; $p < 0.0001$. See Table 2 and Figure 6.

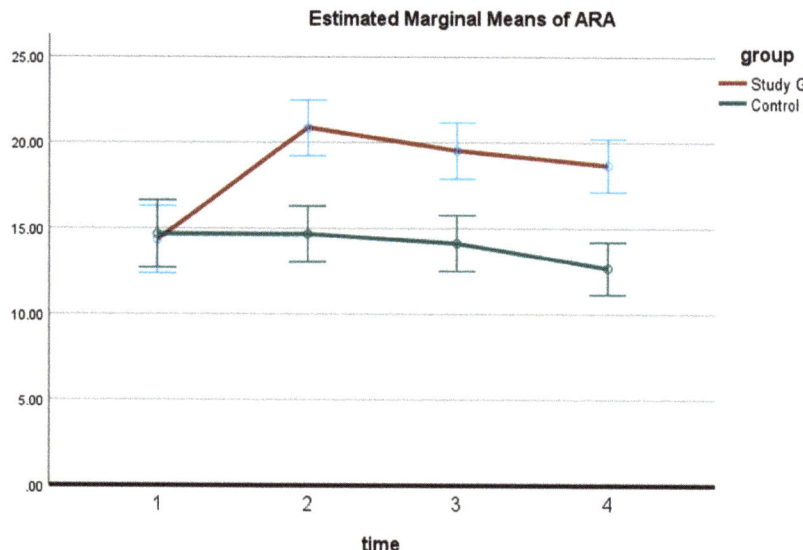

Figure 6. The cervical lordosis absolute rotation angle C2–C7 (ARA) for the control group and study group is shown as the mean ± SD. Four different time periods are shown: baseline or pretreatment, after completion of the 10-week program, the 3-month follow-up, and the 2-year follow-up. 1: pretreatment; 2: 10 weeks post-treatment; 3: at 3 months; 4: at 2-year follow-up.

3.3. DSSEPs

The repeated measures one-way ANOVA, comparing initial DSSEPs to 10-week treatment values, identified statistically significant improvements for both groups ($p < 0.0001$). A Tukey's Multiple Comparison Test revealed significant increases in the mean of the post-test compared with pretreatment values for both the study and controls. However, only in the study group did the post-test reveal insignificant changes in DSSEPs at 3-month and 2-year follow-ups compared to the 10-week data; $p > 0.05$. In contrast, at 3-month and 2-year follow-ups the control groups DSSEP measurements regressed back to baseline values. The between-group analysis identified that the study group had statistically significant improvements in the DSSEPs for all three nerve root levels compared to the control group at each of the three follow-up measurements; $p < 0.0001$. See Table 3 and Figures 7 and 8.

Table 3. The results for the repeated measures one-way analysis of variance (ANOVA) for the DSSEPs amplitudes in the study and control groups for three nerve root levels: C6, C7, and C8.

Measures		Pretreatment	At 10 Weeks	At 3 Months	At 2 Years	p			Post Hoc Test (MD)	
						G	T	G × T		
C6	S C	0.41 ± 0.1 0.42 ± 0.2 0.8 [−0.16–0.13]	0.80 ± 0.19 0.56 ± 0.15 <0.001 [0.11–0.37]	0.79 ± 0.11 0.40 ± 0.15 <0.001 [0.272–0.5]	0.82 ± 0.14 0.42 ± 0.17 <0.001 [0.31–0.48]	<0.001	<0.001	<0.001	1 vs. 2 1 vs. 3 1 vs. 4	−0.267 * −0.18 * −0.21 *
C7	S C	0.4 ± 0.1 0.69 ± 0.2 0.05 [−0.26–0.02]	1.18 ± 0.33 0.7 ± 0.18 <0.001 [0.32–0.72]	1.0 ± 0.37 0.52 ± 0.21 <0.001 [0.30–0.76]	1.1 ± 0.37 0.51 ± 0.18 <0.001 [0.36–0.81]	<0.001	<0.001	<0.001	1 vs. 2 1 vs. 3 1 vs. 4	−0.38 * −0.24 * −0.26 *
C8	S C	0.6 ± 0.2 0.8 ± 0.2 0.15 [−0.33–0.05]	1.3 ± 0.5 0.9 ± 0.3 0.005 [0.17–0.84]	1.4 ± 0.6 0.7 ± 0.3 <0.001 [0.30–1.1]	1.5 ± 0.6 0.7 ± 0.2 <0.001 [0.32–1.08]	<0.001	<0.001	<0.001	1 vs. 2 1 vs. 3 1 vs. 4	−0.35 * −0.32 * −0.33 *

Study group: SG; Control group: CG; * Statistically significant difference: p-value; MD: mean difference; 1: pretreatment; 2: 10 weeks post-treatment; 3: at 3 months; 4: at 2-year follow-up.

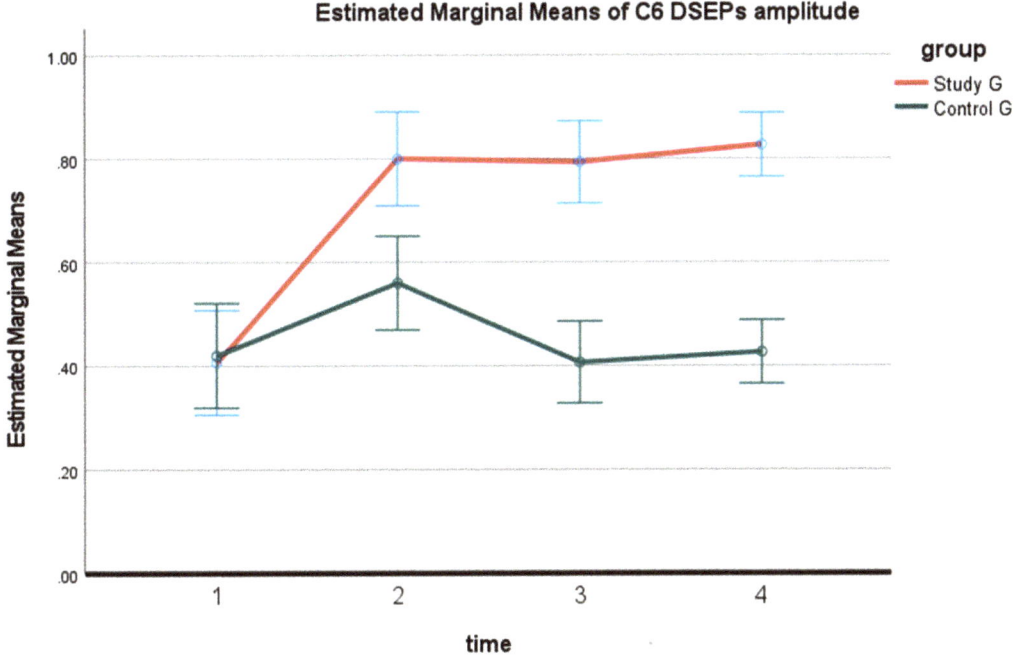

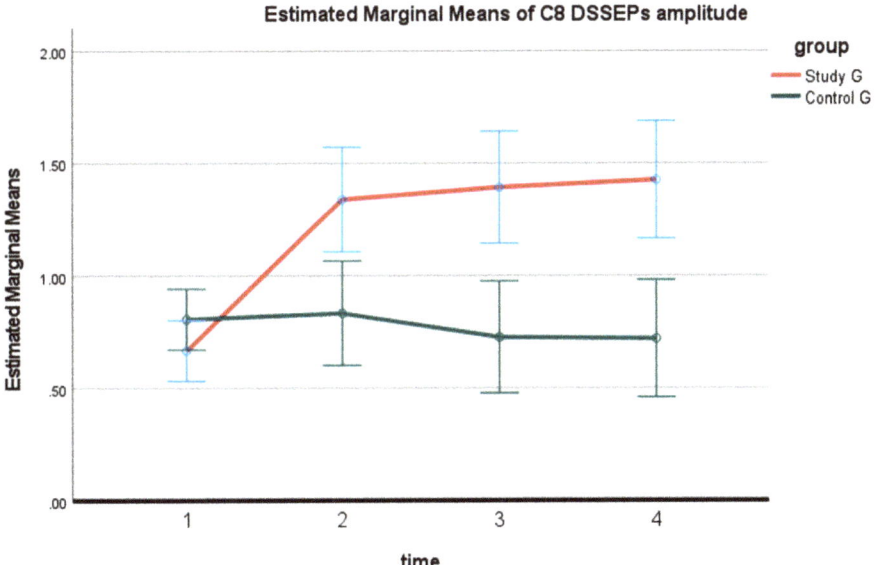

Figure 7. Cont.

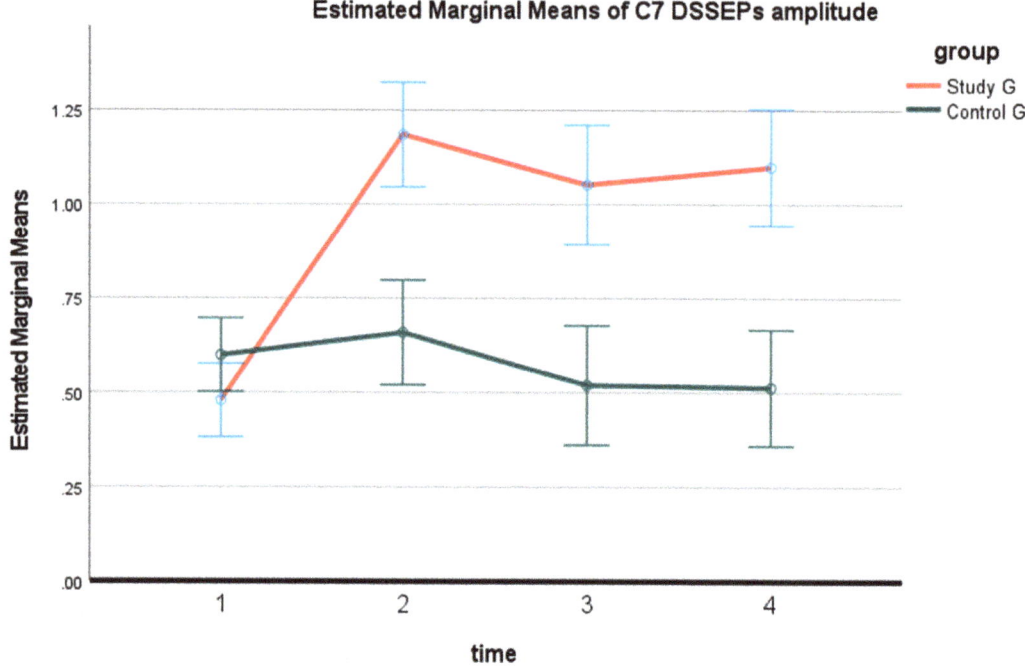

Figure 7. Mean and ± SD of the DSSEPS for study and control groups at four time periods: baseline or pretreatment, after completion of the 10-week program, the 3-month follow-up, and the 2-year follow-up.

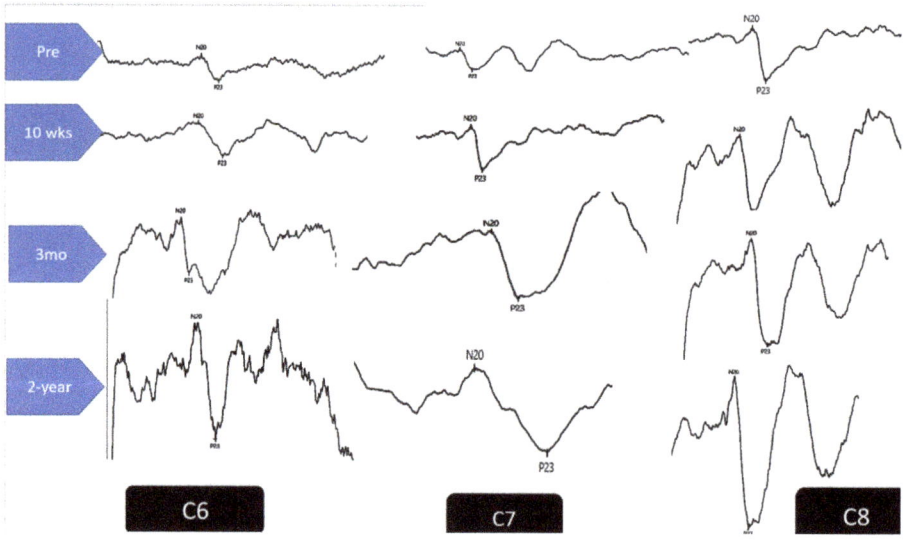

Figure 8. Example of DSSEPs at each of the levels C6–C8 at the four intervals of measurement for the study group (2-way traction).

3.4. Correlations

All correlation results for ARA C2–C7 lordosis and pain and the DSSEPs at each of the three levels are presented as (1) a baseline correlation and (2) for follow-up treatment data at the 2-year mark. At baseline, for both groups, increased cervical lordosis was inversely correlated to pain intensity (r= −0.49; p = 0.005); however, this inverse correlation was only maintained at follow-up for the study group receiving traction (r = −0.6; r= p = 0.01). See Table 4. We identified a linear correlation between initial DSSEPs and ARA C2–C7 for both groups at each of the three nerve root levels C6–C8 (r = 0.65, r= 0.57, r= 0.8, p < 0.0001). Whereas this linear relationship between ARA C2–C7 became insignificant in the control group but was maintained in the study group at a 2-year follow-up at C6 (r = 0.55; p = 0.033). In contrast, both groups were found to have significant correlations at the 2-year mark for C7 and C8 nerve root DSSEPs (p < 0.001). See Table 4

Table 4. Pearson correlation between ARA C2–C7 and DSSEPS and between ARA and pain. Post-manipulating (post-treatment) data are shown for the 2-year follow-up compared to initial baseline data.

	Number of XY Pairs	r	p
ARA & DSSEP (C6) (baseline data)	30	0.65	<0.001 *
ARA & DSSEP (C7) (baseline data)	30	0.57	<0.001 *
ARA & DSSEP (C8) (baseline data)	30	0.8	<0.001 *
Post-manipulating data (C6)	15	0.55	0.033 *
study control	15	0.19	0.49
Post-manipulating data (C7)	15	0.74	<0.001 *
study control	15	0.62	<0.001 *
Post-manipulating data (C8)	15	0.8	<0.001 *
study control	15	0.58	<0.001 *
ARA C2–C7 and pain Baseline data	30	−0.49	0.005 *
Post-treatment data Study group	15	−0.6	0.01 *
Control group	15	−0.17	0.05 *

p: probability value; r: Pearson's correlation coefficient; *: statistically significant difference.

3.5. Medication and Alternative Therapy Usage

At the 2-year follow-up, participants were asked if they were using alternative (non-surgical) therapies and/or medications to aid in managing the frequency and intensity of pains. Table 5 reports these interventional therapies utilized by the participants in the two groups (Study Group and Control Group) tracked at the 2-year follow-up. The data are reported by an individual participant in each group that the information was obtained from and not the number of people in each group using each intervention. Thus, 11 total participants were using medications and therapies (nine participants in the control group and two participants in the study group) indicating alternative services and medications were used by 4.5 times more participants in the control group and they were using a greater number of services. Table 5.

Table 5. Medication and interventional therapies utilized by of the participants in the two groups (Study Group and Control Group) tracked at the 2-year follow-up.

Medication Utilization & Therapy Used
Control Group
• NSAIDs
• Tricyclic antidepressants
• NSAIDs, hydrotherapy

Table 5. *Cont.*

Medication Utilization & Therapy Used
• NSAIDS, Acupuncture
• Tricyclic antidepressants, semi-hard cervical collar
• Tricyclic antidepressants, semi-hard cervical collar
• Tricyclic antidepressants, soft tissue massage
• Opioid medications
• NSAIDS, Ultrasound therapy
Study Group
• NSAIDs
• Cervical spine epidural steroids

The data are reported by an individual participant in each group in each individual row that the information was obtained from and not the number of people in each group using each intervention. Thus, 11 total participants were using medications and therapies (nine participants in the control group and two participants in the study group) indicating alternative services and medications were used by 4.5 times more participants in the control group and they were using a greater number of services.

4. Discussion

This study compared outcomes of cervical spondylotic radiculopathy (CSR) in a group receiving three-point bending cervical extension traction combined with neck stretches and IR to a group receiving neck stretches and IR only. We had hypothesized that the study group receiving traction would show cervical curve correction resulting in short and long-term benefits on neurophysiological findings and improved pain. The differences between our study and control groups' short and long-term radiographic, DSSEPs, and pain parameters indicate that this hypothesis is supported. This study provides objective evidence that sagittal cervical curve malalignment, and not just pathoanatomy, influences nerve root function and pain.

4.1. Cervical Lordosis Improvements

Concerning the cervical lordosis in the study group, a primary finding was a significant increase in the ARA C2–C7 (mean 7.5°) after 10 weeks of three-point bending traction treatment with no significant loss of lordosis at 3-month and 2-year follow-up. In contrast, the control group receiving IR and neck stretches revealed no significant differences in cervical lordosis between baseline, 10 weeks of treatment, 3-month, and 2-year follow-up measurements. Our study group's results are in agreement with a previous non-randomized controlled trial on three-point bending traction conducted by Harrison et al. [24]. Here, [24] three-point bending cervical traction combined with cervical manipulation was found to improve segmental and global cervical lordosis by a mean of 14° in thirty-seven sessions over the course of 8 to 10 weeks. In a pilot randomized trial on cervical radiculopathy due to disc herniation, Moustafa and colleagues [16] demonstrated that their group receiving a novel extension traction device termed the Denneroll, was found to have an improvement in lordosis of approximately 13° after 10 weeks of care. An explanation for the reduced cervical curve improvements (about 50% less) found in the current study compared to the Moustafa et al. [16] and Harrison et al. [24] investigations is likely a result of the different types of spine disorder populations being studied; chronic neck pain vs. CSR patients in the current study and the modification to the extension traction position for CSR patients. Though our trial is the first to assess lordotic improvements in a specific population with CSR receiving three-point bending cervical extension traction, the results are qualitatively comparable to previous investigations reporting cervical curve correction with these types of traction [25].

Loss of cervical lordosis is often attributed to muscles spasm. Thus, it may be speculated that our study group's increased lordosis was attributed to the relief of muscle spasms and or tightness. However, we found no statistically significant differences in the control group's cervical lordosis who were subjected to neck stretches and IR; which should also reduce muscle spasm/tightness. The lack of a cause-and-effect association between muscle spasm and hypo-lordosis in our study is consistent with a study of acute and chronic neck pain patients by Helliwell et al. [35] and with the biomechanical investigation performed by Fedorchuk et al. [36].

4.2. Pain Improvements

Our study findings offer initial encouragement for pain management in CSR patients using conservative care. For our control group, the transient short-term effect of traditional exercises and IR alone are in agreement with Ylinen et al. [1] who conducted a study to compare the effects of manual therapy and stretching exercise on neck pain and disability. The difference in effectiveness between the two treatments was minor and low-cost stretching exercises were recommended in the first instance as an appropriate intervention to relieve pain, at least in the short term. The randomized trial by Levoska and Keinänen-Kiukaanniemi [37] also found that stretching, light exercises, clay, and massage treatments reduced the occurrence of chronic neck pain. Regarding the efficacy of traction therapy on the outcomes of CSR, a recent randomized trial with a 3-month follows up found that distraction traction therapy provided improvements that reached minimally important clinical differences in about 50% of treated patients [38]. However, in a systematic literature review, Colombo and colleagues [13] identified that, compared to matched controls, the reduction in pain intensity after traction was statistically significant but did not reach meaningful clinically important differences at follow-up. The conflicting, transient, and limited effect of conservative therapies for CSR management reported in some trials is likely multi-factorial and may be attributed to the unique variables of the individual patient. For example, sustained postural imbalance, represented by cervical hypolordosis or kyphosis, causes increased and altered mechanical loading [4–8,20–22]. Once abnormal sagittal cervical alignment becomes established and maintained beyond a critical threshold, the result will be an increase in the probability of pathologies in both the soft and hard tissues of the spine [4–7,20–22]. To this point, in both our study and control groups, we identified a statistically significant negative correlation between cervical lordosis and neck pain for the pre-treatment data ($r = -0.49$). In other words, as the cervical lordosis became straighter, the pain intensity increased.

Of importance, comparing the 10-week to the 3-month data, there was a correlation between the amount of change in lordosis and pain intensity for the traction group; while there was an insignificant association for the control group. These findings indicate that the improvement in pain intensity in the study group at 3-month and 2-year follow-up is probably a result of restoring the cervical lordosis. Overall, our findings support a mechanical relationship between loss of lordosis and pain intensity in this CSR population, particularly at long term follow-up. This mechanical relationship between loss of cervical lordosis and neck pain has previously been identified in two separate investigations. Both McAviney et al. [28] and Harrison et al. [29] identified moderate to good sensitivity and specificity for a hypo cervical lordosis (less than 20°) to discriminate between normal controls and chronic neck pain subjects without significant spinal degeneration. In contrast, in a prospective study of 107 volunteers aged over 45 years with moderate-severe degeneration, Grob et al. [39] examined the correlation between the presence of neck pain and alterations in cervical lordosis concluding that the presence of such structural abnormalities in the patient with neck pain is not related to their cause of pain.

The discrepancy and conflict regarding cervical lordosis found in the results obtained by the previous authors [28,29,39] cannot be directly compared with our current study for several reasons. First, the previous studies [28,29,39] were cross-sectional correlation studies without the ability to ascribe cause and effect. Second, the selection criteria for patient inclusion in the previous studies were patients complaining of primary lower extremity pain in the Grob et al. [39] study and acute and chronic neck pain patients without CSR in the McAviney et al. [28] and Harrison et al. [29] study. In the current study, after 30 sessions, the study group's cervical curve closely approximated the 20° benchmark as reported previously [28,29]. However, note-worthy is that over the 2-year time period, the study groups' ARA-lordosis is becoming slightly decreased compared to the 10-week post-treatment value. It is interesting to speculate the need for further corrective interventional care in this group to maintain the ARA above the 20° mark; future studies are needed to evaluate multiple 10-week programs of care and supportive care over the course of 2-year follow-up in an effort to maintain the cervical curve above the 20° mark.

4.3. DSSEPs Improvement

We used DSSEPs to measure depressed and improved nerve root function resulting from CSR. DSSEPs overcome the inherent problems associated with mixed nerve stimulation as in the case of F wave measures and mixed nerve SSEPS will be minimized. At 10 weeks of treatment, we found statistically significant improvements in DSSEPs for both groups (one-way ANOVA, $p < 0.0001$). However, at 3-month and 2-year follow-ups, the control group's values regressed back to baseline values whereas the traction group continued to show statistically significant improvements. Our findings indicate only a transient effect on DSSEPs for stretching exercises and infrared radiation when used alone for the treatment of CSR populations visible at the 10-week immediate post-treatment follow-up. Qualitatively, our findings are in agreement with the clinical trial on CSR by Moustafa and Diab [14] where they used three different cervical traction setups in an attempt to identify the optimum angle of combined distraction traction. The authors identified that distraction combined with slight head extension was found to be associated with the best improvement in neurophysiological measures in patients with cervical radiculopathy and this result was maintained at 1-year follow-up. Though these authors discuss their findings relative to an abnormal cervical lordosis and the extension traction position likely benefits the lordotic configurator; no radiographic data was supplied [14].

Significantly, we identified a linear correlation between initial DSSEPs and cervical lordosis (ARA C2–C7) for both groups at initial evaluation ($r = 0.65$; $p < 0.0001$); whereas, this relationship was only maintained in the study group at the final follow-up for all measured cervical root levels. Thus, our findings support a relationship between abnormal cervical lordosis and altered neurophysiological deficits on the one hand and that the consequent improvement in neurophysiology is related to the restoration of cervical lordosis. Still, it seems logical and, is generally accepted, that ventro-flexion traction (especially for the lower cervical spine) is more beneficial in improving the nerve root function in CSR due to its effects on the intervertebral foramen [12,13,38]. For example, Wainner and Gill [40] evaluated the nonsurgical treatment of cervical disc herniations with flexion distraction and reported that flexion distraction might be an effective therapy in the treatment of cervical disc herniation and improving neural function as indicated by a reduction in pain. Though contradictory as it seems, our findings support a strong correlation between lordosis increases and peak-to-peak amplitude of DSSEPs for pre-and-post manipulating data. To the best of our knowledge, this is the first study to explicitly examine these relationships in detail in a clinical trial on CSR patients.

Mechanically, the current study findings make sense and agree with Schnebel et al. [41] who investigated the role of spinal flexion and extension in changing nerve root compression (transverse load). It was found that the amount of compressive force and tension in the nerve root was increased with flexion of the spine and decreased with the extension of the spine. This tension and compression may adversely affect the CNS and nerve root function due to the absence of any perineurium, the primary load-carrying structure [17,18]. The observations of Abdulwahab and Sabbahi [42] also correlate well with this mechanical explanation. These authors [42] found that neck retraction appeared to increase the H reflex amplitude in patients with radiculopathy; the opposite effect was found with cervical flexion posture.

The conflicts found in the results of the previous investigations and the current study findings regarding nerve root function and flexion distraction vs. two-way extension traction can be explained in two ways. Previous studies have referred to an increase in the volume of the intervertebral foramen as a direct cause of decompression; while simultaneously disregarding the adverse mechanical tension and shear experienced by the spinal cord and nerve roots as they make contact with any infringing pathology [17,18]. This concept is in agreement with Albert et al. [43] and supported by Brian et al. [44] who reported that although foraminal height and foraminal area increase significantly after anterior cervical discectomy and fusion in a patient with cervical radiculopathy, no correlation was found with relief of clinical symptoms. The second reason explaining the above conflict is that many studies [5] refer to the improvement in patient pain as a direct measure for improvement in the nerve root function; ignoring the fact that neurophysiological deficits in CSR often occur without overt pain or symptomatology. Pain seems to have a strong correlation only when there is inflammation, especially when the dorsal root ganglia are involved [45].

4.4. Limitations

The current study has several limitations, each of which points toward directions of future study. The primary limitations were the lack of investigator blinding and the sample was a convenient sample of patients with CSR rather than a random sample of the whole population. Further, the sample size was just above the minimum number for statistical significance with only 15 participants per group; 14 were needed. Larger sample sizes in future RCTs need to be performed to confirm or refute our findings; specifically, the 2-year follow-up in the control group where the sample size of 12 participants' data was just under the minimum of 14 needed for robust statistical claims to be made. Ideally, it would have been beneficial to provide a 5-year follow-up of our population to truly understand the impact of cervical curve restoration in the long term. However, due to the smaller sample size of our trial (15 participants in each group), it was not possible to follow our patients past 2-years as we would not have had enough data for statistical analysis. Additionally, in terms of the existing conservative care literature on CSR outcomes in RCTs, it is clear that studies use 1–2 year follow-ups as their definition of 'long term'. In fact, most CSR RCTs only offer 3-month to 1-year follow-up and it is rare that studies go on for 2 years and longer [2,8–13]. Still, future investigations should provide results at 1, 2, 5-year, and 10-year follow-ups using the type of extension two-way traction as reported in our investigation to truly understand the long-term results of curve correction in CSR. Lastly, biomechanical investigations via computer simulation would be beneficial in future experimental designs to understand the soft tissue deformation and strain/strain effects of three-point-bending extension traction methods for cervical curve restoration in patients with cervical spondylotic radiculopathy.

5. Conclusions

Our investigation identified that the correction of the cervical lordosis, in hypolordotic spines of patients suffering from CSR, had improved pain and neurophysiology. The group receiving three-point bending cervical traction attained a significant increase in cervical lordosis, improvement in their pain intensity, and nerve root function measured with DSSEPs. Follow-up measurement revealed stable improvement in all measured variables. These observed effects of sagittal curve correction offer insights to clinicians working with patients with cervical spine disorders such as chronic CSR. Future trials should continue to investigate the rehabilitation of the abnormal cervical curve in CSR populations focusing on larger sample sizes, who are the optimum candidates, what an adequate curve correction is, and longer follow-up time periods.

Author Contributions: I.M.M. and A.A.D. conceived the research idea and D.E.H. participated in its design. I.M.M., A.A.D. and D.E.H. contributed to the statistical analysis. I.M.M. and A.A.D. participated in the data collection and study supervision. I.M.M., A.A.D. and D.E.H. contributed to the interpretation of the results and wrote the original and final drafts. All authors have read and agreed to the published version of the manuscript.

Funding: This research received no external funding.

Institutional Review Board Statement: The study was conducted in accordance with the Declaration of Helsinki and approved by the Ethics Committee of the Faculty of Physical Therapy, Cairo University with the ethical approval No Cairo23-987-12 M.S. Recruitment began after approval was obtained from the participants and they signed informed consent prior to data collection. The trial was retrospectively registered with ClinicalTrials.gov (NCT05547997) accessed on 20 September 2022. The reason for retrospective trial registration was that legislation in Egypt only required local registration for clinical trials at the time of the study design and this is what was conducted initially by prospectively registration in a non-WHO-approved registry.

Informed Consent Statement: Written informed consent was not obtained for the person depicted in Figure 1 as this is a photo from a model production shoot and the copyright holder is an author (DEH) on the manuscript and has provided consent for this image to be reproduced.

Data Availability Statement: The datasets analyzed in the current study are available from the corresponding author on reasonable request.

Conflicts of Interest: D.E.H. teaches rehabilitation methods and products to physicians for patient care as used in this manuscript. D.E.H. is not a patent holder for the 2-way traction depicted and described herein. All the other authors declare that they have no competing interests.

References

1. Ylinen, J.; Kautiainen, H.; Wirén, K.; Häkkinen, A. A stretching exercises vs manual therapy in treatment of chronic neck pain: A randomized, controlled cross-over trial. *J. Rehabil. Med.* **2007**, *39*, 126–132. [CrossRef]
2. Luyao, H.; Xiaoxiao, Y.; Tianxiao, F.; Yuandong, L.; Wang, P. Management of Cervical Spondylotic Radiculopathy: A Systematic review. *Glob. Spine J.* **2022**, *12*, 1912–1924. [CrossRef]
3. Clark, C.R. Differential diagnosis and non-operative management. In *The Adult Spine: Principles and Practice*, 2nd ed.; Frrymoyer, J.W., Ed.; Lippicott-Raven: Philadelphia, PA, USA, 1997; Volume 21, pp. 2421–2428.
4. Alghamdi, A.; Alqahtani, A. Magnetic Resonance Imaging of the Cervical Spine: Frequency of Abnormal Findings with Relation to Age. *Medicines* **2021**, *8*, 77. [CrossRef]
5. Faldini, C.; Pagkrati, S.; Leonetti, D.; Miscione, M.T.; Giannini, S. Sagittal segmental alignment as predictor of adjacent-level degeneration after a cloward procedure. *Clin. Orthop. Relat. Res.* **2011**, *469*, 674–681. [CrossRef]
6. Li, L.; Li, N.; Zhou, J.; Li, H.; Du, X.; He, H.; Rong, P.; Wang, W.; Liu, Y. Effect of cervical alignment change after anterior cervical fusion on radiological adjacent segment pathology. *Quant. Imaging Med. Surg.* **2022**, *12*, 2464–2473. [CrossRef]
7. Harrison, D.E.; Harrison, D.D.; Janik, T.J.; William Jones, E.; Cailliet, R.; Normand, M. Comparison of axial and flexural stresses in lordosis and three buckled configurations of the cervical spine. *Clin. Biomech.* **2001**, *16*, 276–284. [CrossRef]
8. Mallard, F.; Wong, J.J.; Lemeunier, N.; Côté, P. Effectiveness of Multimodal Rehabilitation Interventions for Management of Cervical Radiculopathy in Adults: An Updated Systematic Review from the Ontario Protocol for Traffic Injury Management (Optima) Collaboration. *J. Rehabil. Med.* **2022**, *54*, jrm00318. [CrossRef]
9. Borrella-Andrés, S.; Marqués-García, I.; Lucha-López, M.O.; Fanlo-Mazas, P.; Hernández-Secorún, M.; Pérez-Bellmunt, A.; Tricás-Moreno, J.M.; Hidalgo-García, C. Manual Therapy as a Management of Cervical Radiculopathy: A Systematic Review. *Biomed. Res. Int.* **2021**, *2021*, 9936981. [CrossRef]
10. Kuligowski, T.; Skrzek, A.; Cieślik, B. Manual Therapy in Cervical and Lumbar Radiculopathy: A Systematic Review of the Literature. *Int. J. Environ. Res. Public Health* **2021**, *18*, 6176. [CrossRef]
11. Zhu, L.; Wei, X.; Wang, S. Does cervical spine manipulation reduce pain in people with degenerative cervical radiculopathy? A systematic review of the evidence, and a meta-analysis. *Clin. Rehabil.* **2016**, *30*, 145–155. [CrossRef]
12. Romeo, A.; Vanti, C.; Boldrini, V.; Ruggeri, M.; Guccione, A.A.; Pillastrini, P.; Bertozzi, L. Cervical Radiculopathy: Effectiveness of Adding Traction to Physical Therapy-A Systematic Review and Meta-Analysis of Randomized Controlled Trials. *Phys. Ther.* **2018**, *98*, 231–242, Erratum in *Phys. Ther.* **2018**, *98*, 727. [CrossRef] [PubMed]
13. Colombo, C.; Salvioli, S.; Gianola, S.; Castellini, G.; Testa, M. Traction Therapy for Cervical Radicular Syndrome is Statistically Significant but not Clinically Relevant for Pain Relief. A Systematic Literature Review with Meta-Analysis and Trial Sequential Analysis. *J. Clin. Med.* **2020**, *9*, 3389. [CrossRef] [PubMed]
14. Moustafa, I.M.; Diab, A.A. Multimodal treatment program comparing 2 different traction approaches for patients with discogenic cervical radiculopathy: A randomized controlled trial. *J. Chiropr. Med.* **2014**, *13*, 157–167. [CrossRef] [PubMed]

15. Murphy, D. Conservative management of cervical spine syndromes. In *Dusfuntion in the Cerival Spine*; Murphy, D., Ed.; McGraw-Hill: New York, NY, USA, 2000; pp. 71–103.
16. Moustafa, I.M.; Diab, A.A.; Taha, S.; Harrison, D.E. Addition of a Sagittal Cervical Posture Corrective Orthotic Device to a Multimodal Rehabilitation Program Improves Short- and Long-Term Outcomes in Patients with Discogenic Cervical Radiculopathy. *Arch. Phys. Med. Rehabil.* **2016**, *97*, 2034–2044. [CrossRef] [PubMed]
17. Harrison, D.E.; Cailliet, R.; Harrison, D.D.; Troyanovich, S.J.; Harrison, S.O. A Review of Biomechanics of the Central Nervous System. PART II: Strains in the Spinal Cord from Postural Loads. *J. Manip. Physiol. Ther.* **1999**, *22*, 322–332. [CrossRef]
18. Breig, A. *Adverse Mechanical Tension in the Central Nervous System: An Analysis of Cause and Effect: Relief by Functional Neurosurgery*; Almqvist and Wiksell International: Stockholm, Sweden, 1978; p. 130.
19. Lin, T.; Wang, Z.; Chen, G.; Liu, W. Predictive Effect of Cervical Sagittal Parameters on Conservative Treatment of Single-Segment Cervical Spondylotic Radiculopathy. *World Neurosurg.* **2020**, *134*, e1028–e1036. [CrossRef]
20. Ames, C.P.; Blondel, B.; Scheer, J.K.; Schwab, F.J.; Le Huec, J.C.; Massicotte, E.M.; Patel, A.A.; Traynelis, V.C.; Kim, H.J.; Shaffrey, C.I.; et al. Cervical radiographical alignment: Comprehensive assessment techniques and potential importance in cervical myelopathy. *Spine* **2013**, *38*, S149–S160. [CrossRef]
21. Scheer, J.K.; Tang, J.A.; Smith, J.S.; Acosta, F.L., Jr.; Protopsaltis, T.S.; Blondel, B.; Bess, S.; Shaffrey, C.I.; Deviren, V.; Lafage, V.; et al. Cervical spine alignment, sagittal deformity, and clinical implications: A review. *J. Neurosurg. Spine* **2013**, *19*, 141–159. [CrossRef]
22. Lin, B.J.; Hong, K.T.; Lin, C.; Chung, T.T.; Tang, C.T.; Hueng, D.Y.; Hsia, C.C.; Ju, D.T.; Ma, H.I.; Liu, M.Y.; et al. Impact of global spine balance and cervical regional alignment on determination of postoperative cerviacl alignment after laminoplasty. *Medicine* **2018**, *97*, e13111. [CrossRef]
23. Pope, M. Case studies. In *Chiropractic the Physics of Spinal Correection*; Harrison, D.D., Ed.; National Library of Medicine: Bethesda, MA, USA, 1988; Volume 92, pp. 12–85.
24. Harrison, D.E.; Cailliet, R.; Harrison, D.D.; Janik, T.J.; Holland, B.A. New 3-point bending traction method for restoring cervical lordosis and cervical manipulation: A non-randomized clinical controlled trial. *Arch. Phys. Med. Rehabil.* **2002**, *83*, 447–453. [CrossRef]
25. Oakley, P.A.; Ehsani, N.N.; Moustafa, I.M.; Harrison, D.E. Restoring cervical lordosis by cervical extension traction methods in the treatment of cervical spine disorders: A systematic review of controlled trials. *J. Phys. Ther. Sci.* **2021**, *33*, 784–794. [CrossRef] [PubMed]
26. Naguszewski, W.K.; Naguszewski, R.K.; Gose, E.E. Dermatomal somatosensory evoked potential demonstration of nerve root decompression after VAX-D therapy. *Neurol. Res.* **2001**, *23*, 706–714. [CrossRef] [PubMed]
27. Pope, P.H.M.; Oepkes, C.T.; Notermans, S.L.H.; Vlek, N.M.T.; Stegeman, D.F. Dermatomal somatosensory evoked potentials of the lumbar and cervical roots. Method and normal values. *Eur. Arch. Psychiatry Clin. Neurosci.* **1988**, *238*, 22–27.
28. McAviney, J.; Schulz, D.; Bock, R.; Harrison, D.E.; Holland, B. Determining the Relationship between Cervical Lordosis and Neck Complaints. *J. Manip. Physiol Ther.* **2005**, *28*, 187–193. [CrossRef] [PubMed]
29. Harrison, D.D.; Harrison, D.E.; Janik, T.J.; Cailliet, R.; Haas, J.W.; Ferrantelli, J.; Holland, B. Modeling of the Sagittal Cervical Spine as a Method to Discriminate Hypo-Lordosis: Results of Elliptical and Circular Modeling in 72 Asymptomatic Subjects, 52 Acute Neck Pain Subjects, and 70 Chronic Neck Pain Subjects. *Spine* **2004**, *29*, 2485–2492. [CrossRef]
30. Mansoori, S.S.; Moustafa, I.M.; Ahbouch, A.; Harrison, D.E. Optimal duration of stretching exercise in patients with chronic myofascial pain syndrome: A randomized controlled trial. *J. Rehabil. Med.* **2021**, *53*, jrm00142. [CrossRef]
31. Kisner, C.; Colby, L.A. Therapeutic exercise foundations and techniques. In *The Spine: Exercise and Manipulation Interventions*; Kisner, C., Thorp, J.N., Eds.; 6th ed.; FA Davis: Philadelphia, PA, USA, 2012; pp. 485–538.
32. Liguori, R.; Taher, G.; Trojaborg, W. Somatosensory evoked potentials from cervical and lumbosacral dermatomes. *Acta Neurol. Scand.* **1991**, *84*, 161–166. [CrossRef]
33. Harrison, D.E.; Harrison, D.D.; Cailliet, R.; Troyanovich, S.J.; Janik, T.J.; Holland, B. Cobb Method or Harrison Posterior Tangent Method: Which is Better for Lateral Cervical Analysis? *Spine* **2000**, *25*, 2072–2078. [CrossRef]
34. Chuds, J.D.; Piva, S.R.; Fritz, J.M. Responsiveness of the numeric pain rating scale in patients with low back pain. *Spine* **2005**, *30*, 1331–1334.
35. Helliwell, P.S.; Evans, P.F.; Wright, V. The straight cervical spine: Does it indicate muscle spasm? *J. Bone Jt. Surg. Br.* **1994**, *76*, 103–106. [CrossRef]
36. Fedorchuk, C.A.; McCoy, M.; Lightstone, D.F.; Bak, D.A.; Moser, J.; Kubricht, B.; Packer, J.; Walton, D.; Binongo, J. Impact of Isometric Contraction of Anterior Cervical Muscles on Cervical Lordosis. *J. Radiol. Case Rep.* **2016**, *10*, 13–25. [CrossRef] [PubMed]
37. Levoska, S.; Keinänen-Kiukaanniemi, S. Active or passive physiotherapy for occupational cervicobrachial disorders? A comparison of two treatment methods with a 1-year follow-up. *Arch. Phys. Med. Rehabil.* **1993**, *74*, 425–430. [PubMed]
38. Rulleau, T.; Abeille, S.; Pastor, L.; Planche, L.; Allary, P.; Chapeleau, C.; Moreau, C.; Cormier, G.; Caulier, M. Effect of an intensive cervical traction protocol on mid-term disability and pain in patients with cervical radiculopathy: An exploratory, prospective, observational pilot study. *PLoS ONE* **2021**, *16*, e0255998. [CrossRef]
39. Grob, D.; Frauenfelder, H.; Mannion, A.F. The association between cervical spine curvature and neck pain. *Eur. Spine J.* **2007**, *16*, 669–678. [CrossRef]
40. Wainner, R.S.; Gill, H. Diagnosis and nonoperative management of cervical radiculopathy. *J. Orthop. Sports Phys. Ther.* **2000**, *30*, 728–744. [CrossRef]

41. Schnebel, B.E.; Watkins, R.G.; Dillin, W. The role of spinal flexion and extension in changing nerve root compression in disc herniations. *Spine* **1989**, *14*, 835–837. [CrossRef]
42. Abdulwahab, S.S.; Sabbahi, M. Neck retractions, cervical root decompression, and radicular pain. *J. Orthop. Sports Phys. Ther.* **2000**, *30*, 4–12.
43. Albert, T.J.; Smith, A.; Bresseler, E. An vivo analysis of dimentional changes of the neuro-foramen after anterior cervical discectomy and fusion: A radiologic investigation. *J. Spinal Disord.* **1997**, *10*, 229–233. [CrossRef]
44. Brian, K.; David, H.K.; Andrea, M.; Louis, G.J. Outcomes Following Anterior Cervical Discectomy and Fusion: The Role of Interbody Disc Height, Angulation, and Spinous Process Distance. *J. Spinal Disord. Tech.* **2005**, *18*, 304–308.
45. Wang, X.; Liu, Y.; Zhang, H.; Jin, J.; Ma, Y.; Leng, Y. Sinomenine alleviates dorsal root ganglia inflammation to inhibit neuropathic pain via the p38 MAPK/CREB signalling pathway. *Eur. J. Pharmacol.* **2021**, *897*, 173945. [CrossRef]

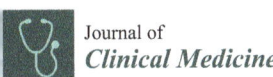

Article

Does Improvement towards a Normal Cervical Sagittal Configuration Aid in the Management of Lumbosacral Radiculopathy: A Randomized Controlled Trial

Ibrahim Moustafa Moustafa [1,2], Aliaa Attiah Mohamed Diab [1,2] and Deed Eric Harrison [3,*]

1 Department of Physiotherapy, College of Health Sciences, University of Sharjah, Sharjah P.O. Box 27272, United Arab Emirates
2 Faculty of Physical Therapy, Cairo University, Giza 12511, Egypt
3 Private Practice and CBP Non-Profit, Inc., Eagle, ID 83616, USA
* Correspondence: drdeed@idealspine.com

Abstract: A randomized controlled study with a six-month follow-up was conducted to investigate the effects of sagittal head posture correction on 3D spinal posture parameters, back and leg pain, disability, and S1 nerve root function in patients with chronic discogenic lumbosacral radiculopathy (CDLR). Participants included 80 (35 female) patients between 40 and 55 years experiencing CDLR with a definite hypolordotic cervical spine and forward head posture (FHP) and were randomly assigned a comparative treatment control group and a study group. Both groups received TENS therapy and hot packs, additionally, the study group received the Denneroll cervical traction orthotic. Interventions were applied at a frequency of 3 x per week for 10 weeks and groups were followed for an additional 6-months. Radiographic measures included cervical lordosis (CL) from C2–C7 and FHP; postural measurements included: lumbar lordosis, thoracic kyphosis, trunk inclination, lateral deviation, trunk imbalance, surface rotation, and pelvic inclination. Leg and back pain scores, Oswestry Disability Index (ODI), and H-reflex latency and amplitude were measured. Statistically significant differences between the groups at 10 weeks were found: for all postural measures, CL ($p = 0.001$), AHT ($p = 0.002$), H-reflex amplitude ($p = 0.007$) and latency ($p = 0.001$). No significant difference for back pain ($p = 0.2$), leg pain ($p = 0.1$) and ODI ($p = 0.6$) at 10 weeks were identified. Only the study group's improvements were maintained at the 6-month follow up while the control groups values regressed back to baseline. At the 6-month follow-up, it was identified in the study group that improved cervical lordosis and reduction of FHP were found to have a positive impact on 3D posture parameters, leg and back pain scores, ODI, and H-reflex latency and amplitude.

Keywords: randomized controlled trial; traction; disc herniation; cervical lordosis; lumbosacral radiculopathy

1. Introduction

Lumbosacral radiculopathy associated with disk herniation is one of the most common health-related complaints [1]. Radiculopathy of the S1 nerve root is a frequent pathology, strongly associated with delayed recovery, persistent disability, and increased health care utilization and costs [2]. Despite the high prevalence of this condition [3], its conservative treatment has long remained a challenge for the clinician [4], since there is no strong evidence of the effectiveness of most treatments, particularly for long-term management outcomes [5].

The challenge clinicians face is merging an understanding of the patient's local pathology (e.g., disc herniation) as an etiological factor of their lower back pain (LBP) with an understanding of how altered regional and full spine alignment and biomechanics play a role in the patient's unique condition. The interaction of tissue pathology and spine dysfunction is clearly ellicudated by Murphy's concept [6], "pathoanatomy and dysfunction

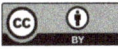

often interact to produce clinical symptoms". In terms of local biomechanical dysfunction, several investigations have identified that altered trunk posture [7,8] and lumbar spine hypolordotic alignment [9,10] are important etiological factors contributing to the development of and with the presence associated LBP.

In the past decade several publications have identified that head and neck alignment plays a role in whole body pain and impairment including LBP and related disorders [11,12]; whether this is a pure mechanical phenomenon remains unclear. Studies have identified that several of the postural upright postural neurophysiological reflexes, are located within the head and neck region [13]. This implies that correction of the altered cervical spine alignment could be required to achieve optimal full spine postural correction, where the rest of the spine orients itself in a top-down fashion [14].

Besides the surgical outcomes of adult spine deformity linking head and neck alignment to health quality of life in thoraco-lumbar deformity patients [11,12], relatively few correlational studies were identified linking cervical spine alignment to thoracic spine ailments and full spine alignment to LBP [15,16]. However, considering the effect that abnormal cervical posture (flexion and translation) has on the stress and strain experienced in the entire spinal cord and nerve roots [17,18], it would seem logical that alterations in cervical spine alignment would influence, at least to some extent, pain and radiculopathy in lumbosacral disorders. It would seem that lumbosacral radiculopathy and LBP conservative treatment today is universally lacking investigations seeking to understand the influence of alignment of the cervical spine relative to pain, disability, and other management outcomes [19,20].

Despite the fact that there is some evidence of a link between lower back pain disorders and head/neck posture [11,12,21], there is limited experimental data to support a cause-and-effect relationship and interventional outcomes. Accordingly, the primary hypothesis of this study was that cervical curve restoration and forward head posture reduction will have short- and long-term effects on three-dimensional (3D) spinal posture parameters as well as lumbar radiculopathy management outcomes such as symptoms, disability, and neurophysiological findings [19,20].

In the current study we used a cervical traction orthotic device termed the Denneroll™ to help restore normal sagittal spinal configuration based on principles of 3-point bending traction methods [22]. The Denneroll device uses sustained cervical spine extension loading in a prone position in order to create visco-elastic creep-deformation in the connective tissues of the spine leading to more consistent and effective correction of the cervical sagittal alignment. This was the primary reason for choosing this device to test our working hypothesis.

2. Methods

A prospective, randomized, controlled study was conducted at a research laboratory of our university. All the patients were conveniently selected from our institution's outpatient clinic. Recruitment began after approval was obtained from the Ethics Committee of the Faculty of Physical Therapy, Cairo University; all participants signed informed consent prior to data collection. Patients were recruited from May 2011 to June 2011 for a 10-week treatment investigation with a six-month follow-up. This trial was retrospectively registered at ClinicalTrials.gov (accessed on 10 September 2022) with registration number: NCT05553002.

- Participant inclusion

Pain, disability, and symptoms: Patients were included if they had a confirmed chronic unilateral lumbosacral radiculopathy associated with L5-S1 lumbar disc prolapse with symptoms lasting longer than 3 months to avoid the acute stage of inflammation. All the patients had unilateral leg pain with mild to moderate disability according to the Oswestry Disability Index (ODI) (up to 40%) [23]. All patients had side-to-side H-reflex latency differences of more than 1 ms. Further, patients were selected with lumbar hyperlordosis (sway back posture), which is considered a common posture aberration in CLBP patients [24].

- Participant exclusion criteria

Exclusion criteria included previous history of lumbosacral surgery, metabolic system disorder, cancer, cardiac problems, peripheral neuropathy, history of upper motor neuron lesion, spinal canal stenosis, rheumatoid arthritis, osteoporosis and any lower extremity deformity that might interfere with global postural alignment. The demographic characteristics of the patients are shown in Table 1.

Table 1. Baseline participant demographics and tests of significance of between group variables.

	Study Group (n = 40)	Control Group (n = 40)	p ‡
Age (y)	46.3 ± 2.05	45.9 ± 2.1	0.391
Height (cm)	172 ± 9	175 ± 10	0.162
Weight (kg)	75 ± 9	80 ± 10	0.021 *
Gender			1.000
Male	22	23	
Female	18	17	
Work			0.087
Sedentary	25	18	
Mobile	11	10	
Sedentary and mobile	4	12	
Previous back pain treatment (yes/no)			0.580
Surgery	0	0	
Medication	29	30	
Physical therapy	5	7	
Other	6	3	

‡: Two-sided 2-sample t test for continuous variables and Fisher's exact test for categorical variables. SD: Standard deviation; values are mean (±SD) for age, height, weight and number for the term 'other'. *: Statistically significant difference between groups for weight.

Radiography: Participants were screened prior to inclusion by measuring their lateral cervical for a cervical absolute rotatory angle (ARA) formed by two lines intersecting from the posterior body margins of C2–C7 and forward head distance (AHT measured as the horizontal displacement of the posterior superior body corner of C2 vertebra relative to a vertical line extending superiorly from the posterior inferior body corner of C7). Lateral cervical X-rays were obtained with the participant in an upright, neutral, standing posture. If the ARA angle was less than 25° and greater than 0, then a participant was included in the study; thus, straightened and kyphotic cervical curvatures were excluded. Also, if the AHT distance was greater than 15 mm then a participant was included in the study. These X-ray cut-points for ARA and AHT were based on the mean values reported in the study by Harrison et al. [25].

- Randomization assignment

The patients were randomly assigned to to either the treatment group (n = 40) or the control group (n = 40). An independent person, blinded to the research protocol and not otherwise involved in the trial, operated the random assignment through picking one of the sealed envelopes which contained numbers chosen by a random number generator. A diagram of patients' retention and randomization throughout the study is shown in Figure 1.

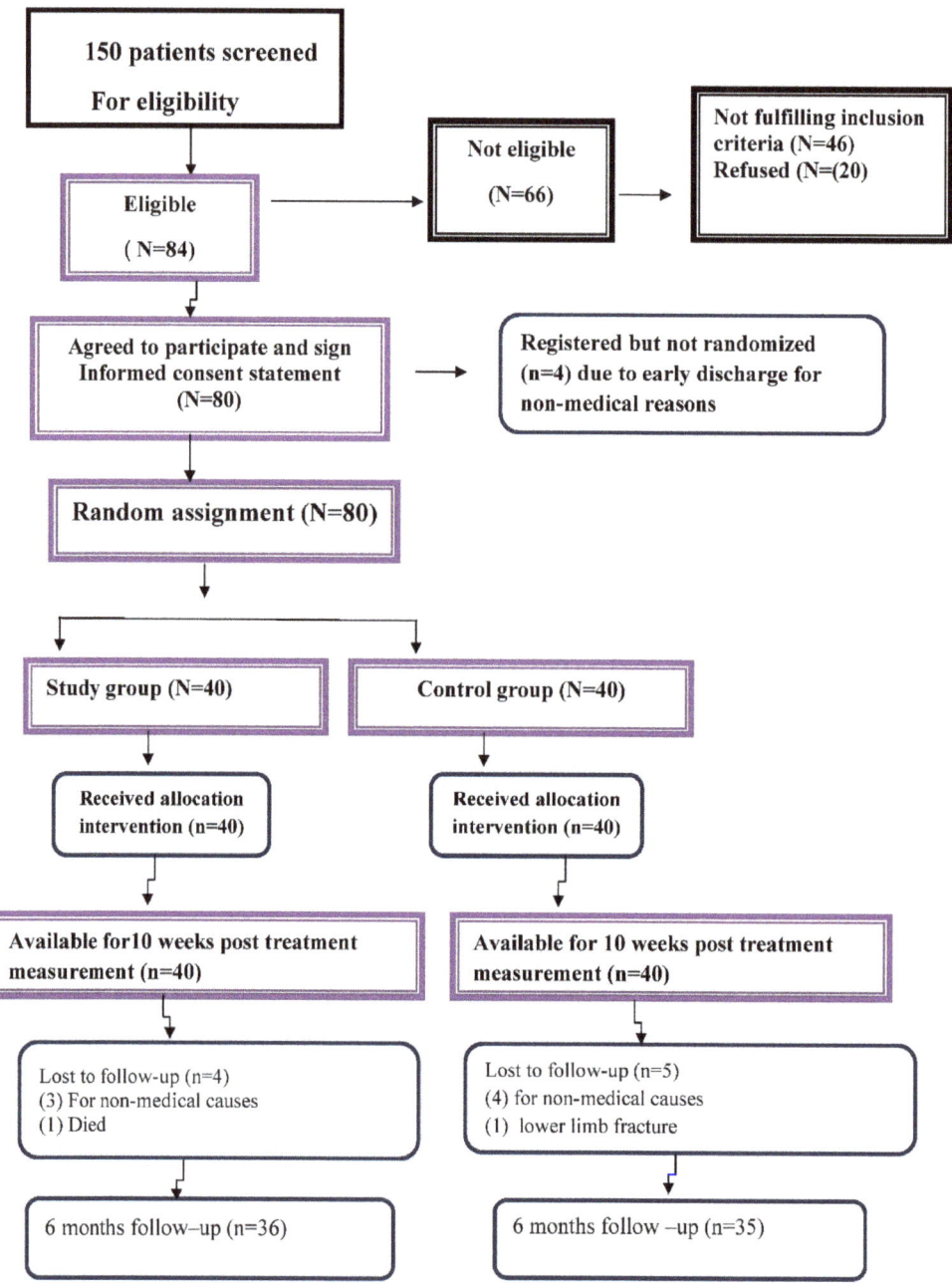

Figure 1. Flow of study participants.

- Interventions

The patients in both groups received hot packs (15 min) and TENS therapy to control pain and eliminate the causal role of muscle spasms and/or tightness in changing the posture parameters; these procedures were applied with the patient in the prone position on an examination bench. The TENS treatment was introduced using an electrotherapy device (Phyaction 787, The Netherlands). The TENS therapy was delivered at the lumbosacral region for 20 min. The frequency was set to 80 Hz and pulse width to 50 μs due to its analgesic effect [26]. These conventional treatments were repeated three times per week over the course of 10 weeks for 30 total sessions. Those in the control group received this conventional treatment only.

The experimental group additionally received Denneroll cervical extension traction (Denneroll Industries (www.denneroll.com (accessed on 10 September 2022)) of Sydney, Australia). Here, the patient lies flat on their back (supine) on the ground with their legs extended and arms by their sides. The patient is encouraged to relax whilst lying on the Denneroll [22]. The Denneroll was placed on the ground and postioned in the posterior aspect of the neck depending on the area needing to be addressed (Figure 2). Participants were screened and tested for tolerance to the extended position on the device to insure they were capable of performing this position; while the Denneroll takes the segments of the cervical spine near the apex of the curve to their end range of extension motion, it does not create hyperextension of the skull relative to the torso. See Figure 2. Patients began with 3 min per session and progressed to a maximum of 20 min per session in an incremental fashion.

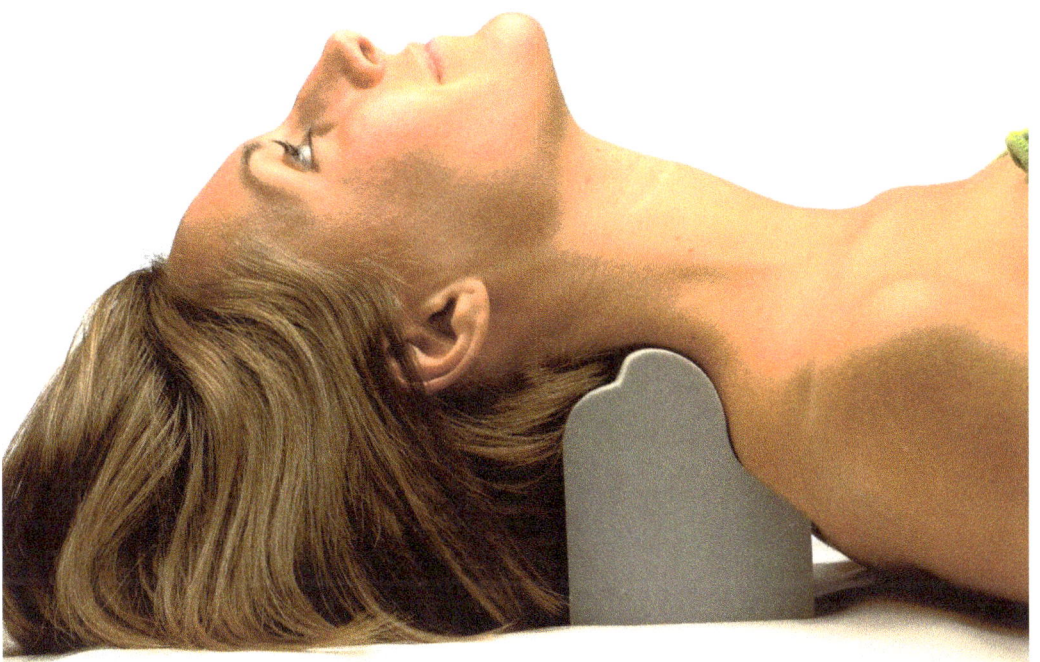

Figure 2. The Denneroll cervical traction orthotic. The participant must lie on a firm surface, such as the floor, and place the peak of the Denneroll just distal to the apex of their cervical lordotic abnormality as shown on the lateral cervical X-ray. Shown is a mid-cervical spine placement. ©Copyright CBP Seminars. Reprinted with permission.

The apex of the Denneroll orthotic was placed in one of three regions based on lateral cervical radiographic displacements:

1. In the upper cervical region (C2–C4) region. This position allows extension bending of the upper cervical segments while causing slight anterior head translation (AHT). One subject received this placement location.
2. The apex of the Denneroll orthotic is placed in the mid-cervical region (C4-C6) region. This position allows extension bending of the mid-upper cervical segments while creating a slight posterior head translation. Ten subjects received this placement location.
3. The apex of the Denneroll orthotic is placed in the upper thoracic lower-cervical region (C6-T1) region. This position allows extension bending of the lower to middle cervical segments while creating a significant posterior head translation. Twenty-nine subjects received this placement location.

- Outcome Measures

A repeatable and reliable method [27,28] was used to quantify the main outcome measurement represented in cervical lordosis (ARA C2–C7) and any amount of anterior head posture AHT (C2–C7). Standard lateral cervical radiographs were obtained at three intervals (pretreatment, 10-weeks post-treatment, and at the six-month follow-up). A representative example of a lateral cervical X-ray in a study group patient at three intervals of measurement is given graphically in Figure 3.

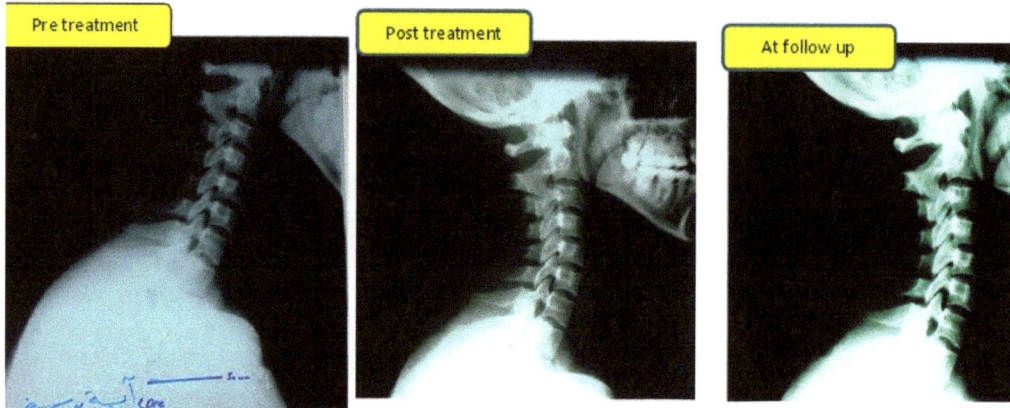

Figure 3. Sample of lateral cervical X-ray findings of a participant in the study group receiving Denneroll traction application at the three intervals of measurement. Pre-treatment prior to study participation, 10-week post-treatment participation, and at the 6-month study follow up radiographs are shown demonstrating improved cervical lordosis and reduced anterior head posture.

Other outcome measures used to compare effectiveness of the treatment between the study and control groups included the 3D spinal posture parameters, disability, and neurophysiological findings.

Rasterstereography (Formetric 2, Diers International GmbH, Schlangenbad, Germany) was used to examine posture and back shape characteristics. All testing procedures were done following Lippold et al.'s protocol [29]. The Formetric scans were taken in a relaxed standing position. The patient was positioned in front of the black background screen at a distance of two meters from the measurement system. The column height was aligned to move the relevant parts of the patient's back into the center of the control monitor by using the column up/down button of the control unit; to ensure the best lateral and longitudinal position of the patient a permanent mark on the floor was used. The patient's back surface (including upper buttocks) was completely bare in order to avoid image disturbing structures.

After the patient and the system were correctly positioned, the system was ready for image recording. The image processing consisted of automatic back surface reconstruction and shape analysis. The sagittale plane parameters (lumbar angles, thoracic angles, and trunk inclination), the frontal plane parameters (trunk imbalance and lateral deviation) and the transversal plane parameters (vertebral surface rotation and pelvis torsion) were selected to cover the posture profile in three planes. A representative example of the Formetric system's print out is given graphically for a study group participant (Figure 4).

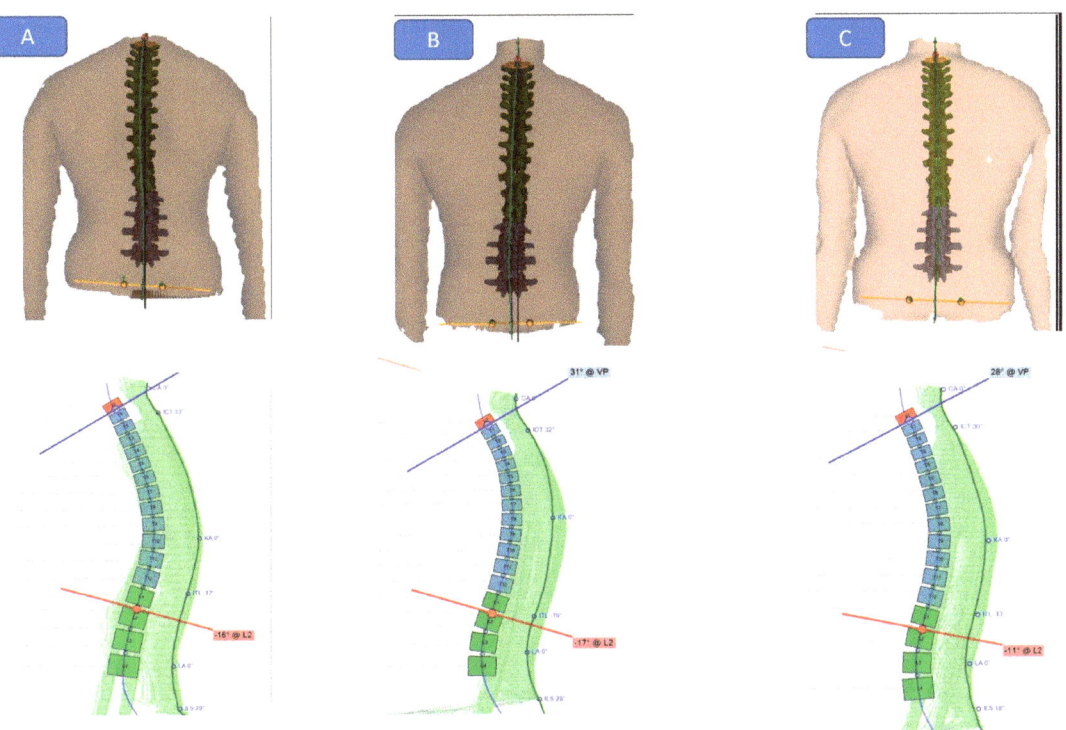

Figure 4. Formetric findings at the three intervals of measurement for a representative patient in the study group: In the left-hand column is the sagittal plane surface profile of the thoracic and lumbar spines while the right-hand column is the posterior view of the coronal and transverse aspects of posture deformity for the thoracic, lumbar, and top of the pelvic regions. (**A**) pre-treatment; (**B**) 10-weeks post-treatment; and (**C**) is the 6-month follow up.

Disability was measured using the Oswestry Disability Index. The total score is transferred onto a scale ranging from 0 to 100, where 0 indicates no disability and 100 indicates worst possible disability [23].

The back and leg pain intensity were measured using the numerical pain rating scale (NPRS), which is considered a valid and reliable scale [30]. The patients were asked to place a mark along a line to denote their pain level; 0 reflecting "no pain" and 10 reflecting the "worst pain".

Latency and peak-to-peak amplitude of the H-reflex, the recommended H-reflex diagnostic criteria for lumbosacral radiculopathy [20], were used in the current study. An electromyogram device (Tonneisneuroscreen plus version 1.59, Germany) was used to measure this variable for all patients before starting the treatment, at the end of 10 weeks, and at the six-month follow-up. All testing procedures were done following Al-Abdulwahab and Al-Jabrb's protocol [31]. The patient was lying supine on a wooden padded table, with arms on the side. The knee was flexed 20 degrees by placing a small cushion under the knee to relax the gastrocnemius muscle. The tibial nerve was stimulated at the popliteal fossa, midway between the tendon of the biceps femoris and semimembranosus, using a silver–silver chloride surface-stimulating bar electrode with the cathode proximal to the anode.

For recording, surface bar electrodes were placed 3 cm distal to the bifurcation of the gastrocnemii and superior to the Achilles tendon. A ground surface metal electrode was positioned midway between the stimulation and recording electrodes to minimize the stimulus artifact. Before attaching the recording electrodes, the underlying skin was shaved and cleaned with a piece of cotton soaked with alcohol. The stimulation parameters were 1.0 ms pulse duration and intensity that elicited H-maximum with minimum and stable M-response at a frequency of 0.2 Hz. Four readings of the maximum H-reflex with minimum and stable M-responses were recorded and averaged from the involved leg. The signals were amplified 500–2000 × using differential amplification and filtered at 3 Hz–10 kHz, digitized (10 kHz) and stored on a computer for analysis.

- Sample size determination

A prior power calculation indicated that 27 patients were needed in each group to detect a difference in cervical lordotic angle between the groups with 90% power and a 5% significance level; a 2-tailed test, and an expected effect size of $d = 0.9$ based on a pilot study consisted of 10 patients who received the same program. The sample size estimation was based on an unpublished pilot randomized controlled clinical trial that used a similar protocol for patients with discogenic lumbosacral radiculopathy. The population was in the same age range with minimal change in the control treatment (stretching vs. hot backs herein). In this pilot, the traditional therapy was TENS, back and lower limb stretching exercises, and ARA C2–C7 cervical lordosis for our primary outcome. The pilot project had no long-term follow-up; therefore, the sample size was calculated based on pre-post lordosis changes. The mean change and standard deviation of the cervical lordosis were estimated at 3.2 and 3.7, respectively. To account for the possibility of significant drop-out rates, the sample size was increased by 40%.

- Data analysis

To compare the experimental group and the control group, statistical analysis was based on the intention-to-treat principle, and p-values less than 0.05 were considered significant. We used multiple imputations to handle missing data. To impute the missing data, we constructed multiple regression models including variables potentially related to the fact that the data were missing and also variables correlated with that outcome. We used Stata (Stata Corp, College Station, TX, USA). The 2-way repeated-measures analysis of covariance was used to compare between groups. The model included one independent factor (group), one repeated measure (time), and an interaction factor (group * time). The baseline values of the outcomes were used as covariates to assess the between-group differences, to center the baseline covariates, everyone's score value was subtracted from the overall mean. A t-test at two follow-up points (after 10 weeks of treatment and at the six-month follow-up) was performed to test the between group differences at the different intervals.

3. Results

A diagram of patients' retention and randomization throughout the study is shown in Figure 1. One hundred and fifty patients were initially screened. After the screening process, 84 patients were eligible to participate in the study and 80 completed the first follow up at 10 weeks, while 71 of them completed the entire study including the 6-month follow up. The study design did not include a pre-determined adverse event protocol. However, participants were formally asked during their treatment sessions if they were experiencing any unusual adverse events or increased pain due to the interventions. No adverse events were documented by the treating therapist aside from minimal and transient discomfort in the neck as the patient acclimatized to using the Denneroll device at the point of cervical spine contact.

Results are summarized and presented as mean (±SD) in Table 2. After 10 weeks of treatment, the analysis of covariance (ANCOVA) revealed a significant difference between the study and control groups adjusted to baseline values for all following variables: ARA ($p = 0.001$), AHT ($p = 0.002$), neurophysiological findings represented in H-reflex amplitude ($p = 0.007$) and H-reflex latency ($p = 0.001$); 3D postural parameters in terms of trunk inclination ($p = 0.001$), lumbar lordosis ($p = 0.002$), thoracic kyphosis ($p = 0.001$), trunk imbalance ($p = 0.001$), pelvic inclination ($p = 0.005$), and surface rotation ($p = 0.01$).

Table 2. Means, standard deviations (±SD), and statistical significance for all outcome variables in the control group versus the study subjects at initial, 10 weeks of treatment, and 6-month follow up.

Dependent Variables		Initial Baseline	10-Weeks Post	6-Month Follow Up	p-Value G	T	G*T
Trunk inclination	Study G	6 ± 1.0	5.1 ± 1.1	5.5 ± 1.4	<0.001	<0.001	<0.001
	Control G	6.7 ± 1.3	6.5 ± 1.1	6.8 ± 1.3			
	Between group analysis		0.01	0.04			
Thoracic kyphosis	Study G	64.9 ± 4.2	62.0 ± 5.3	63.1 ± 5.1	<0.001	<0.001	<0.001
	Control G	62.2 ± 4.9	61.5 ± 4.9	61.9 ± 5.2			
	Between group analysis		0.001	0.001			
Lumbar lordosis	Study G	49.5 ± 3.4	46.7 ± 3.5	47.1 ± 3.3	<0.001	<0.001	<0.001
	Control G	49.1 ± 3.2	48.3 ± 3.2	48.9 ± 3.4			
	Between group analysis		0.002	0.001			
Trunk imbalance	Study G	20.4 ± 2.9	17.4 ± 2.8	17.8 ± 2.7	<0.001	<0.001	<0.001
	Control G	20.1 ± 2.9	19.3 ± 2.4	19.5 ± 2.6			
	Between group analysis		0.001	<0.001			
Pelvic inclination	Study G	3.2 ± 0.6	1.9 ± 0.8	2.0 ± 1	<0.001	<0.001	<0.001
	Control G	3.0 ± 0.6	3.0 ± 0.9	3.3 ± 0.8			
	Between group analysis		0.005	0.02			
Surface rotation	Study G	5.6 ± 1.1	5.01 ± 1.3	5.6 ± 1.6	<0.001	<0.001	<0.001
	Control G	6.4 ± 1.0	6.3 ± 0.9	6.7 ± 1.0			
	Between group analysis		0.01	0.05			
+ Cervical ARA	Study G	13.3 ± 3	18.25 ± 2.6	17.6 ± 2.8	<0.001	<0.001	<0.001
	Control G	13.5 ± 2.7	14 ± 2.8	14 ± 2.9			
	Between group analysis		0.001	0.01			
Functional index	Study G	29 ± 5.6	25.3 ± 5.4	25 ± 5	<0.001	<0.001	<0.001
	Control G	31.9 ± 5.8	31.6 ± 5.5	33 ± 6.2			
	Between group analysis		0.6	<0.001			
H-reflex amplitude	Study G	2.4 ± 0.3	2.8 ± 0.4	2.7 ± 0.3	<0.001	<0.001	<0.001
	Control G	1.9 ± 0.2	2.1 ± 0.4	2 ± 0.6			
	Between group analysis		0.007	<0.001			

Table 2. Cont.

Dependent Variables		Initial Baseline	10-Weeks Post	6-Month Follow Up	p-Value G	T	G*T
H-reflex latency	Study G	33.5 ± 0.7	32.4 ± 0.7	32.5 ± 0.6	<0.001	<0.001	<0.001
	Control G	33.8 ± 0.6	33.5 ± 1.1	34 ± 2.1			
	Between group analysis		0.001	0.004			
Back pain	Study G	5.2 ± 0.8	3.5 ± 1.1	3.3 ± 1.5	<0.001	<0.001	<0.001
	Control G	4.6 ± 1	3.4 ± 1	4.7 ± 1.5			
	Between group analysis		0.27	<0.001			
Leg pain	Study G	6.9 ± 0.7	4.8 ± 1.3	4.7 ± 1.5	<0.001	<0.001	<0.001
	Control G	6.4 ± 1.1	4.7 ± 1.4	6.1 ± 1.6			
	Between group analysis		0.1	<0.001			
++ AHT	Study G	26.5 ± 5.7	21 ± 5.3	22.0 ± 5.3	<0.001	<0.001	<0.001
	Control G	26.1 ± 3.9	24.9 ± 3.8	25.3 ± 3.2			
	Between group analysis		0.002	0.028			

T2-way repeated-measures analysis of covariance was used to compare between groups. The model included one independent factor (group: G), one repeated measure (time: T), and an interaction factor (group * time: G*T). +ARA: Absolute rotation angle for cervical lordosis along the backs of vertebral body margins of C2 and C7. ++AHT: Forward or anterior head translation posture.

At the six-month follow-up, the analysis showed that there were still significant differences between the study and control groups for all the previous variables: radiographic measurements of cervical lordosis ARA ($p = 0.01$), AHT ($p = 0.028$); neurophysiological findings represented in H-reflex amplitude ($p < 0.001$) and H-reflex latency ($p = 0.004$); as well as the 3D postural parameters of trunk inclination ($p = 0.04$), lumbar lordosis ($p = 0.001$), thoracic kyphosis ($p = 0.001$), trunk imbalance ($p < 0.001$), pelvic inclination ($p = 0.02$), and surface rotation ($p = 0.05$). Table 2 presents this data. Figure 3 depicts an example of radiographic changes in the study group across the 3 time periods of evaluation. Figure 4 depicts an example of the 3D posture changes in the study group across the 3 time periods of evaluation.

At the 10-week post-treatment analysis, for back pain, leg pain and the ODI disability index, the between group analysis revealed insignificant difference between the groups at the first measurement interval: back pain, $p = 0.27$; leg pain, $p = 0.1$; and ODI, $p = 0.6$. In contrast, at the 6-month follow up, there was statistically significant differences between the groups for back pain ($p < 0.001$), leg pain ($p < 0.001$), and ODI ($p < 0.001$). These data are reported in Table 2. Specifically, the 6-month follow up data indicated that the control group's scores regressed back to pre-intervention levels while the study groups' improvements in these variables were maintained.

4. Discussion

This study tested the hypothesis that correction of sagittal cervical alignment would influence management outcomes of chronic lumbosacral radiculopathy. We compared TENS and hot packs in a control group to the outcomes of a study group receiving the control interventions plus the addition of an extension cervical traction device (the Denneroll) known to correct sagittal cervical spine alignment. [22] As expected, after 10 weeks of treatment, the study group (traction group) was found to have improvements in the cervical lordosis and anterior head translation compared to no change in the control group. Additionally, at 10 weeks, the study group was found to have improved 3D thoraco-lumbar-pelvic posture as well as improved neurophysiology as measured with the H-reflex.

Unexpectedly, the patient perceptive outcomes of lower back pain, leg pain, and lower back disability showed no differences between the groups; both groups improved equally at

10 weeks of treatment. However, after the 6-month follow-up with no further interventions, the control groups improvements regressed back to baseline values while the study group showed improved lumbar radiculopathy management outcomes for all variables. Thus, the difference in our study groups 6-month outcomes compared to the control group of improved radiographic, 3D postural parameters, clinical, and neurophysiological variables all indicate that our hypothesis is supported; improved cervical sagittal alignment does have a significant effect on the management outcomes of lumbosacral radiculopathy.

- Back pain, leg pain improvements at 10 weeks

The outcomes of back pain, leg pain, and disability for both the study group and control group showed similar improvements at the 10-week post-treatment assessment. The temporal reduction of pain in both our groups can be attributed to the short-term effect of TENS and hotpacks. For instance, Escortell-Mayor et al. [32] reported that the effect of TENS significantly decreased 6 months after the intervention. Similarly, the systematic review of Gaid and Cozens [33] provides evidence to support the use of TENS as a short-term effective treatment modality for chronic lower back pain. This is likely the explanation for the worsening (waning of treatment effect) of pain and disability in our control group at 6 months.

- Sagittal Cervical Alignment

The improvement in the forward head posture and cervical lordotic curve recorded by the study group receiving the Denneroll was anticipated in as much as previous investigations have identified that this device does indeed improve the cervical lordosis and reduce anterior head translation [22]. Sustained extension loading on devices like the Denneroll causes stretching of the visco-elastic tissues (discs, ligaments, muscles) of the cervical spine in the direction of the neutral head and neck posture and increased lordosis; this is the likely explanation and rationale for sustained extension loading restoring the cervical lordosis and improving anterior head translation [22,34,35].

Our study identified a smaller mean improvement in cervical lordosis compared to previous investigations using extension traction devices [22,34,35]. These smaller mean changes are likely a result of our use of only 30 sessions on the Denneroll and the predetermined inclusion criteria of hypolordosis with AHT, thoracic hyperkyphosis, and lumbar hyperlordosis for subject participation. It is possible that if we allowed straight and reversed cervical curves in our population, the corrections would have been greater as the potential for improvement would be more. We suggest it is likely that the improved cervical sagittal alignment played a role in the improved outcomes of lumbosacral radiculopathy in our study group for the reasons discussed below.

- 3-D Posture Changes

The study group receiving the Denneroll traction experienced significant changes in posture parameters occurring in the sagittal, transverse, and coronal planes. These postural changes suggest an important role for the cervical spine on global spinal posture via complex neurophysiological reflex mechanisms [13]. For instance, studies have identified neurological regulation of static upright human posture that is largely dependent on head posture [36,37] and consequently a normal joint afferentation process.

Our results are conceptually in agreement with Lewit [31] who highlighted the association between head posture and the pelvo-ocular reflex, where an anterior pelvic translation to balance the head's center of gravity may occur; this interdependence between body segments has been reported by others as well [38,39]. Additionally, in the study group receiving the Denneroll traction, the resultant changes in the sagittal contour of the whole spine may have contributed to the significant improvements of posture parameters in the transverse and coronal planes as well. For example, the relationship between the sagittal and coronal spinal contours [40–42] and between the sagittal configuration of the spine and axial rotation displacements [43] has been detailed.

It is likely that the continuous asymmetrical loading from altered postures (forward head posture, loss of cervical lordosis, sagittal, transverse and coronal displacements) may be the possible explanation for the decline in the functional status for the control group at the 6-month follow up as supported by predictions from experimental and biomechanical spine-posture modelling studies [44,45], surgical outcomes [11,12] and large cohort investigations [15]. Abnormal posture is considered as a predisposing factor for pain because it elicits abnormal stresses and strains in many structures, including bones, intervertebral discs, facet joints, musculotendinous tissues, and neural elements [11,12,17,18,44,45]. Thus, the 6-month improvement of pain for the study group seems reasonably attributable to the restoration of normal posture.

In contrast to our findings, other studies in the literature have reported that postural abnormalities were of minor importance for LBP and disability [46–48]. The lack of a clear correlation between sagittal spine curves and health was suggested in a systematic review conducted by Christensen and Hartvigsen [47]. However, the contradictory findings between the correlation between posture and pain in previous studies might simply be due to a lack of uniform classification and measures; most of the previous research is based on 2D posture analysis and poor experimental design. Further, when taken as a whole, comprehensive literature reviews including systematic literature reviews and meta-analyses on the topic, suggests a correlation between sagittal plane posture and patient outcomes [11,12,15,49,50]; especially in the cervical spine [51–53].

- Neurophysiological improvements

The current investigation assessed neurophysiological responses at the nerve root by evaluating the H-reflex. Notably, we identified significantly improved H-reflex latency and amplitude in the study group compared with the control group at the 10-week evaluation and this improvement was maintained at the 6-month follow-up. The only explanation that seems reasonable herein, is that improved posture and cervical spine alignment in the study group reduced longitudinal stress and strain in the central nervous system and in the lumbosacral nerve roots. This concept is supported by biomechanical investigations confirming that abnormal posture of any part of the spinal column will induce abnormal stresses in the entire cord and nerve roots while normal posture will minimize these stresses [17,18]. This concept of altered postures of the thoraco-lumbar spine increasing tension on the nerve root and increasing the likelihood of radiculopathy has been documented elsewhere [54].

Specific to the cervical spine, Breig and Marions [18] demonstrated the effect that slight cervical spine flexion (straightening of the cervical lordosis) has on the lumbosacral nerve roots where increased tension was found as far down as the cauda equina and the sacral plexus. With loss of the cervical lordosis causing increased tension in the lumbosacral nerve roots, a disc herniation in the lumbosacral region would be associated with an increased shear load at the interface between the disc and the nerve root [17]. Finally, it has recently been confirmed that improvement of the sagittal cervical radiographic alignment does improve neurophysiological amplitudies and latencies of somatosensory evoked potentials in the cervical spine, both measured in the peripheral (nerve root) and central systems (central condition time) [22,55]. Thus, it seems logical that our study findings indicate that improved cervical sagittal alignment and improved 3D posture were the explanations for the improvements in the H-reflex identified in our study group.

- Study limitations

Our study has some potential limitations, each of which points towards directions of future investigations. The primary limitations were the lack of investigator blinding and the sample was a convenient sample rather than a random sample of the whole population. Further, it remains to be seen what effect a greater frequency and number of traction sessions will produce and what effect the Denneroll would have on improvement of altered cervical curves with other types of primary lumbar disorders.

5. Conclusions

Our study identified that both groups experienced improvement in lower back pain, leg pain and disability levels after 10 weeks (30 sessions) of interventions. However, cervical lordosis, 3D posture of the trunk and the neurophysiological findings, represented in the H-reflex, identified greater improvements in the study group receiving the Denneroll. At the 6-month follow up, the control groups improvement in lower back pain, leg pain and disability reverted back to pre-study values. In contrast, at the 6-month follow-up the Denneroll traction study group showed improvements in all variables, including lower back pain, leg pain, disability, the 3D posture parameters, neurophysiological, and sagittal cervical alignment. These findings suggest that improving the cervical sagittal radiographic alignment offers benefits to this population suffering from chronic lower back pain and lumbosacral radiculopathy.

Author Contributions: I.M.M., A.A.M.D. and D.E.H. conceived the research idea and participated in its design. I.M.M., A.A.M.D. and D.E.H. all contributed to the statistical analysis. I.M.M. and A.A.M.D. participated in the data collection and study supervision. I.M.M., A.A.M.D. and D.E.H. all contributed to the interpretation of the results and wrote the original and final drafts. All authors agree with the order of presentation of the authors. All authors have read and agreed to the published version of the manuscript.

Funding: This research project received funding of the cervical Dennerolls used for the participants from CBP NonProfit, Inc. Eagle, ID, USA (836161).

Institutional Review Board Statement: The study was conducted in accordance with the Declaration of Helsinki and approved by the Ethics Committee of the Faculty of Physical Therapy, Cairo University; all participants signed informed consent prior to data collection. This trial was retrospectively registered at ClinicalTrials.gov (accessed on 10 September 2022) with registration number (NCT05553002).

Informed Consent Statement: Written informed consent was not obtained for the person depicted in Figure 2 as this is a photo from a model production shoot and the copyright holder is an author (D.E.H.) on the manuscript and has provided consent for this image to be reproduced.

Data Availability Statement: The datasets analyzed in the current study are available from the corresponding author on reasonable request.

Conflicts of Interest: D.E.H. teaches rehabilitation methods and sells the Denneroll products to physicians for patient care as used in this manuscript. D.E.H. is not a patent holder for the Denneroll products. All the other authors declare that they have no competing interests.

References

1. Modic, M.; Ross, J.S.; Obuchowski, N.; Browning, K.; Cianflocco, A.; Mazanec, D. Contrast enhanced MR imaging in acute lumbar radiculopathy: A pilot study of the natural history. *Radiology* **1995**, *195*, 429–435. [CrossRef] [PubMed]
2. Tubach, F.; Beaute, J.; Leclerc, A. Natural history and prognostic indicators of sciatica. *J. Clin. Epidemiol.* **2004**, *57*, 174–179. [CrossRef]
3. Anderson, G.B.J. Epidemiology of spinal disorders. In *The Adult Spine: Principles and Practice*; Frymoyer, J.W., Ed.; Raven: New York, NY, USA, 1991; pp. 110–146.
4. Heliovaraa, M.; Helmhout, P.H.; Harts, C.C.; Viechtbauer, W.; Staal, J.B.; de Bie, R.A. Isolated lumbar extensor strengthening versus regular physical therapy in an army working population with nonacute low back pain: A randomized controlled trial. *Arch. Phys. Med. Rehabil.* **2008**, *89*, 1675–1685.
5. Boswell, M.V.; Trescot, A.M.; Datta, S.; Schultz, D.M.; Hansen, H.C.; Abdi, S.; Sehgal, N.; Shah, R.V.; Singh, V.; Benyamin, R.M.; et al. American Society of Interventional Pain Physicians. Interventional techniques: Evidence-based practice guidelines in the management of chronic spinal pain. *Pain Physician* **2007**, *10*, 7–11. [PubMed]
6. Murphy, D. Conservative management of cervical spine syndromes. In *Dysfunction in the Cervical Spine*; Murphy, D., Ed.; McGraw-Hill: New York, NY, USA, 2000; pp. 71–103.
7. Brumagne, S.; Janssens, L.; Knapen, S.; Claeys, K.; Suuden-Johanson, E. Persons with recurrent low back pain exhibit a rigid postural control strategy. *Eur. Spine J.* **2008**, *17*, 1177–1184. [CrossRef] [PubMed]
8. Wong, K.C.; Lee, R.W.; Yeung, S.S. The association between back pain and trunk posture of workers in a special school for the severe handicap. *BMC Musculoskelet. Disord.* **2009**, *10*, 43–50. [CrossRef]

9. Chun, S.W.; Lim, C.Y.; Kim, K.; Hwang, J.; Chung, S.G. The relationships between low back pain and lumbar lordosis: A systematic review and meta-analysis. *Spine J.* **2017**, *17*, 1180–1191. [CrossRef]
10. Sadler, S.G.; Spink, M.J.; Ho, A.; De Jonge, X.J.; Chuter, V.H. Restriction in lateral bending range of motion, lumbar lordosis, and hamstring flexibility predicts the development of low back pain: A systematic review of prospective cohort studies. *BMC Musculoskelet. Disord.* **2017**, *18*, 179. [CrossRef]
11. Protopsaltis, T.S.; Scheer, J.K.; Terran, J.S.; Smith, J.S.; Hamilton, D.K.; Kim, H.J.; Mundis, G.M., Jr.; Hart, R.A.; McCarthy, I.M.; Klineberg, E.; et al. How the neck affects the back: Changes in regional cervical sagittal alignment correlate to HRQOL improvement in adult thoracolumbar deformity patients at 2-year follow-up. *J. Neurosurg. Spine* **2015**, *23*, 153–158. [CrossRef]
12. Scheer, J.K.; Passias, P.G.; Sorocean, A.M.; Boniello, A.J.; Mundis, G.M., Jr.; Klineberg, E.; Kim, H.J.; Protopsaltis, T.S.; Gupta, M.; Bess, S.; et al. Association between preoperative cervical sagittal deformity and inferior outcomes at 2-year follow-up in patients with adult thoracolumbar deformity: Analysis of 182 patients. *J. Neurosurg. Spine* **2016**, *24*, 108–115. [CrossRef]
13. Morningstar, M.W.; Pettibon, B.R.; Schlappi, H.; Schlappi, M.; Ireland, T.V. Reflex control of the spine and posture: A review of the literature from a chiropractic perspective. *Chiropr. Osteopath.* **2005**, *13*, 16–26. [CrossRef] [PubMed]
14. Buchanan, J.J.; Horak, F.B. Emergence of postural patterns as a function of vision and translation frequency. *J. Neurophysiol.* **1999**, *81*, 2325–2339. [CrossRef] [PubMed]
15. Glassman, S.D.; Bridwell, K.; Dimar, J.R.; Horton, W.; Berven, S.; Schwab, F. The impact of positive sagittal balance in adult spinal deformity. *Spine* **2005**, *30*, 2024–2029. [CrossRef] [PubMed]
16. Lau, K.T.; Cheung, K.Y.; Chan, K.B.; Chan, M.H.; Lo, K.Y.; Chiu, T.T. Relationships between sagittal postures of thoracic and cervical spine, presence of neck pain, neck pain severity and disability. *Man. Ther.* **2010**, *15*, 457–462. [CrossRef] [PubMed]
17. Harrison, D.E.; Cailliet, R.; Harrison, D.D.; Troyanovich, S.J.; Harrison, S.O. A review of biomechanics of the central nervous system. Part II: Strains in the spinal cord from postural loads. *J. Manipulative Physiol. Ther.* **1999**, *22*, 322–332. [CrossRef]
18. Breig, A.; Marions, O. Biomechanics of the lumbosacral nerve roots. *Acta Radiol.* **1963**, *1*, 1141–1160. [CrossRef]
19. Atlas, S.J.; Keller, R.B.; Wu, Y.A.; Deyo, R.A.; Singer, D.E. Long-term outcomes of surgical and nonsurgical management of sciatica secondary to a lumbar disc herniation: 10 year results from the maine lumbar spine study. *Spine* **2005**, *30*, 927–935. [CrossRef] [PubMed]
20. Velazquez-Perez, L.; Sanchez-Cruz, G.; Perez-Gonzalez, R.M. Neurophysiological diagnosis of lumbosacral radicular compression syndrome from late responses. *Rev. Neurol.* **2002**, *34*, 819–823. [PubMed]
21. Rocabado, M.; Iglarsh, Z.A. *Musculoskeletal Approach to Maxillofacial Pain*; Lippincott: Philadelphia, PA, USA, 1991; Volume 136–138, pp. 190–191.
22. Moustafa, I.M.; Diab, A.A.; Taha, S.; Harrison, D.E. Addition of a Sagittal Cervical Posture Corrective Orthotic Device to a Multimodal Rehabilitation Program Improves Short- and Long-Term Outcomes in Patients with Discogenic Cervical Radiculopathy. *Arch Phys. Med. Rehabil.* **2016**, *97*, 2034–2044. [CrossRef]
23. Fairbank, J.C.; Couper, J.; Davies, J.B.; O'Brien, J.P. The Oswestry low back pain disability questionnaire. *Physiotherapy* **1980**, *66*, 271–273.
24. Christie, H.J.; Kuma, R.S.; Warren, S.A. Postural aberrations in low back pain. *Arch Phys. Med. Rehabil.* **1995**, *76*, 218–224. [CrossRef]
25. Harrison, D.D.; Janik, T.J.; Troyanovich, S.J.; Holland, B. Comparisons of Lordotic Cervical Spine Curvatures to a Theoretical Ideal Model of the Static Sagittal Cervical Spine. *Spine* **1996**, *21*, 667–675. [CrossRef] [PubMed]
26. Shanahan, C.; Ward, A.R.; Robertson, V.J. Comparison of the analgesic efficacy of interferential therapy and transcutaneous electrical nerve stimulation. *Physiotherapy* **2006**, *92*, 247–253. [CrossRef]
27. Harrison, D.E.; Harrison, D.D.; Cailliet, R.; Troyanovich, S.J.; Janik, T.J.; Holland, B. Cobb mor Harrison posterior tangent method: Which is better for lateral cervical analysis? *Spine* **2000**, *25*, 2072–2078. [CrossRef] [PubMed]
28. Jackson, B.L.; Harrison, D.D.; Robertson, G.A.; Barker, W.F. Chiropractic biophysics lateral cervical film analysis reliability. *J. Manipulative Physiol. Ther.* **1993**, *16*, 384–391.
29. Lippold, C.; Danesh, G.; Hoppe, G.; Drerup, B.; Hackenberg, L. Trunk inclination, pelvic tilt and Pelvic rotation in relation to the craniofacial morphology in Adult. *Angle Orthodontist.* **2007**, *77*, 29–35. [CrossRef]
30. Chuds, J.D.; Piva, S.R.; Fritz, J.M. Responsiveness of the numeric pain rating scale in patients with low back pain. *Spine* **2005**, *30*, 1331–1334.
31. Lewit, K. Muscular and articular factors in movement restriction. *Man. Med.* **1985**, *1*, 83–85.
32. Escortell-Mayor, E.; Riesgo-Fuertes, R.; Garrido-Elustondo, S.; Asúnsolo-del Barco, A.; Díaz-Pulido, B.; Blanco-Díaz, M.; Bejerano-Álvarez, E. Primary care randomized clinical trial: Manual therapy effectiveness in comparison with TENS in patients with neck pain. *Man. Ther.* **2011**, *16*, 66–73. [CrossRef]
33. Gaid, M.; Cozens, A. The role of transcutaneous electric nerve stimulation (TENS) for the management of chronic low back pain. *Int. Musculoskelet. Med.* **2009**, *31*, 19.
34. Harrison, D.E.; Harrison, D.D.; Betz, J.; Janik, T.J.; Holland, B.; Colloca, C. Increasing the Cervical Lordosis with CBP Seated Combined Extension-Compression and Transverse Load Cervical Traction with Cervical Manipulation: Non-randomized Clinical Control Trial. *J. Manipulative Physiol. Ther.* **2003**, *26*, 139–151. [CrossRef]

35. Harrison, D.E.; Cailliet, R.; Harrison, D.D.; Janik, T.J.; Holland, B. A new 3-point bending traction method for restoring cervical lordosis and cervical manipulation: A nonrandomized clinical controlled trial. *Arch Phys. Med. Rehabil.* **2002**, *83*, 447–453. [CrossRef] [PubMed]
36. Ledin, T.; Hafstrom, A.; Fransson, P.A.; Magnusson, M. Influence of neck proprioception on vibration-induced postural sway. *Acta Oto-Laryngol.* **2003**, *123*, 594–599. [CrossRef] [PubMed]
37. Karnath, H.O.; Konczak, J.; Dichgans, J. Effect of prolonged neck muscle vibration on lateral head tilt in severe spasmodic torticollis. *J. Neurol. Neurosurg. Psychiatry* **2000**, *69*, 658–660. [CrossRef]
38. Carlson, M. Clinical Biomechanics of Orthotic Treatment of Thoracic Hyperkyphosis. *JPO* **2003**, *15*, 31–35. [CrossRef]
39. Sato, K.; Kikuchi, S.; Yonezawa, T. In vivo intradiscal pressure measurement in healthy individuals and in patient with ongoing back problems. *Spine* **2001**, *24*, 2468–2474. [CrossRef]
40. Rigo, M.; Quera-Salvá, G.; Villagers, M. Sagittal configuration of the spine in girls with idiopathic scoliosis: Progressing rather than initiating factor. *Stud. Health Technol. Inform.* **2006**, *123*, 90.
41. Dobosiewicz, K.; Durmala, J.; Jendrzejek, H.; Czernicki, K. Influence of method of asymmetric trunk mobilization on shaping of a physiological thoracic kyphosis in children and youth suffering from progressive idiopathic scoliosis. *Stud. Health Technol. Inform.* **2002**, *91*, 348–351.
42. Kadoury, S.; Cheriet, F.; Labelle, H. Prediction of the T2-T12 kyphosis in adolescent idiopathic scoliosis using a multivariate regression model. *Stud. Health Technol. Inform.* **2008**, *140*, 269–272.
43. Vuillerme, N.; Danion, F.; Forestier, N.; Nougier, V. Postural sway under muscle vibration and muscle fatigue in humans. *Neurosci. Lett.* **2002**, *333*, 131–135. [CrossRef]
44. Harrison, D.E.; Colloca, C.J.; Keller, T.S.; Harrison, D.D.; Janik, T.J. Anterior thoracic posture increases thoracolumbar disc loading. *Eur. Spine J.* **2005**, *14*, 234–242. [CrossRef] [PubMed]
45. Keller, T.S.; Colloca, C.J.; Harrison, D.E.; Harrison, D.D.; Janik, T.J. Morphological and Biomechanical Modeling of the Thoracolumbar Spine: Implications for the Ideal Spine. *Spine J.* **2005**, *5*, 297–305. [CrossRef] [PubMed]
46. Balague, F.; Troussier, B.; Salminen, J.J. Non-specific low back pain in children and adolescents: Risk factors. *Eur. Spine J.* **1999**, *8*, 429–438. [CrossRef]
47. Christensen, S.T.; Hartvigsen, J. Spinal curves and health: A systematic critical review of the epidemiological literature dealing with associations between sagittal spinal curves and health. *J. Manipulative Physiol. Ther.* **2008**, *31*, 690–714. [CrossRef] [PubMed]
48. Corso, M.; Cancelliere, C.; Mior, S.; Kumar, V.; Smith, A.; Côté, P. The clinical utility of routine spinal radiographs by chiropractors: A rapid review of the literature. *Chiropr. Man. Therap.* **2020**, *28*, 33. [CrossRef]
49. Harrison, D.E.; Betz, J.; Ferrantelli, J.F. Sagittal spinal curves and health. *J. Vertebr. Subluxation Res.* **2009**. Available online: https://vertebralsubluxationresearch.com/2009/07/31/sagittal-spinal-curves-and-health/ (accessed on 12 September 2022).
50. Oakley, P.A.; Betz, J.W.; Harrison, D.E.; Siskin, L.A.; Hirsh, D.W. International Chiropractors Association Rapid Response Research Review Subcommittee. Radiophobia Overreaction: College of Chiropractors of British Columbia Revoke Full X-ray Rights Based on Flawed Study and Radiation Fear-Mongering. *Dose Response* **2021**, *19*, 15593258211033142.
51. Ling, F.P.; Chevillotte, T.; Leglise, A.; Thompson, W.; Bouthors, C.; Le Huec, J.C. Which parameters are relevant in sagittal balance analysis of the cervical spine? A literature review. *Eur. Spine J.* **2018**, *27* (Suppl. S1), 8–15. [CrossRef]
52. Azimi, P.; Yazdanian, T.; Benzel, E.C.; Hai, Y.; Montazeri, A. Sagittal balance of the cervical spine: A systematic review and meta-analysis. *Eur. Spine J.* **2021**, *30*, 1411–1439. [CrossRef] [PubMed]
53. Oakley, P.A.; Ehsani, N.N.; Moustafa, I.M.; Harrison, D.E. Restoring cervical lordosis by cervical extension traction methods in the treatment of cervical spine disorders: A systematic review of controlled trials. *J. Phys. Ther. Sci.* **2021**, *33*, 784–794. [CrossRef]
54. Ten Brinke, A.; Van der Aa, H.E.; Van der Palen, J.; Oosterveld, F. Is leg length discrepancy associated with the side of radiating pain in patients with a lumbar herniated disc? *Spine* **1999**, *24*, 684–686. [CrossRef]
55. Moustafa, I.M.; Diab, A.A.; Hegazy, F.; Harrison, D.E. Demonstration of central conduction time and neuroplastic changes after cervical lordosis rehabilitation in asymptomatic subjects: A randomized, placebo-controlled trial. *Sci. Rep.* **2021**, *11*, 15379. [CrossRef] [PubMed]

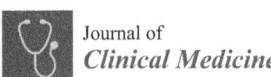

Article

Randomized Feasibility Pilot Trial of Adding a New Three-Dimensional Adjustable Posture-Corrective Orthotic to a Multi-Modal Program for the Treatment of Nonspecific Neck Pain

Ahmed S. A. Youssef [1,2], Ibrahim M. Moustafa [3], Ahmed M. El Melhat [4,5], Xiaolin Huang [1], Paul A. Oakley [6] and Deed E. Harrison [7,*]

1. Department of Rehabilitation Medicine, Tongji Hospital, Tongji Medical College, Huazhong University of Science and Technology, 1095#, Jiefang Avenue, Wuhan 430030, China
2. Basic Science Department, Faculty of Physical Therapy, Beni-Suef University, Beni-Suef 62521, Egypt
3. Department of Physiotherapy, College of Health Sciences, University of Sharjah, University City, Sharjah 27272, United Arab Emirates
4. Department of Physical Therapy for Musculoskeletal Disorders and their Surgeries, Faculty of Physical Therapy, Cairo University, Cairo 12613, Egypt
5. Department of Physical Therapy, Faculty of Health Sciences, Beirut Arab University, Beirut P.O. Box 11-5020, Lebanon
6. Independent Researcher, Newmarket, ON L3Y 8Y8, Canada
7. CBP NonProfit, Inc., Eagle, ID 83616, USA
* Correspondence: drdeed@idealspine.com

Abstract: The aim of this study was to investigate the feasibility and effect of a multimodal program for the management of chronic nonspecific neck pain CNSNP with the addition of a 3D adjustable posture corrective orthotic (PCO), with a focus on patient recruitment and retention. This report describes a prospective, randomized controlled pilot study with twenty-four participants with CNSNP and definite 3D postural deviations who were randomly assigned to control and study groups. Both groups received the same multimodal program; additionally, the study group received a 3D PCO to perform mirror image® therapy for 20–30 min while the patient was walking on a treadmill 2–3 times per week for 10 weeks. Primary outcomes included feasibility, recruitment, adherence, safety, and sample size calculation. Secondary outcomes included neck pain intensity by numeric pain rating scale (NPRS), neck disability index (NDI), active cervical ROM, and 3D posture parameters of the head in relation to the thoracic region. Measures were assessed at baseline and after 10 weeks of intervention. Overall, 54 participants were screened for eligibility, and 24 (100%) were enrolled for study participation. Three participants (12.5%) were lost to reassessment before finishing 10 weeks of treatment. The between-group mean differences in change scores indicated greater improvements in the study group receiving the new PCO intervention. Using an effect size of 0.797, α > 0.05, β = 80% between-group improvements for NDI identified that 42 participants were required for a full-scale RCT. This pilot study demonstrated the feasibility of recruitment, compliance, and safety for the treatment of CNSNP using a 3D PCO to a multimodal program to positively affect CNSNP management.

Keywords: neck pain; orthotic; mirror image® therapy; reverse posture training

Citation: Youssef, A.S.A.; Moustafa, I.M.; El Melhat, A.M.; Huang, X.; Oakley, P.A.; Harrison, D.E. Randomized Feasibility Pilot Trial of Adding a New Three-Dimensional Adjustable Posture-Corrective Orthotic to a Multi-Modal Program for the Treatment of Nonspecific Neck Pain. *J. Clin. Med.* **2022**, *11*, 7028. https://doi.org/10.3390/jcm11237028

Academic Editor: Hiroshi Horiuchi

Received: 12 September 2022
Accepted: 21 November 2022
Published: 28 November 2022

Publisher's Note: MDPI stays neutral with regard to jurisdictional claims in published maps and institutional affiliations.

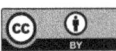

Copyright: © 2022 by the authors. Licensee MDPI, Basel, Switzerland. This article is an open access article distributed under the terms and conditions of the Creative Commons Attribution (CC BY) license (https://creativecommons.org/licenses/by/4.0/).

1. Introduction

Chronic nonspecific neck pain (CNSNP) is a common musculoskeletal disorder worldwide. Because of CNSNP, disability-adjusted life years increased from 17 million (95% confidence interval (CI), 11.4–23.7) in 1990 to 29 million (95% CI, 19.5–40.5) in 2016 [1,2]. Treatment of CNSNP according to the clinical guidelines of APTA [3] includes manual therapy, therapeutic exercises, and posture education or correction. A study by Bernal-Utrera et al.,

2020 concluded that manual therapy achieved a faster reduction in pain perception than therapeutic exercise, but therapeutic exercise reduced disability faster than manual therapy [4].

Although the exact relationship between posture and CNSNP is unsettled, poor posture of the cervical spine appears to influence dorsal neck muscle activity at rest and during movement [5]. Additionally, forward head posture (FHP) is associated with thoracic hyper-kyphosis and indirectly affects cervical flexion and the rotational range of motion (ROM) [6]. In addition, sustained computer work and prolonged use of smartphones appear to modify neck posture, as well as scapular positioning and upper trapezius muscle activity [7,8].

A recent systematic review conducted by Szczygieł et al., 2020 found that the posture of the head has a significant effect on the human body [9]. Abnormal head positions affect muscle activity, proprioception, and respiratory patterns and contribute to neck pain [9]. Another review, by Anabela et al., 2009 [10], concluded that head posture assessment is useful for neck patients, but it must be considered in relation to the patient's symptoms and related functional problems [11–13].

Harrison [14,15] detailed posture displacements of the head, ribcage, and pelvis in three dimensions (3D) as translations and rotational displacements. Therefore, 3D postural assessment and correction during the treatment of CNSNP or postural neck pain should be considered [9,11]. There is also a growing body of research regarding patients with spinal dysfunction using mirror image® therapy, which is prescribed specifically to help normalize the patient's neuromuscular dysfunction and postural deformation by reflecting the patient's posture across different planes [14–17]. The majority of interventions for improvement of abnormal posture focus on single or double combination movements (e.g., 1 or 2 movements at a time) as it is difficult to maneuver a patient's head and neck in multiple planes and postures at once [14–17].

In the current investigation, we designed an adjustable 3D posture corrective orthotic (PCO) for the patient to wear for a short time (patent number CN201921929736.1). The PCO has the ability to reflect all translation and rotational displacements of the head in combination (3D planes). This mirror image therapy is designed to be delivered via the use of the adjustable PCO while the patient is walking at approximately 2–3 miles per hour on a standard, motorized treadmill. The PCO reverses the poor posture according to the 3D posture analysis data.

To the best of our knowledge, no randomized controlled trial (RCT) has evaluated the addition of a 3D adjustable PCO to a care program and investigated the short-term improvement effects on CNSNP management outcomes. The primary aim of our study was to perform a pilot RCT investigation to evaluate the feasibility of conducting a full-scale RCT considering recruitment, compliance to study protocols, adverse events, adherence, sample size calculation, and safety. The secondary aim was to investigate the effect size of adding the 3D PCO for mirror image therapy (reverse posture training) while the patient is walking on a motorized treadmill compared to a control group receiving standard interventions for neck pain intensity, disability, active ROM and 3D posture parameters after 10 weeks of intervention.

2. Methods

2.1. Study Design

This study was a double-blind (the different investigators and outcome assessor were blinded to group allocation) superiority pilot RCT with 2 parallel groups. The study was performed according to CONSORT guidelines. The ethics committee of Tongji Hospital, Tongji Medical College, Huazhong University of Science and Technology (HUST), Wuhan, China, approved the study protocol (certificate of approval number TJ-IRB20170703), which was prospectively registered at clinicaltrials.gov (Id: NCT03331120). The study was performed in the rehabilitation department at Tongji Hospital, affiliated with HUST, China.

2.2. Procedures

Participants were recruited through advertisements in orthopedic and rehabilitation department clinics and via mobile applications, such as WeChat (Tencent Ltd., Shenzhen, China). Participants first completed a written informed consent form, provided demographic data, and completed patient-reported outcome measures, including numeric pain rating scale score (NPRS) and neck disability index (NDI). Then, the outcome assessor measured the rotational and translational displacements of the head in relation to the thoracic region using a global postural system (GPS) device. After eligibility confirmation, another research assistant randomized participants to either a study or a control group receiving standard interventions only using sealed numbered envelopes using a randomization list generated by a random integer generator (www.random.org). A blinded investigator performed all outcome assessments at baseline and after 10 weeks of intervention. Participants were not blinded to their group allocation because of the difference in interventions between the two groups.

2.3. Participants

2.3.1. Inclusion Criteria

Male and female participants aged 17–40; Ability to continue treatment for 10 weeks; Signature on informed consent form; Neck pain that was equal to or greater than 3/10 on the NPRS and pain lasting more than 3 months (chronic neck pain) [18,19]; A neck disability score on the NDI of at least 5 from a total score of 50 [20]; A 3D postural assessment, known as the Global Posture System (GPS) 600, (Chinesport, Udine, Italy).

2.3.2. Posture Translations Displacements Included the Following

Anterior head translation (T_z) more than 2.5 cm [21,22]; Side shifting of the head (T_x) in relation to the thoracic region of more than 0.5 cm [16].

2.3.3. Posture Rotations Displacements Included the Following

Rotation of head about vertical gravity (R_y) more than or equal to 3° [23]; Side bending of head (R_z) more than or equal to 3° [10]; Flexion or extension position of head (R_x). The average angle is 18°; if the angle was greater than this, it means extension in the upper cervical region, and if it is less, it means flexion in the upper cervical region [10]. Participants were included if they had at least two posture displacements, whether they were translations or rotations. We included more obvious amounts of translations of the head posture related to the thoracic region to avoid variability of measurement between participants such that the posture deviations could be visually examined. The mean absolute differences within examiners' measurements (MADOMs) were 0.4 cm or less for lateral translations (T_x Head, T_x Thoracic, and T_x Pelvic) and 0.71 cm or less for forward translational measurements (T_z Head, T_z Thoracic, and T_z Pelvic). The MADOMs were 3.2° or less for flexion-extension rotational measurements (R_x Head, R_x Thoracic, and R_x Pelvic) and 1.4° or less for all axial rotations (R_y Head, R_y Thoracic, and R_y Pelvic) and lateral bending rotations (R_z Head, R_z Thoracic, and R_z Pelvic) [23].

2.3.4. Exclusion Criteria

Neck pain associated with whiplash injuries, medical red flag history (such as tumor, fracture, metabolic diseases, rheumatoid arthritis, or osteoporosis) [19]; Neck pain with cervical radiculopathy or associated with externalized cervical disc herniation [19]; Fibromyalgia syndrome, because its diagnosis is similar to that of CNSNP [24]; Surgery in the neck area, regardless of the cause neck pain accompanied by vertigo caused by vertebra-basilar insufficiency or accompanied by non-cervicogenic headaches [19]; Current pain treatment, psychiatric disorders, or another problem that would contraindicate the use of the techniques in this study [19]; Any of the following conditions: (1) history of cervical or facial trauma or surgery, (2) congenital anomalies involving the spine (cervical, thoracic, or lumbar), (3) bony abnormalities, such as scoliosis, (4) any systemic arthritis,

(5) recurrent middle ear infections over the last 5 years or any hearing impairment requiring the use of a hearing aid, (6) persistent respiratory difficulties over the last 5 years that necessitated absence from work, required long-term medication, or interfered with daily activities, (7) any visual impairment not corrected by glasses, (8) any disorder of the central nervous system, or (9) pregnancy or breast-feeding because these conditions affect head posture [25–28]; Inability to attend a 10-week treatment program.

2.4. Examination Procedures

All participants had histories taken. The history included demographic variables (age, sex, the mode of onset, duration of symptoms, nature and location of symptoms, and mechanism of injury, if it happened previously), as well as questions regarding aggravating and relieving factors, such as posture modifications and changed positions and any prior history of NP. All patients had a recent MRI study, no more than two weeks before the start of the study. In addition to the MRI. In addition to the MRI, other tests were performed to rule out the presence of space-occupying masses such as tumors, extruded intervertebral disks, osteophytes, nerve root irritation, or radiculopathy (specific neck pain), such as the Valsalva test, Spurling test (Foraminal compression test), distraction test, and Jackson compression test, followed by reflexes, cutaneous distribution, joint play movements, palpation, and diagnostic imaging. All participants underwent a physical examination. Pain level, neck function, and 3D posture analysis of the head in relation to the thoracic region and active cervical range of motion were measured before and after treatment [3,29].

2.4.1. Primary Outcomes

The primary outcome of our study was to determine the feasibility of conducting an RCT; thus, we monitored the integrity of the study protocol, recruitment and retention, randomization procedures, primary outcome measures, and the sample-size calculation [30–32]. Further details and the results of each aspect of the primary outcomes are provided in the results section.

2.4.2. Secondary Outcomes

(1) Numeric pain rating scale (NPRS)

The NPRS is an 11-point numeric pain intensity scale ranging from 0 ("no pain") to 10 ("as much pain as possible or intolerable pain"). A change of 2 points or more was identified as the minimal clinically important difference (MCID) in participants with chronic neck pain [33].

(2) Neck disability index (NDI)

The NDI is a patient-completed, condition-specific functional status questionnaire with 10 items. The total score of this questionnaire ranges between 0 and 50 points, with higher scores indicating higher levels of disability, which is expressed as a raw score with a maximum score of 50. The MCID of the NDI is 5.5 [20,33,34].

(3) Active cervical range of motion (CROM)

Active CROM was measured in a sitting position using a CROM goniometer (CROM Deluxe model; Performance Attainment Associates, Roseville, MN, USA). The CROM allows measurement of ROM in three planes (flexion/ extension, lateral flexion, and rotation about gravity). Participants sat upright and were asked to move their necks in each direction 3 times. Documentation of cervical ROM was expressed in the form of full range, a total value for the sagittal (flexion and extension), frontal (lateral flexion right and left), or transverse plane (rotation right and left), in the form of 3 measurements [35,36].

(4) Three-dimensional posture parameters of the head in relation to the thoracic region

A 3D postural assessment, known as the Global Posture System (GPS) 600, (Chinesport, Udine, Italy), was used to examine the postural displacement variables [37–39]. This device was used per the manufacturer's instructions [37]. The device has a unit for podoscopic analysis, a unit for postural analysis, and a stability measuring platform, and it comes with an image acquisition system and custom software. The camera of the image acquisition system was positioned 107 cm from the ground and 190 cm from the subject. The reliability and validity of this device have been verified previously where measurements demonstrated excellent within-rater reliability (ICC = 0.89) and standard error of measurement (SEM) = 1.5 degrees with a minimum detectable change (MDC) = 1.9 degrees; while inter-rater reliability is good to excellent (ICC= 0.7) [40,41]. We analyzed the posture of the head in relation to the thoracic region in terms of translations and rotations.

2.4.3. Assessment Procedures

A. Preparation of patients:

The patients were asked to wear tight-fitting clothes to allow the examiners to find various anatomical sites. The examiners placed 13 markers on each patient before taking the four photographs.

B. Marker placement:

Antero-posterior and lateral view marker locations are shown in Figure 1. The points over which the markers were fixed were well-cleaned with alcohol to remove any moisture and to ensure good fixation. Four photographs or four views were obtained for every patient, one anterior and one posterior view and two lateral (right, Rt, and left, Lt) views.

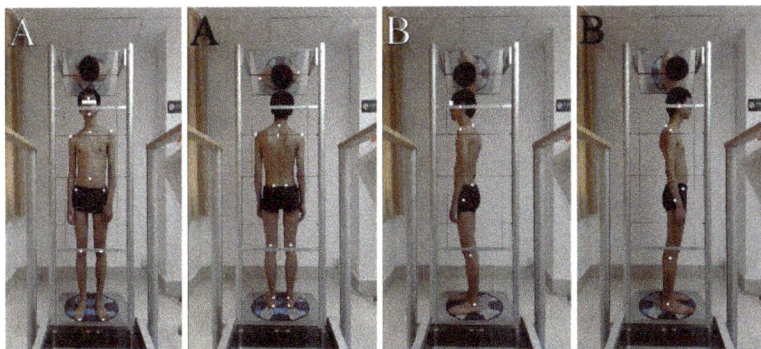

Figure 1. The photographs taken using the Global Posture System (GPS). (**A**) Anterior and posterior views. (**B**) Sagittal plane or lateral views. The six reflective markers used in the analysis are: acromion, anterior superior iliac spine, posterior superior iliac spine, glabella, tragus, C7, and middle sternal notch.

C. Starting position of the patients:

For the photographs, patients were instructed to stand on the lux postural analyzer part of the GPS, to take a deep breath 3–5 times for full relaxation, to nod their head up and down twice with their eyes closed, and to assume what they felt to be a neutral body posture then participants' eyes were opened, and they remained still, without any motion, during this stance. Four digital photographs were taken using a computer mouse. The set of photographs was processed through secure software analysis using GPS.

2.4.4. Measured Items (the Postural Parameters) of the Head Region in Relation to the Thoracic Region

A right-handed Cartesian coordinate system with x-axis positive to the left, y-axis positive vertically, and z-axis positive to the anterior was used to describe postures of the head as translation displacements in centimeters (T_x, T_y, and T_z) along these axes and, in addition, as rotation displacements (R_x, R_y, and R_z) in degrees from a normal upright stance. Vertical translations (T_y), which would require radiographic analysis of hypo- or hyper-lordosis, were not calculated in the present study as is shown in Figure 2 [23].

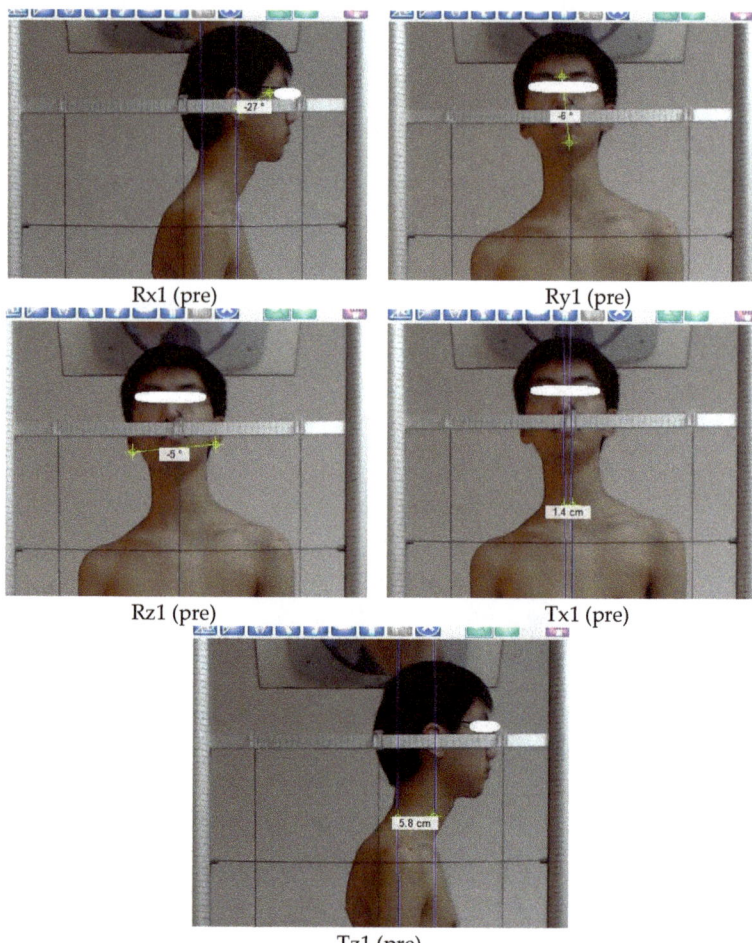

Figure 2. Three-dimensional postural parameters of the head region in relation to the thoracic region. Postural rotations (**Rx**, **Ry**, **Rz**). Postural translations (**Tx**, **Tz**).

2.4.5. Postural Translations of the Head in Relation to the Thoracic Region

Tx (Rt. or Lt. side shifting or lateral translation), is the measure of the horizontal distance from the vertical line passing through the middle sternal notch to the vertical line passing through the nose [16].

Tz (anterior head translation), is the measure of the horizontal distance from the vertical line crossing the middle acromion process to the vertical line crossing the tragus of the ear [22].

2.4.6. Postural Rotations of the Head in Relation to the Thoracic Region

Rx (flexion or extension position of upper cervical), is the measurement of the angle between the tragus of the ear, the canthus of the eye, and the horizontal line [10].

Ry (Rt. or Lt. rotation), is the measurement of the angle between the glabella of the forehead or tip of the nose, the middle point of the chin, and the vertical line [23].

Rz (Rt. or Lt. side bending), is the measurement of the angle between the inferior margins of the right and the left ear and the horizontal line [10].

2.5. Interventions

Both groups received conventional or local treatment consisting of a moist hot pack, soft tissue mobilization, manual therapy, and therapeutic exercises [42–45] (Table 1). Only the study group received 3D PCO to perform the mirror image therapy (reverse posture training) for 20–30 min while the patient was walking on a motorized treadmill 2–3 times per week for 10 weeks. The CONSORT flow chart diagram for this trial is presented in Figure 3.

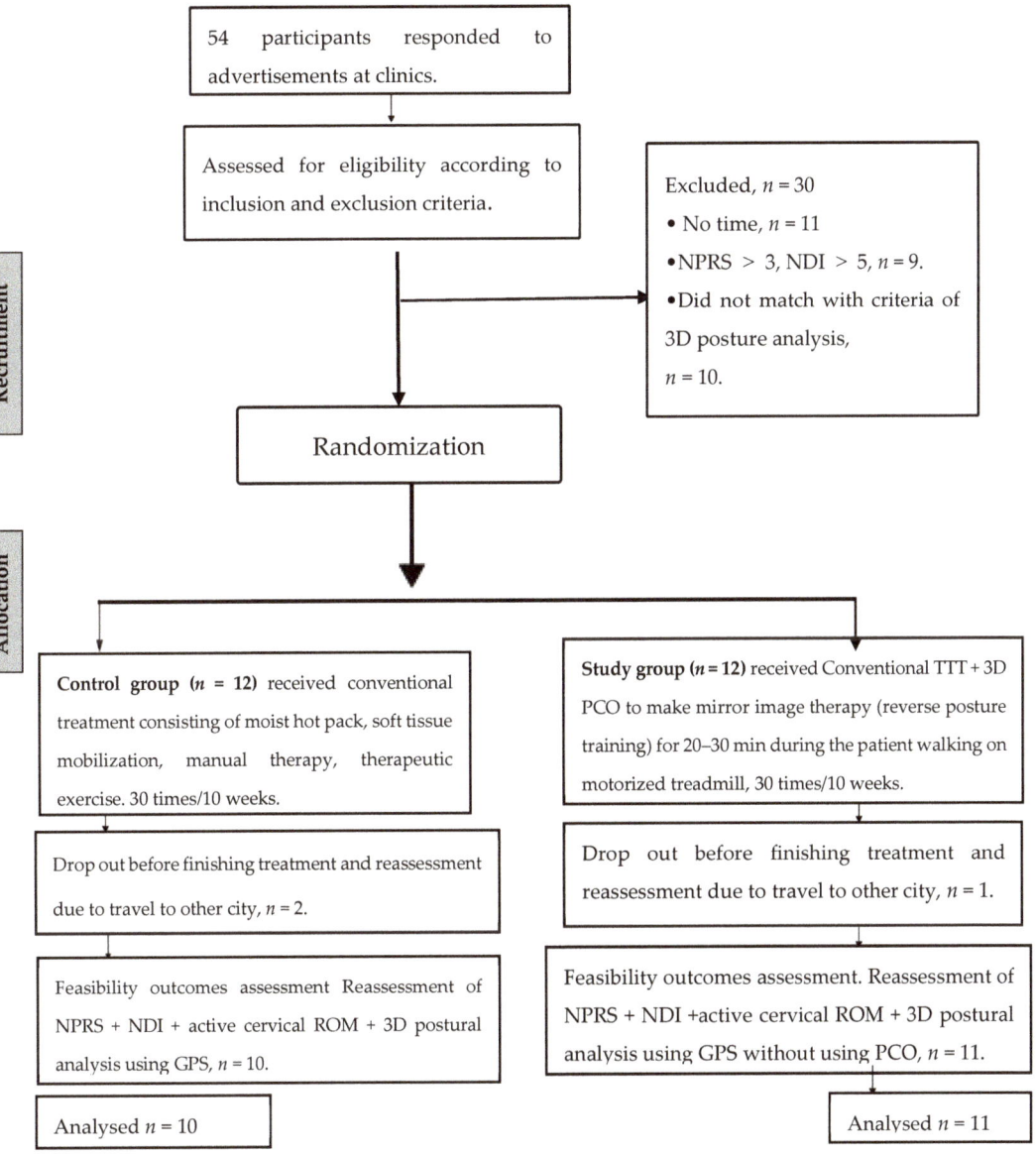

Figure 3. The CONSORT flow chart diagram for the trial.

Table 1. Both the study and control groups received conventional or local treatment consisting of a moist hot pack, soft tissue mobilization, manual therapy, and therapeutic exercises. Description of this conventional treatment, exercise prescription, and progression are presented herein. Participants in both groups attended 30 physical therapy treatment sessions over a 10-week period at 3 sessions per week. See methods section for complete details of progressions.

Conventional Treatment	Description
Moist hot pack	Applied to the area of pain at neck region muscles, such as the upper part of the trapezius, levator scapulae, splenius capitis, and cervicis muscles, for 15 min.
Soft tissue mobilization	Deep stroking massage performed along the entire length of the taut band within the painful or tight muscles.
Cervical mobilization	Low-velocity passive mobilization techniques to the symptomatic cervical segments as determined by the physiotherapist's clinical examination. Physiotherapists could be able to select from what were termed passive accessory and physiological movement techniques as believed appropriate to the individual participant based on the initial and progressive reassessments.
Therapeutic exercises Cervical flexors	Level 1 Re-education of CCF movement pattern 1. Supine, knees bent -Gentle and controlled nodding action facilitated with eye movement 10 reps Holding. 2. Supine, knees bent -Repeated and sustained CCF 10 s holds × 10 reps Level 2 Interaction between the deep/superficial cervical flexors 1. Sitting -Controlled head movement through range of extension and return to neutral 10 reps Co-contraction of the deep cervical flexors/extensors. Level 3 Strength/endurance of the cervical flexors 1. Sitting -Isometric CCF in a range of cervical extension 10 s holds × 10 reps -Lifting the head off the wall (with the chair up to 30 cm away from the wall) 10 s holds × 10 reps 2. Supine -Lifting the head off a pillow (2 or 1 then 0 pillows as per participant's capacity) 10 s holds × 10 reps.
Cervical extensors	Level 1 Re-education of extension movement pattern 1. Prone on elbows/four-point kneeling positions -Cranio cervical extension 3 sets of 5 reps. -Cranio cervical rotation (<45°) 3 sets of 5 reps. -Cervical extension while keeping the cranio cervical region in a neutral position 3 sets of 5 reps. Level 2 Co-contraction of the deep cervical flexors/extensors 1. Sitting -Isometric cervical rotation facilitated with eye movement (left/right sides) 5 s holds × 5 reps. Level 3 Strength/endurance of the cervical extensors 1. Prone on elbows/four-point kneeling positions -Isometric hold in range of cervical extension 10 s holds × 10 reps.
Cervico Scapular control	Level 1-Re-education of scapular movement control Cervico scapular muscle control 1. Sitting -Arm movement without load (external rotation/abduction/flexion < 30°) 10 reps -Arm movement without load throughout range 10 reps 2. Prone on elbows/four-point kneeling position -Thoracic lift (serratus anterior) and isometric hold 5 s holds × 5 reps. Level 2 Strength/endurance of cervico scapular muscles 1. Sitting -Arm movement with load using Thera-band (external rotation/abduction/flexion < 30°) 10 reps. -Arm movement with load throughout the range 10 reps. 2. Prone -Lift the shoulder off the bed and hold without arm load 10 s holds × 10 reps. -Lift the shoulder off the bed and hold with arm load using Thera-band 10 s holds × 10 reps.

Table 1. *Cont.*

Conventional Treatment	Description
Postural correction	Level 1 Correction of spinal posture Sitting -Active upright sitting initiated with lumbo-pelvic movement 10 s holds × 10 reps Level 2 Correction of spinal posture and scapular orientation Sitting -Actively positioning the scapular in a neutral posture while maintaining spinal posture 10 s holds × 10 reps Level 3 Spinal and scapular correction plus occipital lift Sitting -Actively lengthen the back of the neck while maintaining spinal and scapular posture 10 s holds × 10 reps. Standing on wall Actively extend spine then chin in cervical with squeezing abdomen 10 s holds × 10 reps.

CCF: craniocervical flexion; reps: repetitions.

Study Group 3D PCO Performed the Mirror Image® Therapy (Reverse Posture Training) While the Patient Was Walking on Motorized Treadmill

Mirror image therapy (reverse posture training) was delivered via the use of the adjustable PCO (patent number CN201921929736.1), as shown in Figure 4. The PCO was applied, to reverse the abnormal posture according to the 3D posture analysis data, while the patient was walking at approximately 2–3 miles per hour on a standard motorized treadmill for 20–30 min per session. To facilitate tissue remodeling and to stretch ligamentous tissues reverse posture training was applied in the mirror image traction or therapeutic position; an example of participant data is shown in Table 2. Then, walking training using the treadmill was performed during which the participant's mirror image traction could be held by the adjustable PCO based on mirror image therapy, which has been previously used in other studies based on Harrison et al., 2004 [16,17,46]. The rationale for walking on the treadmill while maintaining a patient's mirror image position is based on the concept of neuromuscular retraining of motor patterns that have developed over time in both static and dynamic posture tasks and is based on the earlier randomized trial by Diab and Moustafa [17]. This program was repeated 2–3 times/week for 10 weeks, as in Figure 5 (as shown in the Supplementary Video File).

Table 2. Example of 3D posture analysis data and mirror image therapy (reverse posture training) using the posture corrective orthotic PCO.

3D Posture Analysis of Head in Relation to Thoracic	Reverse 3D Posture Data by PCO (Mirror Image Therapy)
1. Rx (extension position of the head) = 25° − 18° = 7° extension.	7° flexion of the head.
2. Ry (right or left rotation of the head) = 6° left rotation.	6° right rotation of the head.
3. Tz (anterior head translation = 5.8 cm anterior head translation.	5.8 cm posterior head translation.
4. Rz (right or left side bending) = 5° right side bending.	5° left side bending.
5. Tx (side shifting of the head = 1.4 cm right side shifting.	1.4 cm left side shifting.

Participants in both groups attended 30 physical therapy treatment sessions over a 10-week period at 2–3 sessions per week. Short-term follow-up evaluations were performed after 10 weeks of interventions. To minimize therapist variation and to increase consistency, the same physiotherapist independently delivered the entire intervention program for every participant. Every physiotherapist had 10 years of experience and received training for the application of the specific interventions for one week before starting the study. Participants in both groups were advised to perform all therapeutic exercises once daily as their home routine during non-treatment days and to follow the posture correction advice. Record sheets were collected every week and were subsequently analyzed to calculate the mean exercise frequency per week and the mean exercise time per day. To monitor the exercise times and the number of sets performed during the study accurately, videos of the exercises, photos of postural correction, and a record sheet were distributed to the participants.

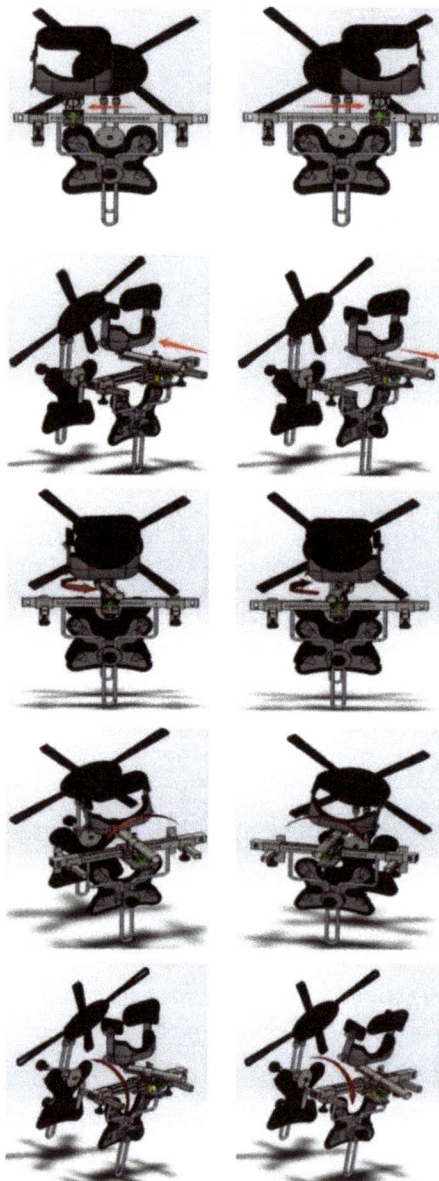

Figure 4. Posture corrective orthotic (PCO) demonstrating the availability to move in different directions and lock the head in its opposition position. Top row: lateral translation of the head left and right (Tx). Second row: anterior and posterior translation of the head (Tz). Third row: rotation of the head about vertical gravity left and right (Ry). Fourth row: side bending of the head left and right (Rz). Bottom row: extension and flexion of the head (Rx). See Figure 5 for a sample patient setup.

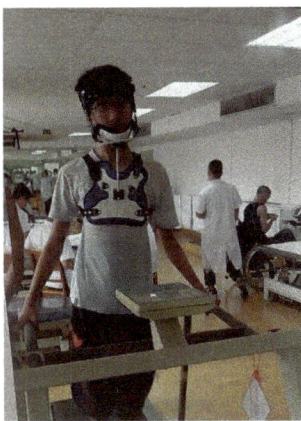 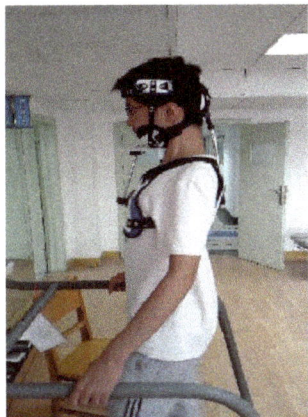

Figure 5. Three-dimensional PCO to perform the mirror image therapy (reverse posture training) while the patient was walking on motorized treadmill.

2.6. Statistical Analysis

Primary outcome measures and their results described in our study protocol [47] are discussed descriptively in Table 3. To estimate the sample size for a future full-scale RCT, between-group effect sizes and 95% confidence intervals (CIs) with Hedges' correction were calculated for the change in the secondary outcomes of NPRS, NDI, active cervical ROM, and 3D posture parameters. The mean ± standard deviation (SD) value for each of the secondary outcomes was used in the calculation of the effect size. The estimated sample size was then determined using the between-group effect size with a minimum of 80% power ($\alpha = 0.01$ or 3D posture parameters and $\alpha = 0.05$ for other secondary outcomes) using G power software. The sample size will be increased by 20% to allow for an estimated dropout rate in the future RCT. Statistical methods for the secondary outcome measures were evaluated by comparing the change within groups (from baseline to post-treatment) and then estimating the within-group effect size. Complete analyses were conducted to include outcomes from all participants who completed baseline and post-treatment evaluations as recommended in CONSORT guidelines [48]. The between-group difference in change scores for each outcome measure from baseline to post-treatment was calculated as the mean and 95% CI. All statistical analyses were performed with SPSS Version 2.2 software (IBM Corporation, Armonk, NY, USA). Correlations (Pearson's r) were used to examine the relationships between the 3D postural parameters and all measured outcomes.

Table 3. Results of primary aim (feasibility).

Primary Aim/Criteria	Description
Integrity of the study protocol • Recruitment: minimum requirement of 80% of eligible participants entering study.	With 45% of interested participants being eligible. 100% of eligible participants enrolled in the study. Inclusion criteria of the study protocol appeared acceptable.
Validity of eligibility criteria	The eligibility criteria were followed with another published paper [19], and our protocol that was published previously [47].
Understanding and integrity of intervention for treating physical therapists	During the post-study interview, physical therapists said that one-week training before study was appropriate and enough, continuous communication with the study authors was essential to ensure that the protocol was followed throughout the study.
Convenience of intervention for participants	During the post-study interview, participants upraised the concern that with one treating physical therapist, appointments availability were limited. They felt that more availability of appointments would enhance recruitment and retention or more than treating physical therapist for every participant.

Table 3. Cont.

Primary Aim/Criteria	Description
Integrity and suitability of intervention to participants	During the post-study interview, participants in both groups said that they believed the intervention was valuable, and they would participate in the study again. Only one issue was that the treatment period was too long and, hope to reduce treatment period of intervention in the future, and none expressed offense about being randomized to the control intervention.
Feasibility of study time requirement and study facilities for participants	During the post-study interview, while participants stated that a large time commitment was required to participate in the study, they all acknowledged that this was necessary for improvement. However, they advised us to reduce treatment sessions to less than 30 times although ten weeks was good time to make improvement in posture deviations. All participants felt that the services in which the interventions were delivered were appropriate.
Recruitment and retention procedures • Goals for minimum requirement for adequate recruitment and retention: at least 80% of participants attended 75% of appointments and completed 75% of the prescribed exercises	Fifty-four people responded to recruitment at rehabilitation clinic over a 9-months inclusion period. Of these, 45% fulfilled inclusion criteria, and all were included in the study at rehabilitation clinic. Of the 24 participants, 21 attended all treatment sessions and 3 lost before finishing treatment. No adverse events were recorded. Exercise intervention compliance was measured using either record sheet diaries or via WeChat application.
Testing of outcome measurement collection • Determined by completeness of outcome data collected, and through post-study interview	At the end of the study, all 21 participants who finished the study completed patient-reported outcome questionnaires, neck ROM and 3D posture parameters. The blinded outcome assessor, with no missing data, collected it for all participants.
Suitability of randomization procedure and methods used to ensure blinding • Determined during post-study interviews of treating physical therapist, blinded outcome assessor. Selection of the most appropriate primary outcome measure for a full-scale RCT Determined based on outcome measure with largest between group effect size	The randomization procedure was appropriate, with the treating physical therapist informed of group allocation but outcome measurement assessor was not aware of group allocation of any participants. All participants knew group allocation because of heterogeneity of interventions. NDI (0.79), as a measure of neck disability and quality of life, and 3D posture parameters of head in relation to thoracic (T_x, T_z, R_x, R_z, R_y) were selected.
Estimation of required sample size for a fully powered study • Based on NDI	A sample size of 42 participants (21 in each group) provides a minimum of 80% power ($\alpha = 0.05$) and is required for an effect size of 0.79. To account for an estimated 20% dropout, the recommended sample size is 50 participants (25 in each group).

NDI: neck disability index; ROM: range of motion; 3D: three-dimensional.

3. Results

Of 54 people who responded to advertisements in orthopedic and rehabilitation department clinics and were interested in participating in the study, 11 people did not have time to complete the intervention, 9 people had NPRS less than 3 and NDI less than 5, and 10 people did not meet the inclusion criteria of 3D posture measurements of the head in relation to the thoracic region. In the end, 30 people were excluded and 24 people were included (45% who fulfilled inclusion criteria and 100% of included participants enrolled in the study), as shown in Figure 3. Those 24 participants fulfilled all procedures of assessment and interventions, but 3 (12.5%) participants were lost and did not make the final assessment (2 from the control group and 1 from the study group). Complete demographic characteristic data of participants are shown in Table 4.

The results of the primary outcome aspects related to feasibility are provided in Table 3. Using the extension of the CONSORT statement for pilot and feasibility studies when developing the protocol our findings were informed by our previously published protocol. The recruitment into our study was achieved in an acceptable period, and less than 15% of participants were lost to follow-up before the final assessment because they had to travel to other cities and did not have time to continue the treatment and assessment. We used complete case analyses, where 12.5 % (3 of 24) of participants were excluded because of missing data.

Table 4. Demographic characteristic data of participants.

	Study Group (n = 12)	Control Group (n = 12)	p-Value
Age (y) mean ± SD	27.4 ± 5.5	27.2 ± 4.7	0.7
Weight (kg) mean ± SD	64.58 ± 6.9	67.2 ± 5.8	0.3
Height (m) mean ± SD	1.65 ± 0.5	1.67 ± 0.6	0.6
BMI (kg/m^2), mean ± SD	23.5 ± 1.2	24.2 ± 0.97	0.2
Male, n (%)	8 (66.7%)	7 (58%)	0.5
Female, n (%)	4 (33.3%)	5 (42%)	0.5
Participants Employment			
University student, n (%)	7 (58%)	6 (50%)	0.6
Desk office worker n (%)	4 (33.3%)	4 (33.3%)	0.5
House wife, n (%)	1 (8.3%)	2 (16.7%)	0.6
Married, n (%)	4 (33.3%)	3 (25%)	0.7
Duration of Pain, n (%)			
3–24 months	8 (66.7%)	9 (75%)	0.6
>24 months	4 (33.3%)	3 (25%)	0.7
Current use of Medications, n (%)			
Yes	2	3	0.6
No	10	9	0.7
Referred pain, n (%)	6 (50%)	7 (58%)	0.5
Current smoker, n (%)	2 (16.7%)	3 (25%)	0.6

Mean ± SD: standard deviation; BMI: body mass index.

Table 5 shows the within-group change in each of the secondary outcome measures for each group. In general, larger improvements and greater effect sizes were found in the study group for pain, disability, postural measures, and cervical spine range of motion.

Between-group differences in change scores, effect size, and estimated sample size for each of the secondary outcome measures of NDI, NPRS, and range of motion are shown in Table 6. While Table 7 presents the between-group differences in change scores, effect size, and estimated sample size for each of the secondary outcome measures of 3D posture displacements of Tx, Tz, Rx, Ry, and Rz. In general, larger improvements and greater effect sizes were found in the study group for pain, disability, postural measures, and cervical spine range of motion in Tables 6 and 7. Sample size estimates for the full-scale RCT indicated that a minimum of 14 participants (ROM for flexion and extension) and a maximum of 80 participants (ROM y-axis rotation) would be needed for full statistical evaluation. A full-scale RCT using our multimodal program for participants with CNSNP related to poor posture would require a sample of 42 participants (without calculating any dropout) to demonstrate a clinically meaningful functional improvement based on the NDI. Table 6.

We found a moderately positive correlation between pre- and post-treatment changes in 3D postural parameters and pre- and post-treatment changes in pain and NDI, indicating that as posture displacement decreased in our population, so did pain intensity and NDI scores. However, as shown in Table 8, we discovered a moderately negative correlation between cervical ROM values and pre- and post-treatment changes in 3D postural parameters.

Table 5. Within-group change in secondary outcome measures for each group. Postural translations (Tx and Tz) are measured in centimeters, postural rotations (Rx, Ry, Rz), and ranges of motion (ROM) are measured in degrees. The mean difference (MD) is the difference between the baseline and after-treatment values. A negative value for the change (MD) in range of motion indicates an increase in the overall motion for the variable.

	Baseline	Post Intervention	MD [†]	ES
	Mean ± SD	Mean ± SD	(p Value 95% CI)	(d)
NDI (0–50) Study G	12.42 ± 4.54	3.33 ± 2.42	9.1 ± 4.3 <0.001 * (6.4, 11.8)	2.5
Control G	12.41 ± 3.02	5.41 ± 2.35	7 ± 1.13 <0.001 * (6.4, 7.7)	2.5
NPRS (0–10) Study G	5 ± 1.4	1.8 ± 1.03	3.2 ± 1.26 <0.001 * (2.4, 3.9)	2.6
Control G	4.91 ± 1.2	2.29 ± 0.87	2.6 ± 0.4 <0.001 * (2.4, 2.9)	2.49
Tx Study G	0.97 ± 0.4	0.41 ± 0.13	0.56 ± 0.37 <0.001 * (0.3, 0.8)	1.87
Tx Control G	0.75 ± 0.35	0.68 ± 0.31	0.075 ± 0.05 0.29 (0.04, 0.1)	0.2
Tz Study G	3 ± 1.3	1.34 ± 1.1	1.6 ± 1.05 <0.001 * (0.9, 2.4)	1.2
Tz Control G	3.1 ± 1.4	2.85 ± 1.6	0.24 ± 0.28 0.23 (0.06, 0.4)	0.15
Rx Study G	24.8 ± 4.17	19.41 ± 2.54	5.4 ± 3.2 <0.001 * (3.4, 7.45)	1.56
Control G	23.8 ± 3.95	22.3 ± 3.98	1.5 ± 2.3 0.013 (0.03, 2.96)	0.38
Ry Study G	3.5 ± 1.6	1.58 ± 0.67	2 ± 1.88 <0.001 * (0.7, 3.1)	1.35
Ry Control G	3 ± 1.3	2.33 ± 1.4	0.5 ± 0.52 0.16 (0.2, 0.8)	0.29
Rz Study G	3.3 ± 1.5	1.5 ± 0.79	1.83 ± 1.8 <0.001 * (0.7, 2.97)	1.34
Rz Control G	3 ± 1.4	2.33 ± 1.4	0.5 ± 0.52 0.2 (0.2, 0.8)	0.29
ROM flex and extension Study G	87.1 ± 4.18	108.1 ± 4	−21 ± 0.18 <0.001 * (−21.3, −20.7)	5
Control G	86.7 ± 4.37	100.6 ± 4	−13.9 ± 0.37 <0.001 * (−14.4, −13.5)	3.3
ROM lateral flexion Study G	65.75 ± 4.5	80.25 ± 4	−14.5 ± 0.5 <0.001 * (−14.7, −14.3)	3.4
Control G	63.91 ± 4.6	73.41 ± 4.2	−9.5 ± 0.4 <0.001 * (−9.8, −9.4)	2.1
ROM rotation Study G	101.8 ± 2.33	118.8 ± 2	−17 ± 0.33 <0.001 * (−17.1, −16.96)	7.8
Control G	101.58 ± 2.2	117.48 ± 2	−15.9 ± 0.02 <0.001 * (−16, −15.8)	7.5

Mean. MD, mean difference NDI, neck disability index. NPRS, numeric pain rating scale. ROM, range of motion. Flex. flexion. ES (d), effect size (Cohen's d), Tx, side shifting of head. Tz, Ant. head translation. Rx, upper extension of head. Ry, R.t or l.t rotation of head. Rz, side bending R.t or l.t of head. [†] Values in parentheses are 95% confidence interval. G, group. Sig.; significant, 001, Sig; 0.01. * Significant for TZ, TX, Rx, Ry, Rz. Sig; 0.05, * significant for all other outcomes.

Table 6. Between-group differences in change scores, effect size, and estimated sample size for each of the secondary outcome measures with significance level of 0.05. The mean difference (MD) is the difference between the two groups' change score values. A negative value for the change (MD) in range of motion indicates an increase in the overall motion for the variable for that group whereas the difference between the group is a positive number indicating greater improvement for the study group. Ranges of motion (ROM) are measured in degrees.

	Study Group Change Score * (Baseline to Posttreatment)	Control Group Change Score * (Baseline to Posttreatment)	MD † (p Value 95% CI)	ES (d)	Estimated Total Sample Size for Outcome Measure, n ‡
NDI (0–50)	9.1 ± 4.3	7 ± 1.13	2.08 <0.001 * (4.11, 0.06)	0.79	42
NPRS (0–10)	3.2 ± 1.26	2.6 ± 0.4	0.458 <0.001 * (1.26, 0.35)	0.58	76
ROM flex and exten.	−21 ± 0.18	−13.9 ± 0.37	7.42 <0.001 * (3.79, 11.1)	1.78	14
ROM lateral flexion	−14.5 ± 0.5	−9.5 ± 0.4	6.8 <0.001 * (2.97, 10.7)	1.26	22
ROM rotation	−17 ± 0.33	−15.9 ± 0.02	1.35 <0.001 * (−0.49, 3.2)	0.56	80

NDI, neck disability index. NPRS, numeric pain rating scale. ROM, range of motion. Flex and exten., flexion and extension. MD, mean difference. * Values are mean ± SD. † Values in parentheses are 95% confidence interval. ‡ Estimated sample size determined using Student t test sample size calculation, without adjusting for anticipated dropouts and losses to follow-up ($\alpha = 0.05$, $\beta = 0.80$). Sig; 0.05. ES (d), effect size (Cohen's d).

Table 7. Between-group differences in change scores, effect size, and estimated sample size for 3D posture parameters of head related to thoracic with significance level 0.01. Postural translations (Tx and Tz) are measured in centimeters and postural rotations (Rx, Ry, Rz) are measured in degrees.

	Study Group Change Score *	Control Group Change Score *	MD † (p Value 95% CI)	ES (d)	Estimated Total Sample Size for Outcome Measure, n ‡
Tx (side shifting of head)	0.56 ± 0.37	0.07 ± 0.04	.48 <0.001 * (−0.48, −0.05)	1.70	18
Tz (Ant. H. Translation)	1.6 ± 1.05	0.24 ± 0.28	1.36 <0.001 * (−2.6, −0.28)	1.1	38
Rx (upper extension of head)	5.4 ± 3.2	1.5 ± 2.3	3.9 <0.001 * (−5.75, −0.09)	1.12	36
Ry (rot. R.t or l.t of head)	2 ± 1.88	0.5 ± 0.52	1.5 <0.001 * (−1.72, 0.22)	0.96	48
Rz (side bending R.t or l.t of head)	1.83 ± 1.8	0.5 ± 0.52	1.33 <0.001 * (−1.8, 0.15)	0.90	52

H, head. rot., rotation. * Values are mean ± SD. † Values in parentheses are 95% confidence interval. ‡ Estimated sample size determined using Student t test sample size calculation, without adjusting for anticipated dropouts and losses to follow-up ($\alpha = 0.01$, $\beta = 0.80$). Sig; 0.01. ES (d), Effect size (Cohen's d).

Table 8. Correlations (Pearson's r) were used to examine the relationships between the 3D postural parameters and all measured outcomes for the entire sample. * Indicates a statistically significant difference at $p < 0.001$.

	Change in Neck Pain	Changes in NDI	Changes in ROM Flex and Exten	Changes in ROM Lateral Flexion	Changes in ROM Rotation
Change in Tx (side shifting of head)	0.5 <0.001 *	0.5	−0.48 <0.001 *	−0.51 <0.001 *	−0.41 0.01
Change in Tz (Ant. H. Translation)	0.6 <0.001 *	0.31 0.06	−0.53 <0.001 *	−0.43 0.04	−0.33 0.05
Change in Rx (upper extension of head)	0.3 0.06	0.49 <0.001 *	−0.51 <0.001 *	−0.32 0.05	−0.3 0.06
Change in Ry (rot. R.t or l.t of head)	0.5 <0.001 *	0.62 <0.001 *	−0.4 0.01	−0.56 <0.001 *	−0.71 <0.001 *
Change in Rz (side bending R.t or l.t of head)	0.4 0.01	0.46 <0.001 *	−0.3 0.06	−0.51 <0.001 *	−0.54 <0.001 *

4. Discussion

Our promising results suggest that it is feasible to conduct a full-scale RCT using a 3D PCO to perform mirror image therapy (reverse posture training) while a patient is walking on a motorized treadmill. Based on our data, a full-scale RCT using our multimodal program for participants with neck pain related to poor posture or postural neck pain would require a sample of 42 participants (without calculating any dropout) to demonstrate a clinically meaningful functional improvement based on the NDI. While feasible, our results also suggest that some modifications to the protocol may enhance participant enrolment, including access to the intervention and the effectiveness of various aspects of the intervention in future studies. Furthermore, since study participants indicated that the treatment sessions were quite lengthy, a reduction in treatment time is needed in a future full-scale trial. This can be accomplished by reducing the number of interventions (hot packs and one of the mobilization procedures) and reducing the walking time on the treadmill to 15–20 min instead of 20–30 min.

In our pilot study, 54 people responded to advertisements, 24 (45%) of whom were eligible. Therefore, at least 93 potential participants would be required to respond to advertisements to obtain a sample of 42 participants. This information will assist in planning the extent of the intervention, timelines for recruitment, and budgets for future studies.

The diagnosis was based on physical examination, including history, demographic variables, the mode of onset, duration of symptoms, nature, and location of symptoms, as well as questions regarding aggravating and relieving factors, such as posture modifications and change positions and any prior history of neck pain (3). The assessment also depended on pain level, neck disability, 3D posture analysis of the head in relation to the thoracic region, and active cervical range of motion. We subsequently used an X-ray to exclude any specific cause of pain. Notably, a large number (30/54, 55%) of participants were excluded; they had neck pain, but their NPRS was less than 3 and NDI was less than 5, and posture modifications or poor posture were not the risk factor for the problem occurring. Those symptoms were diagnosed as myofascial pain syndrome. Other participants had NPRS and NDI and a score of more than 3 and 5, respectively, but did not match the 3D posture analysis criteria; the cause of the problem was not due to posture modifications or poor posture. We tried to include participants who had poor posture according to the 3D analysis, and to modify poor posture, which affects participant symptoms and function; ultimately, we attempted to include only participants with postural components to their neck pain [10,13].

We included neck pain and a disability score from moderate to severe on the NPRS and NDI. Most participants had a fixed position during smartphone use or in the workplace for long periods or had a monotonous constrained vision-related task such as computer programming. Only three participants were housewives using smartphones for extended times in the flexed neck position; the other participants were university students and desk office workers who were often using computers in a slumped seated position in FHP for a prolonged time.

To the best of our knowledge, this intervention was the first to use a 3D PCO for mirror image therapy (reverse posture training) of the cervical spine while the patient is walking on a motorized treadmill and to utilize a supervised, tailored brace for each participant according to 3D posture analysis, as well as functional walking training for at least 20 min using the PCO as active not passive therapy. Within-group effect sizes for improvement of 3D posture analysis data of the head, in relation to the thoracic region (five posture variables, two translation displacements, and three rotational displacements), in the study group were very large (1.19–1.87). Interestingly, the control group also had small to medium gains in 3D posture analysis data (effect size, 0.15–0.38). Likely speaking, the larger changes in the study groups' postures are due to the targeted mirror image therapy using the PCO with functional walking training on a treadmill. The training was thus tailored according to each participant's 3D analysis data. Because both groups practiced a therapeutic exercise program as shown in Table 1, this might explain the posture improvement in some parameters (Rx, Ry, and Rz) of 3D posture analysis in the control group. In addition, the study group reported large within-group improvements in pain, function, and quality of life, but due to the limitation in the sample size, we can only infer that this was due to the PCO training and postural correction.

Future fully powered RCTs should explore whether greater improvements in pain and quality of life are associated with improvements in 3D posture parameters and whether or not these continue to improve after follow-up for 3 to 6 months or longer. Our future RCT will include these specifications, especially a follow-up period of 6 months (ClinicalTrials.gov ID: NCT04263883), and will use a sham or a placebo brace for the control group.

In our pilot study, the effect size for between-group differences in change scores is moderately large in the study group for all secondary outcomes, such as NDI, NPRS, and all active neck ROM, as well as all parameters of 3D posture analysis. The changes visualized on photographic measurements would be due to the application of traction forces to the lateral cervical structures or the reverse posture traction (reverse posture training) on 3D planes. The muscles and ligamentous structures of the spine are viscoelastic. The deformation of these structures is, mechanically, time-dependent and force-dependent [16]. When under loading, spinal ligaments complete a stress relaxation process in approximately 500 s (8.33 min). However, the intervertebral disc will continue to deform for 20 min to 60 min [16,49,50]. For this reason, we progressively increased the PCO therapy up to 20 min in the form of functional training, such as walking, to attain the maximum amount of deformation to the paraspinal structures in a clinically efficient time.

The strengths of our study included using the extension of the CONSORT statement for pilot and feasibility studies when developing the protocol [48,51]. In addition, our findings were informed by our previously published protocol [47]. The recruitment into our study was achieved in an acceptable period, and less than 15% of participants were lost to follow-up before the final assessment because they had to travel to other cities and did not have time to continue the treatment and assessment. We used complete case analyses, where 12.5% (3 of 24) of participants were excluded because of missing data. Despite options for the statistical imputation of missing data, minimizing the dropout rate should be a priority in our future studies.

5. Limitations

The study had some potential limitations, each of which points toward directions for future study. The first limitation of our study was the lack of blinding of participants and physiotherapists because of the nature and difference of the interventions. It was difficult to blind participants and healthcare providers. However, the investigator, outcome assessor, and data analyst were blinded to the participant allocation group. We can overcome this issue in future studies by adding a placebo-treated group for mirror image traction using another orthotic intervention, such as another cervicothoracic brace without adjustment according to 3D posture analysis. Additionally, our study results are limited to the outcome measurements chosen to evaluate CNSNP. It is possible that using different outcome measures of neck pain, such as muscle endurance, motor control, and proprioceptive tasks, would produce different findings between the intervention and control groups. Third, the assessment of psychosocial models, such as depression and fearful avoidance of movement, were not included in our pilot, and we will assess them in a future RCT. Fourth, our study did not include a true natural history group with chronic neck pain and participants must not have had physical therapy treatment in the previous 6 months, but it was unknown which other treatment they might have received prior to the previous 6 months.

The last limitation was the small sample size, which weakens any strong interpretation regarding the effectiveness of our intervention. We could not solve all these limitations at the same time in one study because the PCO used in the study is a new device for therapeutic use. Instead, we focused on the design of a new postural mirror image brace and first assess its feasibility, the pilot study outcomes, and the secondary assessment of its direct effect on 3D posture parameters and its indirect effect on neck pain, disability, and active neck ROM.

6. Conclusions

It was demonstrated that a full-scale RCT of a 3D PCO to perform mirror image therapy (reverse posture training) is feasible. Adding a 3D PCO to a multimodal program positively affected neck pain management outcomes by reducing neck pain, improving neck function, and increasing active ROM, which was likely due to improved 3D posture alignment of the head. Adequately powered and improved studies are needed to confirm or refute this association.

Supplementary Materials: The following supporting information can be downloaded at: https://www.mdpi.com/article/10.3390/jcm11237028/s1, Video S1: Mirror image postural neuromuscular retraining of motor patterns.

Author Contributions: A.S.A.Y., I.M.M., A.M.E.M., X.H. and D.E.H. conceived the research idea and participated in its design; A.S.A.Y., I.M.M., A.M.E.M. and X.H. contributed to the statistical analysis; A.S.A.Y., I.M.M., A.M.E.M. and X.H. participated in the data collection, A.S.A.Y., I.M.M., A.M.E.M., D.E.H. and P.A.O. contributed to the interpretation of the results and wrote the original and final drafts. All authors have read and agreed to the published version of the manuscript.

Funding: This research received no external funding.

Institutional Review Board Statement: The study was conducted in accordance with the Declaration of Helsinki and approved by the Institutional Review Board from the Ethical Committee of Tongji Hospital, Tongji Medical College, Huazhong University of Science and Technology (HUST), Wuhan, China (certificate of approval number TJ-IRB20170703) approval date 3 July 2017. All participants provided written informed consent before the beginning of the study.

Informed Consent Statement: Written informed consent was obtained from the person depicted in Figures 1, 2 and 5, and the supplementary video for the publication of picture and video in the manuscript. A copy of the written consent is available for review by the Editor-in-Chief of this journal.

Data Availability Statement: The datasets analyzed in the current study are available from the corresponding author upon reasonable request.

Conflicts of Interest: P.A.O. is a paid consultant for CBP NonProfit, Inc. D.E.H. teaches rehabilitation methods and sells products to physicians for patient care similar to that used in this manuscript. All the other authors declare that they have no competing interests.

Trial Registration: ClinicalTrials.gov Identifier: NCT03331120. Registered 6 November 2017, https://clinicaltrials.gov/ct2/show/NCT03331120.

Abbreviations

CNSNP: chronic nonspecific neck pain; 3D: three-dimensional; PCO: posture corrective orthotic; ROM: range of motion; NPRS: numeric pain rating scale; NDI: neck disability index; GPS: global posture system; RCT: randomized control trial; Tx: r.t or l.t side shifting of head; Tz: anterior head translation; Rx: extension of upper cervical; Ry: r.t or l.t rot. of head; Rz: R.t or l.t side bending of head; Ant.: anterior; Rot.: rotation; FHP: forward head posture; SD: standard deviation; CI: confidence interval.

References

1. Hay, S.I.; Abajobir, A.A.; Abate, K.H.; Abbafati, C.; Abbas, K.M.; Abd-Allah, F.; Abdulle, A.M.; Abebo, T.A.; Abera, S.F.; Aboyans, V.; et al. Global, regional, and national disability-adjusted life-years (DALYs) for 333 diseases and injuries and healthy life expectancy (HALE) for 195 countries and territories, 1990-2016: A systematic analysis for the Global Burden of Disease Study 2016. *Lancet* **2017**, *390*, 1260–1344. [CrossRef]
2. Salomon, J.A.; Haagsma, J.A.; Davis, A.; de Noordhout, C.M.; Polinder, S.; Havelaar, A.H.; Cassini, A.; Devleesschauwer, B.; Kretzschmar, M.; Speybroeck, N.; et al. Disability weights for the Global Burden of Disease 2013 study. *Lancet Glob. Health* **2015**, *3*, e712–e723. [CrossRef]

3. Childs, J.D.; Cleland, J.A.; Elliott, J.M.; Teyhen, D.S.; Wainner, R.S.; Whitman, J.M.; Sopky, B.J.; Godges, J.J.; Flynn, T.W. Neck pain: Clinical practice guidelines linked to the international classification of functioning, disability, and health from the orthopaedic section of the american physical therapy association. *J. Orthop. Sports Phys. Ther.* **2008**, *38*, A1–A34. [CrossRef] [PubMed]
4. Bernal-Utrera, C.; Gonzalez-Gerez, J.J.; Anarte-Lazo, E.; Rodriguez-Blanco, C. Manual therapy versus therapeutic exercise in non-specific chronic neck pain: A randomized controlled trial. *Trials* **2020**, *21*, 682. [CrossRef]
5. Peolsson, A.; Marstein, E.; McNamara, T.; Nolan, D.; Sjaaberg, E.; Peolsson, M.; Jull, G.; O'Leary, S. Does posture of the cervical spine influence dorsal neck muscle activity when lifting? *Man. Ther.* **2014**, *19*, 32–36. [CrossRef]
6. Quek, J.; Pua, Y.H.; Clark, R.A.; Bryant, A.L. Effects of thoracic kyphosis and forward head posture on cervical range of motion in older adults. *Man. Ther.* **2013**, *18*, 65–71. [CrossRef]
7. Park, S.Y.; Yoo, W.G. Effect of sustained typing work on changes in scapular position, pressure pain sensitivity and upper trapezius activity. *J. Occup. Health* **2013**, *55*, 167–172. [CrossRef]
8. Park, J.-H.; Kang, S.-Y.; Lee, S.-G.; Jeon, H.-S. The effects of smart phone gaming duration on muscle activation and spinal posture: Pilot study. *Physiother. Theory Pract.* **2017**, *33*, 661–669. [CrossRef]
9. Szczygieł, E.; Fudacz, N.; Golec, J.; Golec, E. The impact of the position of the head on the functioning of the human body: A systematic review. *Int. J. Occup. Med. Environ. Health* **2020**, *33*, 559–568. [CrossRef] [PubMed]
10. Silva, A.G.; Punt, T.D.; Sharples, P.; Vilas-Boas, J.P.; Johnson, M.I. Head posture assessment for patients with neck pain: Is it useful? *Int. J. Ther. Rehabil.* **2009**, *16*, 43–53. [CrossRef]
11. Edmondston, S.J.; Chan, H.Y.; Chi Wing Ngai, G.; Warren, M.L.R.; Williams, J.M.; Glennon, S.; Netto, K. Postural neck pain: An investigation of habitual sitting posture, perception of "good" posture and cervicothoracic kinaesthesia. *Man. Ther.* **2007**, *12*, 363–371. [CrossRef] [PubMed]
12. Szeto, G.P.Y.; Straker, L.M.; O'Sullivan, P.B. A comparison of symptomatic and asymptomatic office workers performing monotonous keyboard work-2: Neck and shoulder kinematics. *Man. Ther.* **2005**, *10*, 281–291. [CrossRef]
13. Straker, L.; Smith, A.; Campbell, A.; O'Sullivan, P. Are neck pain and posture related? *Phys. Ther. Rev.* **2010**, *15*, 115–116. [CrossRef]
14. Harrison, D.D.; Janik, T.J.; Harrison, G.R.; Troyanovich, S.; Harrison, D.E.; Harrison, S.O. Chiropractic biophysics technique: A linear algebra approach to posture in chiropractic. *J. Manip. Physiol. Ther.* **1996**, *19*, 525–535.
15. Harrison, D.D. Abnormal postural permutations calculated as rotations and translations from an ideal normal upright static spine. In *Chiropractic Family Practice*; Sweere, J., Ed.; Aspen Publishers: Gaithersburg, MD, USA, 1992.
16. Harrison, D.E.; Cailliet, R.; Betz, J.; Haas, J.W.; Harrison, D.D.; Janik, T.J.; Holland, B. Conservative methods for reducing lateral translation postures of the head: A nonrandomized clinical control trial. *J. Rehabil. Res. Dev.* **2004**, *41*, 631–639. [CrossRef]
17. Diab, A.A.; Moustafa, I.M. New Bracing Concept in the Treatment of Chronic Mechanical Low Back Pain: A Randomized Trial. *Bull. Fac. Phys. Ther.* **2009**, *14*, 63–74.
18. Kovacs, F.M.; Abraira, V.; Royuela, A.; Corcoll, J.; Alegre, L.; Tomás, M.; Mir, M.A.; Cano, A.; Muriel, A.; Zamora, J.; et al. Minimum detectable and minimal clinically important changes for pain in patients with nonspecific neck pain. *BMC Musculoskelet. Disord.* **2008**, *9*, 43. [CrossRef] [PubMed]
19. Beltran-Alacreu, H.; López-de-Uralde-Villanueva, I.; Fernández-Carnero, J.; La Touche, R. Manual therapy, therapeutic patient education, and therapeutic exercise, an effective multimodal treatment of nonspecific chronic neck pain: A randomized controlled trial. *Am. J. Phys. Med. Rehabil.* **2015**, *94*, 887–897. [CrossRef]
20. MacDermid, J.C.; Walton, D.M.; Avery, S.; Blanchard, A.; Etruw, E.; McAlpine, C.; Goldsmith, C.H. Measurement Properties of the Neck Disability Index: A Systematic Review. *J. Orthop. Sport. Phys. Ther.* **2009**, *39*, 400–417. [CrossRef]
21. Lee, H.S.; Chung, H.K.; Park, S.W. Correlation between trunk posture and neck reposition sense among subjects with forward head neck postures. *Biomed Res. Int.* **2015**, *2015*, 689610. [CrossRef]
22. Yeom, H.; Lim, J.; Yoo, S.H.; Lee, W. A new posture-correcting system using a vector angle model for preventing forward head posture. *Biotechnol. Biotechnol. Equip.* **2014**, *28*, S6–S13. [CrossRef]
23. Normand, M.C.; Descarreaux, M.; Harrison, D.D.; Harrison, D.E.; Perron, D.L.; Ferrantelli, J.R.; Janik, T.J. Three dimensional evaluation of posture in standing with the PosturePrint: An intra- and inter-examiner reliability study. *Chiropr. Osteopat.* **2007**, *15*, 15. [CrossRef] [PubMed]
24. Wolfe, F.; Clauw, D.J.; Fitzcharles, M.A.; Goldenberg, D.L.; Katz, R.S.; Mease, P.; Yunus, M.B. The American College of Rheumatology Preliminary Diagnostic Criteria for Fibromyalgia and Measurement of Symptom Severity. *Arthritis Care Res.* **2010**, *62*, 600–610. [CrossRef]
25. Silva, A.G.; Punt, T.D.; Sharples, P.; Vilas-Boas, J.P.; Johnson, M.I. Head Posture and Neck Pain of Chronic Nontraumatic Origin: A Comparison Between Patients and Pain-Free Persons. *Arch. Phys. Med. Rehabil.* **2009**, *90*, 669–674. [CrossRef] [PubMed]
26. Solow, B.; Ovesen, J.; Nielsen, P.W.; Wildschiødtz, G.; Tallgren, A. Head posture in obstructive sleep apnoea. *Eur. J. Orthod.* **1993**, *15*, 107–114. [CrossRef] [PubMed]
27. Fruhmann Berger, M.; Proß, R.; Ilg, U.; Karnath, H.-O. Deviation of eyes and head in acute cerebral stroke. *BMC Neurol.* **2006**, *6*, 23. [CrossRef]
28. Scientifique, B.B.-K. Undefined Posture Normale et Postures Pathologiques. 2004. Available online: ciesitaliaposturology.it (accessed on 1 September 2022).
29. Magee, D. *Orthopedic Physical Assessment*; Saunders: Philadelphia, PA, USA, 2007; 1152p.

30. Bowen, D.J.; Kreuter, M.; Spring, B.; Cofta-Woerpel, L.; Linnan, L.; Weiner, D.; Bakken, S.; Kaplan, C.P.; Squiers, L.; Fabrizio, C.; et al. How We Design Feasibility Studies. *Am. J. Prev. Med.* **2009**, *36*, 452–457. [CrossRef] [PubMed]
31. Lancaster, G.A.; Dodd, S.; Williamson, P.R. Design and analysis of pilot studies: Recommendations for good practice. *J. Eval. Clin. Pract.* **2004**, *10*, 307–312. [CrossRef] [PubMed]
32. Julious, S.A. Sample size of 12 per group rule of thumb for a pilot study. *Pharm. Stat.* **2005**, *4*, 287–291. [CrossRef]
33. Young, I.A.; Dunning, J.; Butts, R.; Mourad, F.; Cleland, J.A. Reliability, construct validity, and responsiveness of the neck disability index and numeric pain rating scale in patients with mechanical neck pain without upper extremity symptoms. *Physiother. Theory Pract.* **2019**, *35*, 1328–1335. [CrossRef]
34. Wu, S.; Ma, C.; Wu, S. Validity and reliability of the neck disability index for cervical spondylopathy patients. *Chin. J. Rehabil. Med.* **2008**, *23*, 625–628.
35. Prushansky, T.; Dvir, Z. Cervical Motion Testing: Methodology and Clinical Implications. *J. Manip. Physiol. Ther.* **2008**, *31*, 503–508. [CrossRef]
36. Audette, I.; Dumas, J.P.; Côté, J.N.; De Serres, S.J. Validity and between-day reliability of the cervical range of motion (CROM) device. *J. Orthop. Sports Phys. Ther.* **2010**, *40*, 318–323. [CrossRef] [PubMed]
37. Gps 600 Postural Lab. Available online: http://www.globalposturalsystem.com/hardware/03008-gps-600-postural-lab/ (accessed on 1 September 2022).
38. Gobbi, G.; Galli, D.; Carubbi, C.; Pelosi, A.; Lillia, M.; Gatti, R.; Queirolo, V.; Costantino, C.; Vitale, M.; Saccavini, M.; et al. Assessment of body plantar pressure in elite athletes: An observational study. *Sport Sci. Health* **2013**, *9*, 13–18. [CrossRef]
39. Toprak, M.; Alptekin, H.K.; Turhan, D. Correction to: P-12 Assessment of Symmetrigraph and Global Postural System Results for the Posture Analysis of the Healthy Individuals. *Chiropr. Man. Therap.* **2018**, *26*, 20. [CrossRef] [PubMed]
40. Xia, N.; Zhang, T.; Wang, C.; Zheng, Q.; Huang, J. Three indicators from two-dimensional body surface photographic measurements to assess the posture of patients with non- specific neck pain: A reliability and validity research. *Chin. J. Rehabil. Med.* **2019**, *34*, 1168–1172.
41. Zheng, Q.; Huang, X.L.; Wang, L.; Xie, L.F. A preliminary study on the reliability of quantitative evaluation of static upright posture. *Chin. J. Rehabil. Med.* **2019**, *34*, 1178–1182.
42. Maitland, G.D.; Hengeveld, E.; Banks, K.; English, K. *Maitland's Vertebral Manipulation*, 7th ed.; Elsevier Butterworth-Heinemann: New York, NY, USA, 2005; pp. 320–321.
43. Jull, G.; Trott, P.; Potter, H.; Zito, G.; Niere, K.; Shirley, D.; Emberson, J.; Marschner, I.; Richardson, C. A randomized controlled trial of exercise and manipulative therapy for cervicogenic headache. *Spine* **2002**, *27*, 1835–1842. [CrossRef]
44. Beer, A.; Treleaven, J.; Jull, G. Can a functional postural exercise improve performance in the cranio-cervical flexion test?-A preliminary study. *Man. Ther.* **2012**, *17*, 219–224. [CrossRef]
45. Jull, G.; Sterling, M.; Falla, D.; Treleaven, J.; O'Leary, S. *Whiplash, Headache, and Neck Pain*, 1st ed.; Elsevier: Amsterdam, The Netherlands, 2008; ISBN 9780443100475.
46. Harrison, D.E.; Cailliet, R.; Betz, J.W.; Harrison, D.D.; Colloca, C.J.; Haas, J.W.; Janik, T.J.; Holland, B. A non-randomized clinical control trial of Harrison mirror image methods for correcting trunk list (lateral translations of the thoracic cage) in patients with chronic low back pain. *Eur. Spine J.* **2005**, *14*, 155–162. [CrossRef]
47. Youssef, A.S.A.; Xia, N.; Emara, S.T.E.; Moustafa, I.M.; Huang, X. Addition of a new three-dimensional adjustable cervical thoracic orthosis to a multi-modal program in the treatment of nonspecific neck pain: Study protocol for a randomised pilot trial. *Trials* **2019**, *20*, 248. [CrossRef] [PubMed]
48. Moher, D.; Hopewell, S.; Schulz, K.F.; Montori, V.; Gøtzsche, P.C.; Devereaux, P.J.; Elbourne, D.; Egger, M.; Altman, D.G. CONSORT 2010 explanation and elaboration: Updated guidelines for reporting parallel group randomised trials. *Int. J. Surg.* **2012**, *10*, 28–55. [CrossRef] [PubMed]
49. Oliver, M.J.; Twomey, L.T. Extension creep in the lumbar spine. *Clin. Biomech.* **1995**, *10*, 363–368. [CrossRef]
50. Burstein, A.H. *Biomechanics in the Musculoskeletal System*; Churchill Livingstone: London, UK, 2001; Volume 83, ISBN 0443065853.
51. Eldridge, S.M.; Chan, C.L.; Campbell, M.J.; Bond, C.M.; Hopewell, S.; Thabane, L.; Lancaster, G.A.; O'Cathain, A.; Altman, D.; Bretz, F.; et al. CONSORT 2010 statement: Extension to randomised pilot and feasibility trials. *Pilot Feasibility Stud.* **2016**, *2*, 64. [CrossRef] [PubMed]

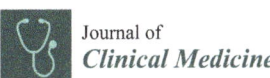

Article

Reduction of Thoracic Hyper-Kyphosis Improves Short and Long Term Outcomes in Patients with Chronic Nonspecific Neck Pain: A Randomized Controlled Trial

Ibrahim Moustafa Moustafa [1,2], Tamer Mohamed Shousha [1,2], Lori M. Walton [1], Veena Raigangar [1] and Deed E. Harrison [3,*]

1 Department of Physiotherapy, College of Health Sciences, University of Sharjah, Sharjah P.O. Box 27272, United Arab Emirates
2 Faculty of Physical Therapy, Cairo University, Giza 12511, Egypt
3 Private Practice and CBP Non-Profit, Inc., Eagle, ID 83616, USA
* Correspondence: drdeed@idealspine.com

Abstract: This study investigates thoracic hyper kyphosis (THK) rehabilitation using the Denneroll™ thoracic traction orthosis (DTTO). Eighty participants, with chronic non-specific neck pain (CNSNP) and THK were randomly assigned to the control or intervention group (IG). Both groups received the multimodal program; IG received the DTTO. Outcomes included formetric thoracic kyphotic angle ICT—ITL, neck pain and disability (NDI), head repositioning accuracy (HRA), smooth pursuit neck torsion test (SPNT) and overall stability index (OSI). Measures were assessed at baseline, after 30 treatment sessions over the course of 10 weeks, and 1-year after cessation of treatment. After 10 weeks, the IG improved more in neck pain intensity ($p < 0.0001$) and NDI ($p < 0.001$). No differences were found for SPNT ($p = 0.48$) and left-sided HRA ($p = 0.3$). IG improved greater for OSI ($p = 0.047$) and right sided HRA ($p = 0.02$). Only the IG improved in THK ($p < 0.001$). At 1-year follow-up, a regression back to baseline values for the control group was found for pain and disability such that all outcomes favored improvement in the IG receiving the DTTO; all outcomes ($p < 0.001$). The addition of the DTTO to a multimodal program positively affected CNSNP outcomes at both the short and 1-year follow-up.

Keywords: neck pain; thoracic kyphosis; randomized trial; postural kyphosis; sensorimotor control

Citation: Moustafa, I.M.; Shousha, T.M.; Walton, L.M.; Raigangar, V.; Harrison, D.E. Reduction of Thoracic Hyper-Kyphosis Improves Short and Long Term Outcomes in Patients with Chronic Nonspecific Neck Pain: A Randomized Controlled Trial. *J. Clin. Med.* 2022, 11, 6028. https://doi.org/10.3390/jcm11206028

Academic Editor: Hiroshi Horiuchi

Received: 13 September 2022
Accepted: 10 October 2022
Published: 13 October 2022

Publisher's Note: MDPI stays neutral with regard to jurisdictional claims in published maps and institutional affiliations.

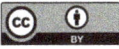

Copyright: © 2022 by the authors. Licensee MDPI, Basel, Switzerland. This article is an open access article distributed under the terms and conditions of the Creative Commons Attribution (CC BY) license (https://creativecommons.org/licenses/by/4.0/).

1. Introduction

Neck pain is the fourth leading cause for sustaining years of disability with an annual prevalence exceeding 30%, most often in females [1]. Biomechanically, the cervical, thoracic, and lumbar spines are interrelated [2]. Although structural causes of neck pain are not completely understood, they are believed to be related to the interrelated functions of anatomical structures connected to the cervical spine [3]. Potentially, any event leading to altered joint mechanics or muscle functions can cause neck pain [4].

The thoracic spine acts as a base of support for the cervical spine and influences its kinematics through the cervicothoracic junction [3]. Several studies have highlighted the effect of thoracic spine abnormalities on the kinematics of the cervical spine [5–7]. Specifically, mobility restrictions in the cervico-thoracic and upper thoracic regions were reported to be associated with neck pain [5,6]. Furthermore, it has been reported that the incidence of neck disorders is increased in older adults with a concomitant higher prevalence of thoracic hyper-kyphosis [6]. This would implicate postural impairments in the thoracic spine leading to a dysfunction of cervico-thoracic musculature such as serratus anterior, levator scapulae, and trapezius [8–10].

Lau et al. reported a positive correlation between a higher upper thoracic angle and neck pain, but failed to link this to neck pain intensity [3]. In addition, Kaya and Çelenay reported a positive correlation between thoracic curvature and neck pain and reported a negative correlation with neck pain intensity [11]. Furthermore, neck pain populations have been reported to have reduced trunk rotations during different speeds of walking [12].

Because changes in sagittal thoracic alignment have been reported to alter the mechanical loading of the cervical spine [10,13] and decreased thoracic mobility has been identified as one of the predictors for neck and shoulder pain [3], it makes sense that thoracic articular treatment improves local kinematics and that simultaneously neck pain improves [7,8,14].

Thoracic kyphosis has not been uniformly correlated with neck pain intensity and there is a general lack of investigations determining the role that rehabilitation of thoracic kyphosis plays in improving chronic cervical spine disorders. The purpose of this study was to investigate the immediate and 1-year effects of a multimodal program, with thoracic hyper kyphosis rehabilitation using the Denneroll™ thoracic traction orthosis (DTTO), applied to participants with chronic non-specific neck pain and thoracic hyper-kyphosis. Regarding the DTTO, it is likely that a significant reduction in thoracic kyphosis will occur due to the visco-elastic effect of the three-point bending extension traction during sustained supine loading while on the DTTO; this has been previously reported for extension traction devices for all regions of the sagittal plane of the spine [15–17].

The study hypothesis is two-fold: (1) the DTTO, as a three-point bending thoracic extension device, will cause a significant reduction in thoracic kyphosis; and (2) that the reduction in thoracic kyphosis will improve the short and long-term outcomes of participants with chronic non-specific neck pain.

2. Methods

A prospective, investigator-blinded, parallel-group, pilot randomized clinical trial was conducted at a research laboratory of our university and was retrospectively registered with the Pan African Clinical Trial Registry (PACTR2019107484227). Recruitment began after approval was obtained from the Ethics Committee of the Faculty of Physical Therapy, Cairo University with the ethical approval No. Cairo-6-2018-11M.S. Following Ethics Committee approval, participant recruitment began in September 2018. The participants were followed up for 1 year (till 2019 October); all participants signed informed consent prior to data collection. The reason behind the retrospective registration was that legislation in Egypt only requires local registration for clinical trials and this what was completed at the outset by prospectively registering in a non-WHO-approved registry.

We recruited a sample of 80 patients from our outpatient facility at the University of Cairo. The Consort participant flow diagram for our study is shown in Figure 1. Participants were screened prior to inclusion by measuring the sagittal thoracic kyphotic angle ICT-ITL (max) using a 4D formetric device (Figure 2). After being screened by a physiotherapist, all potential participants were invited to undergo comprehensive assessment by an orthopedist where other causes of thoracic kyphosis were excluded. Participants were included if the angle measured more 55 degrees. Furthermore, the patients were included if they had chronic nonspecific NP lasting for at least 3 months, and were able to read and speak English.

Exclusion criteria included the presence of any signs or symptoms of medical "red flags", a history of previous spine surgery, signs or symptoms of upper motor neuron disease, vestibular basilar insufficiency, amyotrophic lateral sclerosis, bilateral upper extremity radicular symptoms, a history of spinal column fracture, spinal tumors and related malignancies, congenital spinal anomalies, cancer, or rheumatoid arthritis. Furthermore, individuals with spinal scoliosis were excluded.

Participants were randomly assigned to an intervention group ($n = 40$) or control group ($n = 40$) according to a random number generator and restricted to permuted blocks of different sizes, with the researcher blinded to the sequence designated for each person. The participants in both groups completed a 10-week, 3× per week, 30 sessions total multimodal program consisting of physical pain relief methods, thoracic spine manipulation, myofascial release, and therapeutic exercises. The beneficial effects for this multimodal program have been previously reported [1,14,18–20].

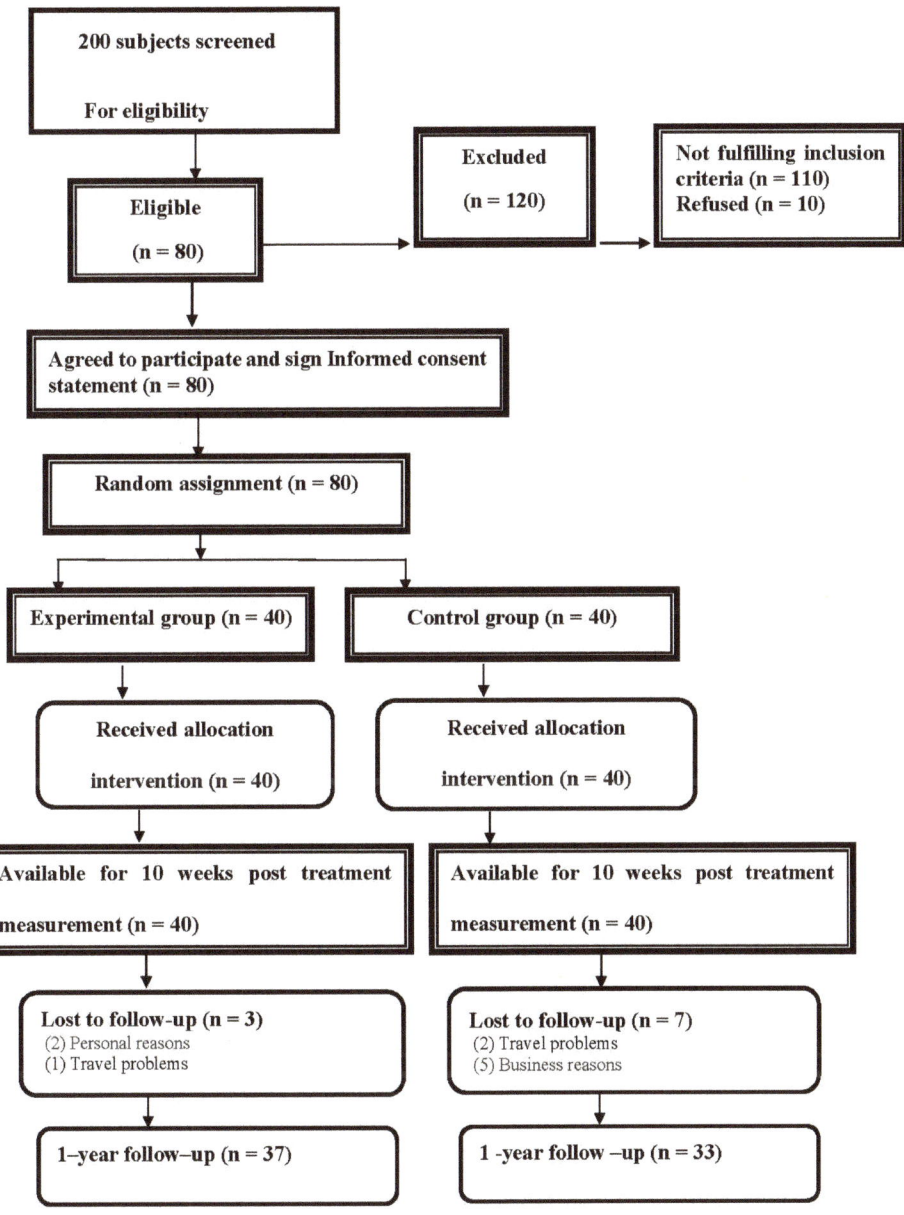

Figure 1. Flow chart of participants in the study over time.

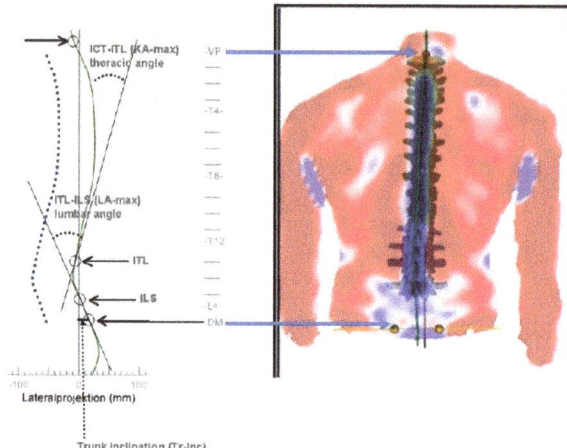

Figure 2. The 4D Formetric device measurement of Thoracic Kyphosis and Trunk Inclination where kyphotic angle ICT-ITL (max) is measured between tangents of cervicothoracic junction (ICT) and of thoracolumbar junction (ITL). ICT: Inflectional points from cervical to thoracic spine. ITL: Inflectional points from thoracic to lumbar spine. KA: kyphosis angle. LA: lordosis angle. VP: Vertebra prominence. DM: Dimple.

2.1. Multimodal Program

The multimodal program was delivered by the same physiotherapist, with 10 years of experience and training in the specific manual techniques in order to minimize inter-therapist variation and enhance fidelity. The participants in both the control and intervention groups received the multimodal program. Both groups received the same length of multimodal treatments and the sessions lasted 30–45 min each. However, the participants in the intervention group received an extra intervention (and time) using the Denneroll™ traction device. Thus, we attempted to provide the same time of attention equivalence in each group provided by the treating therapist during the intervention sessions.

2.2. TENS and Heat Therapy

The participants in both groups received conventional TENS therapy (20 min). TENS was applied over the painful area, using a frequency of 80 Hz; pulse width of 50 μs; intensity (mA) set at the person's sensorial threshold; modulation up to 50% of variation frequency; symmetrical, and rectangular biphasic waveform. These parameters were set for an optimum analgesic effect [18]. Moist hot packs (15 min) were applied prior to electrical stimulation. The TENS and heat therapy were repeated three times per week for 10 weeks.

2.3. Soft Tissue Mobilization

Soft tissue mobilization was performed on the muscles of the upper quarter with the involved upper extremity positioned in abduction and external rotation to preload the neural structures of the upper limb [19]. Manual pressure was applied to the soft tissues of the upper quadrant in a deep, stroking manner. The therapist concentrated on any tissues on the cervical and scapular region and upper extremity that were graded as tight or tender in the evaluation. This soft tissue mobilization was repeated three times per week for 10 weeks (30 sessions, 20 min face-to-face sessions)

2.4. Thoracic Spine Manipulation

Following the protocol previously outlined by Flynn [21], the participants were placed in the supine position with their arms crossed and with one hand, the clinician established a hand contact over the inferior vertebra of the identified hypomobile motion segment. With their second hand, a downward high velocity thrust was applied with the weight of the clinician's body through the patient's elbows or forearms. This procedure was performed at each identified segment with extension restriction range of motion determined clinically.

The initial treatment for all patients included thrust manipulation procedures consisting of a high-velocity, low amplitude end-range procedure, directed at the upper, mid, and lower spines of spinal segments identified as hypomobile during segmental mobility testing. Therapists were required to perform at least 1 technique targeting the upper thoracic spine, 1 technique targeting the mid thoracic spine, and 1 technique targeting the lower thoracic spine during each visit for each patient. If a pop (cavitation) occurred, then the therapist moved on to the next procedure. If not, the participant was repositioned, and the technique was performed again. This procedure was performed for a maximum of 2 attempts.

2.5. Functional Exercises

A functional and strengthening exercise program was administered that focused on deep cervical flexors, shoulder retractors, and serratus anterior activation and was conducted according to the protocol described in Harman et al. [20].

Strengthening deep cervical flexors through chin tucks in supine lying with the head in contact with the floor, the progression of this exercise was to lift the head off the floor in a tucked position and hold it for varying lengths of time (this was to progress by two second holds starting at two second i.e., 2, 4, 6, and 8 s). Shoulder retractors were strengthened first while standing using a TheraBand™ by pulling the shoulders back; then the participant was progressed to shoulder retraction in the prone position using weights. In the standing position, the patient was asked to pinch their scapulae together without elevation or extension in the shoulder holding this position for at least six second then relaxing. Participants performed each of these progressive exercises for two weeks prior to advancing to a more difficult version. At the consultation, if they could complete 3 sets of 12 repetitions correctly for the strengthening, they were progressed to the next exercise.

The progression of exercises was as follows:

(1) TheraBand™;
(2) 3 lbs;
(3) 3 lbs and TheraBand™;
(4) 5 lbs;
(5) 5 lbs and TheraBand™;
(6) 8 lbs;
(7) Using 8 lbs and TheraBand™.

The dynamic hug was performed to strengthen the serratus anterior while standing with the back toward the wall. The participant began with the elbow flexed 45°, the arm abducted 60°, and the shoulder internally rotated. The participant then horizontally flexed the humerus by following an arc described by his hands. Once the participant's hands touched together, they slowly returned to the starting position. Participants were instructed to complete three sets of 12 repetitions of the dynamic hug exercises. The complete functional exercise program was to be repeated three times per week for 10 weeks.

The participants in both groups were instructed to perform neck retraction/extension, scapular retraction, and deep upper cervical flexor strengthening exercises at home, twice daily as their home routine. To monitor the exercise frequency performed during the study, participants were given a pamphlet illustrating the exercises and a record sheet and were instructed to record the time and sets of the home exercises. Mean exercise frequency per week and mean exercise duration per day were recorded. Participants were encouraged to perform all exercises at least twice a week for up to one year after treatment. All persons were contacted by telephone every three months to collect the record sheets and encouraged to maintain the training.

2.6. Denneroll™ Thoracic Traction Orthotic (DTTO)

In addition, the participants in the intervention group received the DTTO (Denneroll Industries, Sydney, NSW, Australia), solely during the clinical setting. Thus, the only difference in treatments between the intervention and the control group was the application of the DTTO Figure 3. The participants were instructed to lie flat on their back on the ground with their knees slightly bent at 20–30° for comfort and arms gently folded across their stomach. The examiner positioned the apex of the DTTO in one of three regions: lower thoracic (T9–T12); mid-thoracic (T5–T8); and upper-thoracic (T1–T4) depending on the apex of each participant's thoracic kyphosis deformity. For lower thoracic kyphosis (T9–T12) the DTTO is turned 180° so the peak contacts the lower thoracic spine (T10) while the tapered end supports the mid thoracic region (Figure 3). For persons with mild–moderate posterior thoracic or backwards tilt translation postures with more of an upper thoracic kyphosis and anterior head translation, the DTTO is placed centered on top of a 20 mm block in order to cause anterior shift of the thoracic spine; set up not shown. All participants began at 3-min per session of DTTO application; at each visit they were encouraged to increase the duration by 2–3 min, until such time they were able to reach the goal of 15–20 min per session.

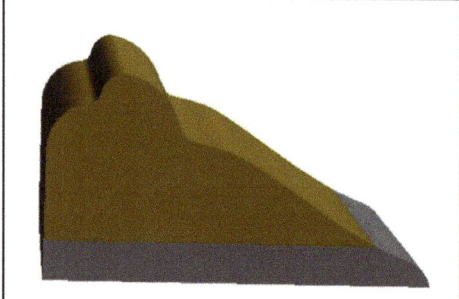 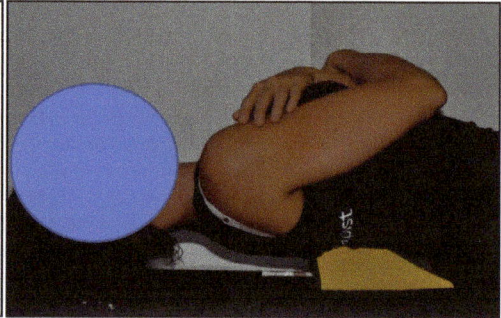

Figure 3. Denneroll™ Thoracic Traction Orthosis (DTTO). The DTTO can be placed in the upper (T3–T4), mid thoracic spine (T5–T8)-shown in B; or lower thoracic region (T9–T12) pending the apex of a participant's thoracic kyphosis and sagittal balance alignment. Each participant began lying supine over the apex of the DTTO for 1–3 min and progress 1–3 min per session until the target of 15–20 min per session was reached. Images copyright CBP Seminars, Inc. Reprinted with permission. Note: The individual used in the figures in this manuscript was a paid model and provided consent for commercial use.

2.7. Outcome Measures

A series of outcome measures were obtained at three intervals: (1) baseline; (2) one day following the completion of 30 visits after 10 weeks of treatment; and (3) one year after the participants' 30 session re-evaluation. The sequence of measurements was identical for all persons. Outcome measures included: (1) kyphotic angle ICT-ITL (max) as a primary outcome; (2) neck pain and disability (NDI); (3) sensorimotor control outcomes; (4) head repositioning accuracy (HRA); (5) smooth pursuit neck torsion test (SPNT); and (6) overall stability index (OSI) as secondary outcomes. All outcome assessments were carried out with two data collectors who were blinded to group allocation to prevent potential recorder and ascertainment bias. Participants were blinded to their measurement scores to address potential expectation bias and were instructed not to inform the assessors of their intervention status.

2.8. ICT-ITL (Max)

Thoracic kyphosis was assessed using a valid and reliable [22], 4D formetric device where determination of thoracic kyphosis angle ICT-ITL (max) is measured between tangents from the cervicothoracic junction (ICT-T1) and that of the thoracolumbar junction (ITL-T12). Participants were included if the angle measured 55° or more [23]. There was a good correlation between the formetric vs. Cobb angle of thoracic kyphosis (Pearson's r correlation = 0.799) but formetric measurements consistently over-estimate thoracic kyphosis by an average of 7° [23]; indicating that the T1–T12 radiographic would be a minimum of 48°, which is the upper end of normal in young adults, when the formetric angle is 55° [24]. See Figures 2 and 4 for the formetric analysis in our participants.

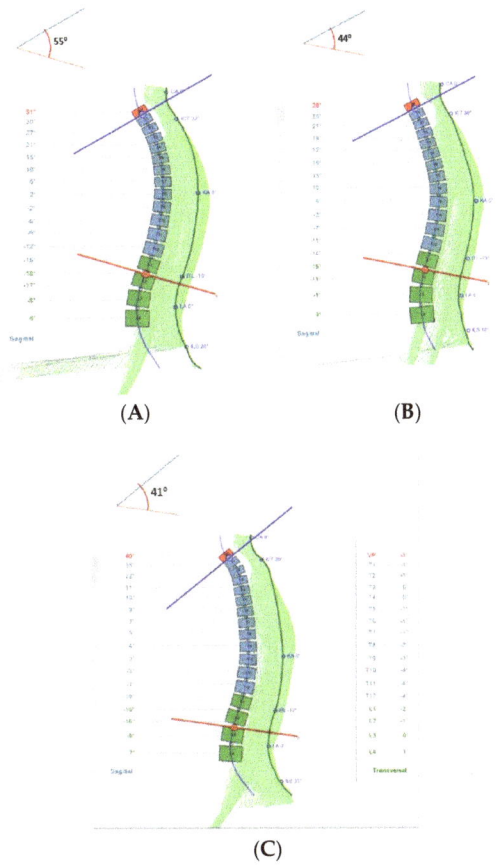

Figure 4. Kyphosis formetric posture alignment outcomes for a sample intervention group participant receiving the DTTO. (**A**) Initial baseline; (**B**) after 10-weeks and 30-sessions of intervention; and (**C**) the 1-year follow-up assessment where no further treatment was provided over the course of one year.

2.9. Neck Disability Index

The neck disability index (NDI) to assess activities of daily living impact was administered. The NDI has good reliability, validity, and responsiveness to change [25].

2.10. Numerical Rating Score (NRS)

Neck pain average intensity over the previous week was assessed using a 0–10 NRS where 0 = no pain, ... , 10 = bed ridden and incapacitated. The reliability [26] and validity [27] of the NRS is good to high.

2.11. Sensorimotor Control Measures

Assessment of sensorimotor function included: (1) cervical joint position sense testing; (2) head and eye movement control; and (3) evaluation of postural stability.

2.12. Cervical Joint Position Sense Testing

The valid and reliable technique [28] of head repositioning accuracy (HRA) assessment with the CROM device was performed according to a previous protocol [29]. In an upright seated posture on a stool with no backrest, the CROM device was placed on the participant's head, both feet were firmly on the floor with knees bent at an approximate 90° angle. The neutral head position (NHP) was established as the beginning and reference positions where the CROM device was adjusted to zero for the primary plane of rotational movement. Individuals were instructed to close their eyes, memorize the starting position, actively rotate their head 30° about the vertical axis, and reposition their head to the starting position with no requirements for speed, only accuracy was encouraged. HRA was measured as the difference in degrees in the primary plane of movement between the origin and the return positions [30]. Participants performed three repetitions within 60 sec in each rotational left and right directions, for a total of six sessions.

2.13. Head and Eye Movement Control: Smooth Pursuit Neck Torsion Test (SPNT)

Electro-oculography was used for the SPNT, which is an accurate means of assessing disturbances in eye movement control [31]. The method has been described elsewhere in detail [32]. The test was performed with the participant's head and trunk in a neutral forward position and then a trunk rotation position (head neutral, trunk in 45° rotation). The participants were instructed to perform three blinks (for recognition and elimination in data analysis) and then to follow the path of a light as closely as possible with their eyes. The SPNT test value was calculated as the difference between the average gain in the neutral and torsion positions for both left vs. right rotation.

2.14. Postural Stability

Postural stability was evaluated with a Biodex Balance System SD (BBS) (Biodex Medical Systems, Inc., Shirley, NY, USA). Dynamic balance testing was assessed allowing simultaneous displacements in both the anterior/posterior (AP) and medial/lateral (ML) directions. BBS measures the deviation of each axis in the horizontal plane of the platform during dynamic balance assessments and reports indices for ML, AP, and an overall stability index (OSI) whereby a reduced balance correlates with large variance. Balance indices were calculated over three 10-s trials, with 20 s of rest between trials; the average of the three trials was recorded. The BBS was set to a dynamic position of 4 out of 8 [33]. Several studies have used the device and have been proven to be reliable and valid for clinical studies [34–36].

All outcome assessments were carried out by 2 assessors blinded to group allocation. The: kyphotic angle ICT-ITL (max); neck pain and disability (NDI); sensorimotor control outcomes; head repositioning accuracy (HRA); and overall stability index (OSI) were performed by a physiotherapist with 20 years of experience in these measurement techniques (T.S.). The SPNT was conducted by an ophthalmologist (not an author) with 5 years of experience (R. W., MD).

3. Statistical Analysis

3.1. Sample Size

A priori sample size calculation based on a non-published pilot study conducted for 9 patients, indicated that 35 participants per each group were required to detect an effect size of 0.7 at 80% power and a significance level of 0.05 (5% chance of type 1 error). The mean difference of the primary outcome thoracic kyphosis angle ICT-ITL (max) was 11 and the standard deviation of this differences was 15. To account for possible drop-outs, the sample size was increased by 10% to 40 per group.

3.2. Data Analysis

Variance homogeneity was tested with Levene's test, obtaining a 95% confidence level and p-value > 0.05, and confirming variance equality. Descriptive statistics (means ± SD unless otherwise stated) were summarized at each time point. Student's t-test for continuous variables or chi-squared for categorical variables were performed.

The design used an intention-to-treat approach with alpha set at 0.05 level of significance for all analyses. Comparative treatment effects of the two alternative treatments over the course of the 1-year follow-up were examined with two-way analysis of covariance with repeated measures, followed by the Bonferroni post hoc test. The models included one independent factor (group), one repeated measure (time), and an interaction factor (group × time) and gender as covariate If interactions were found ($p < 0.05$), the baseline value of the outcome as covariates was used to assess between group differences. Cohen's d was calculated to examine the average impact of the intervention [37].

All data were analyzed using SPSS version 20.0 software (SPSS Inc., Chicago, IL, USA) with normality and equal variance assumptions ensured prior to the analysis.

3.3. Imputation of Missing Values

To impute any missing values for the intervention and control groups, we constructed models that included the variables related to the missing data and the variables correlated with that outcome. The main cause of the missing data was patient dropout at the long-term follow-up measurement interval at 1 year. The outcome measures at 1-year follow up were missing for three patients from the experimental group and seven patients from the control group (reasons for dropout are depicted in Figure 1). As the missing data were at the end of the trial, the last present value was carried forward. Imputation models included corresponding outcome values measured at baseline, then at 10 weeks. Other variables included in the imputation model were selected based on maximizing the correlation with the variable imputed. The characteristics which were associated with the variable imputed in the regression analysis were age, sex, and smoking status. This imputation created five complete datasets according to Rubin's method [38]. Pooled results were used for data analysis. We conducted a sensitivity analysis comparing the results from the imputed data to the original dataset, and the results were similar.

4. Results

Two hundred participants were initially recruited and screened, of whom 80 met the inclusion criteria and agreed to participate in the study. Three persons in the intervention group and seven in the control group resigned at 1-year follow-up for business and personal reasons. Figure 1 presents this information.

4.1. Baseline Demographics and Characteristics

The intervention and control groups were comparable for age, weight, sex, marital status, pain duration, and smoking status, indicating randomization was successful for these variables. Table 1 reports this data.

Table 1. Baseline participant demographics. Interventional group (Int.) is the group receiving standard care plus the Denneroll™ thoracic traction orthotic (DTTO). Control group (Con.) is the group receiving standard care only. Values are expressed as means ± standard deviation where indicated.

	Int. Group (n = 40)	Con. Group (n = 40)
Age (y)	25.05 ± 3	24 ± 4.2
Weight (kg)	66 ± 10	60 ± 9
Sex		
Male	28 (70%)	30 (75%)
Female	12 (30%)	10 (25%)
Single	31 (77.5%)	29 (72.5%)
Married	9 (22.5%)	11 (27.5%)

Table 1. Cont.

	Int. Group (n = 40)	Con. Group (n = 40)
Separated, divorced, or widowed	0	0
Pain duration (%) [Mean ± SD]		
1–3 y	11 (27.5%) [5.3 ± 2]	9 (22.5%) [5.8 ± 1]
3–5 y	16 (40%) [4.9 ± 1.5]	18 (45%) [5.4 ± 1.3]
>5 y	13 (32.5%) [4.8 ± 2]	15 (37.5%) [5.7 ± 0.9]
Smoking		
Light smoker	15 (37.5%)	18 (45%)
Heavy smoker	4 (10%)	2 (5%)
No Smoker	21 (52.5%)	20 (50%)

4.2. Between Group Analysis

A general linear model using repeated measurements identified significant group × time effects in favor of the intervention DTTO group for the following outcomes: thoracic kyphosis angle (ICT-ITL (max); NDI, NRS pain intensity; HRA for right and left rotation repositioning accuracy; SPENT, posture stability measured as the OSI. Table 2 reports the thoracic kyphosis outcomes, Table 3 reports the NDI and pain intensity while Table 4 reports the sensorimotor control outcomes.

Table 2. The changes in sagittal alignment management outcomes in experimental and control groups vs. time. Kyphotic angle ICT-ITL max = angle of kyphosis between tangents of cervicothoracic junction (ICT) and of thoracolumbar junction (ITL). Values are mean ± standard deviation. G = group; T = time; I = intervention group; C = control group; C.I. [] = 95% confidence interval; p = statistical significance; C.I. [] = 95% confidence interval; Cohen's d value = d; * indicates statistically significant difference.

		Baseline	10-Weeks	1-Year Follow up	Cohen's d 10-Weeks vs. Baseline	Cohen's d 1-Year vs. Baseline	p-Value		
							G	T	G vs. T
ICT-ITL max	I	82.15 ± 5.3	63.40 ± 6.2	64.6 ± 5.7	d = 3.2	d = 3.18	<0.001 *	<0.001 *	<0.001 *
	C	83.15 ± 4.9	82.2 ± 4.5	83.8 ± 3.8	d = 0.2	d = −0.14			
p-value C.I.		0.5 [−4.3, 2.3]	<0.001 * [−22.9, −15.8]	<0.001 * [−22.3, −16.1]					

Table 3. The changes in pain and disability outcomes in interventional (DTTO) and control groups vs. time. NDI = neck disability index; Pain intensity is 0–10 where 0 is no pain and 10 is incapacitated; I = interventional group; C = control group; G = group; T = time; G vs. T = group vs. time; all values are expressed as means ± standard deviation; C.I. [] = 95% confidence interval; Cohen's d value = d; * indicates statistically significant difference.

		Baseline	10-Weeks	1-Year Follow up	Cohen's d 10-Weeks vs. Baseline	Cohen's d 1-Year vs. Baseline	p-Value		
							G	T	G vs. T
NDI	I	31.1 ± 3.2	20.6 ± 4.5	10.9 ± 2.4	d = 2.6	d = 7.14	<0.001 *	<0.001 *	<0.001 *
	C	32.2 ± 2	29 ± 3.9	28.1 ± 5.1	d = 1.03	d = 1.05			
p-Value 95% C.I.		0.6 [−2.28, 0.08]	<0.001 * [−10.27, −6.52]	<0.001 * [−18.9, −15.4]					
Pain intensity	I	5 ± 1.5	1.4 ± 1.2	0.5 ± 1	d = 2.65	d = 3.53	<0.001 *	<0.001 *	<0.001 *
	C	5.6 ± 1	2.9 ± 0.9	3.2 ± 1.6	d = 2.8	d = 1.7			
p-Value 95% C.I.		0.04 [−1.16, −0.03]	<0.001 * [−1.07, −0.12]	<0.001 * [−3.29, −2.1]					

Table 4. The changes in posture control outcomes in experimental and control groups vs. time. SPENT = smooth pursuit neck torsion test; OSI = biodex balance test; HRA = head repositioning error in rotation right and left side; I = interventional group; C = control group; G = group; T = time; G vs. T = group vs. time; all values are expressed as means ± standard deviation; C.I. [] = 95% confidence interval; Cohen's d value = d; * indicates statistically significant difference.

		Baseline	10-Weeks	1-Year Follow-up	Cohen's d 10-Weeks vs. Baseline	Cohen's d 1-Year vs. Baseline	p-Value G	p-Value T	p-Value G vs. T
HRA Right	I	3.4 ± 1.4	2.1 ± 1.3	2 ± 1.5	d = 1.4	d = 1.3	<0.001 *	<0.001 *	<0.001 *
	C	4 ± 1.5	2.7 ± 1.1	3.2 ± 1.6	d = 0.9	d = 0.51			
p-value C.I.		0.06 [−1.24, 0.04]	0.02 * [−1.13, −0.06]	<0.001 * [−1.89, −0.5]					
HRA Left	I	4.3 ± 1.4	2.6 ± 1.4	1.8 ± 1.1	d = 1.21	d = 1.98	<0.001 *	<0.001 *	<0.001 *
	C	3.7 ± 1.6	2.9 ± 1.6	2.8 ± 1.2	d = 0.5	d = 0.63			
p-value C.I.		0.07 [−0.06, 1.26]	0.3 [−0.96, 0.36]	<0.001 * [−1.51, −0.48]					
SPENT	I	0.41 ± 0.17	0.28 ± 0.1	0.18 ± 0.09	d = 0.93	d = 1.6	<0.001 *	<0.001 *	<0.001 *
	C	0.34 ± 0.16	0.3 ± 0.06	0.29 ± 0.12	d = 0.09	d = 0.35			
p-value C.I.		0.06 [−0.003, 0.14]	0.48 [−0.06, 0.02]	<0.001 * [−0.15, −0.06]					
OSI	I	0.62 ± 0.13	0.46 ± 0.1	0.41 ± 0.2	d = 1.37	d = 1.24	<0.001 *	<0.001 *	<0.001 *
	C	0.57 ± 0.11	0.52 ± 0.16	0.58 ± 0.19	d = 0.364	d = −0.06			
p-value C.I.		0.06 [−0.003, 0.103]	0.047 * [−0.11, −0.0007]	<0.001 * [−0.25, −0.08]					

4.3. The 10-Week Evaluation

- Thoracic kyphotic angle

Significant differences were found between groups, favoring the intervention group for kyphotic angle ICT-ITL (max) ($p < 0.001$) with an approximate 19° reduction in kyphosis angle for the DTTO group. These data, including effect sizes for both groups, are reported in Table 2. See also Figure 4 for a representative example of the changes.

- NDI and Pain Intensity

Following 30 treatment sessions, the between-group statistical analysis, showed better improvements for the intervention vs. control group in NDI ($p < 0.001$) and pain intensity ($p < 0.001$). These data, including effect sizes for both groups, are reported in Table 3.

- Sensori-motor control

Both groups improved similarly for two sensori-motor control outcomes where no group differences were found for: left sided HRA ($p = 0.3$) and SPENT ($p = 0.48$). In contrast, the intervention group had significantly greater improvements for two sensori-motor control measurements: right sided HRA ($p = 0.02$) and OSI ($p = 0.047$). These data, including effect sizes for both groups, are reported in Table 4.

4.4. One-Year Follow-up

Between group analysis identified a regression back to baseline values for the control group outcomes. Thus, all variables were significantly different favoring the intervention group at 1-year follow-up. Kyphotic angle ICT-ITL (max) maintained its improvement ($p < 0.001$), with an 18° overall improvement from baseline in the DTTO group; see Table 2. Pain and disability were significantly improved in the intervention group vs. the control group: NDI ($p < 0.001$); neck pain intensity ($p < 0.001$). Sensori-motor measures were also significantly improved in the intervention group compared to the control: HRA-right

($p < 0.001$); HRA-left ($p < 0.001$); SPNT ($p < 0.001$); OSI ($p < 0.001$); see Tables 3 and 4. Cohen's d and effect size (r) for both groups for all variables are reported in Tables 2–4.

5. Discussion

The current study presented a two-fold hypothesis: first, that the DTTO would cause a significant reduction in thoracic kyphosis, and two, that the reduction in thoracic kyphosis would improve the short and long-term outcomes of participants with chronic non-specific neck pain with concomitant hyper thoracic kyphosis. The differences between our intervention and control groups identified an 18–19° reduction in thoracic kyphosis in the group receiving the DTTO at both the 10-week and 1-year follow-up, while the control group's kyphosis angle remained unchanged. Concerning the sensorimotor control group's measurements at 10-weeks, two out of the four assessments identified a significant difference in favor of the DTTO group (OSI-balance and Right HRA) and at the 1-year follow-up all of the measures were significantly different in favor of the DTTO group. Thus, both of the hypotheses of our investigation were confirmed by these findings. To our knowledge, this is the first study to provide clear evidence that rehabilitation of thoracic hyper-kyphosis influences these specific outcomes in chronic neck pain sufferers with hyper-kyphosis.

5.1. Thoracic Kyphosis Improvement

Thoracic hyper-kyphosis represents one of the top four spine abnormalities associated with adult spine deformity (ASD), a world-wide, known set of disabilities affecting adults over the age of 18 years [39–41]. For example, Pellise et al. [39]. identified that patients with thoracic kyphosis over 60° had significantly lower health-related quality of life scores compared to patients afflicted with four other major health disorders (Type II diabetes, rheumatoid arthritis, heart disease, pulmonary disease). While 60° is the recommended cut-point for thoracic hyper-kyphosis in ASD populations, other investigations have identified that the cut-point between those with pain, lower self-image, and decreased function is 45° [42–44].

Due to the volume of investigations, identifying thoracic kyphosis is a considerable cause of pain, disability, and reduced quality of life outcomes, conservative treatment strategies to reduce its magnitude are critically necessary. To this end, it is generally considered that effective interventions for postural thoracic hyper-kyphosis should include specific rehabilitation exercises and practiced forced idealized posture alignment in stance and in sitting [44–46]. In more severe cases, or in cases with Scheuermann's kyphosis, a sagittal plane corrective orthosis brace is recommended [45].

A recent systematic literature review with meta-analysis identified that strengthening exercises have a considerable effect on thoracic kyphosis reduction when applied over the course of an average of 12.5 weeks with three sessions per week [44]. Considering only the homogenous exercise studies, an approximate reduction in thoracic kyphosis of 5° or less was identified [44]. More recently, in a small scale RCT with low power, Bezalel et al. [46]. identified a significant reduction in thoracic kyphosis (9°–10° reduction) in patients with Scheuermann's kyphosis receiving the Schroth series of exercises and stretches to reduce kyphosis. Initially, patients had a 60° kyphosis on X-ray (Cobb T3–T10) and inclinometry (T1–T12) that was reduced to approximately 50°.

In the current investigation, we used a four-D formetric scanner to evaluate thoracic kyphosis and our average participant's kyphosis was 82° which was reduced by 18° down to 64° in the group receiving the DTTO. For comparison, it is known that the formetric and inclinometry measures of external thoracic kyphosis overestimate the radiographic determined thoracic kyphosis by approximately 7° and maybe more depending on the unique population [23,46,47]. It is likely that our current participant population had a radiographic determined thoracic kyphosis that averaged at least 60° depending on the vertebral levels of measurement. Further, we estimated our radiographic kyphosis reduction to be between 12°–15° based on existing comparative population data; making our results one of the largest conservative reductions in thoracic kyphosis reported in an RCT in the literature to date [44,46].

Arguably, adults with a large increased thoracic kyphosis (60°–80°) that is 'fixed' (Scheuermann's kyphosis and other deformities) would seem not to be amenable to physical maneuvers (exercise and manipulation); however, they are able to be reduced with three-point bending thoraco-lumbar braces [45]. Similarly, extension traction devices such as the DTTO use the principles of three-point bending as in braces; although extension traction devices are shorter duration applications with higher loading [15–17]. Though we did not specifically investigate the difference between more rigid vs. more flexible thoracic kyphotic deformities, our population did indeed have a large increase in thoracic kyphosis compared to that found in a healthy population [24,42–44]. We speculate that the large and significant reduction in thoracic kyphosis found in our DTTO group is due to the visco-elastic effect of three-point bending extension traction during sustained supine loading while on the DTTO. Our results are generally consistent with previous investigations looking at patients treated with different types of thoracic spine three-point bending extension traction devices; however, these previous investigations suffer from a lack of controls and small sample sizes [15]. Future investigations should use radiography to determine the type of thoracic hyper-kyphosis, its flexibility, and its amenability to three-point bending extension devices such as the DTTO.

5.2. Pain, Disability, and Sensorimotor Control

The assumption that restoring thoracic sagittal plane posture should improve cervical spine pain and kinematics has evidence in the literature. For instance, it has been proposed that upper thoracic kyphosis increases the T1-slope into a more flexed posture and this, in turn, creates a situation of forward head posture, increased strain on the cervical-thoracic muscles and ligaments [15,39,40]. For example, Kaya and Çelenay reported a positive correlation between thoracic curvature and neck pain [11]. Furthermore, abnormal head posture can result in altered joint position and dysfunction that can lead to pain and abnormal afferent information [10,48].

Forward head translation causes both a reduced range of movement and an altered segmental cervical spine kinematic pattern [10]. Thus, altered sagittal cervical spine alignment from thoracic hyper-kyphosis could potentially result in abnormal sensorimotor integration through changes in afferent input as a direct consequence of altered cervical spine kinematics and altered soft tissue strains [48]. The current study's findings of reduced neck pain, disability, and improved sensorimotor control in the DTTO group add credence to the above biomechanical and clinical investigations detailing the effects of thoracic spine abnormalities on the cervical spine. Treating the spine as a synchronized kinetic chain should be considered the standard particularly in cases of chronic non-specific neck pain with concomitant thoracic hyper-kyphosis.

5.3. Limitations and Summary

The current study has limitations to consider which should lead to future investigations. First, we did not use participant and treatment provider blinding. However, examiners did not discuss the clinical importance of correcting the thoracic kyphosis in either group in order to account for the placebo effect in the DTTO group and a possible nocebo effect in the control group at long term follow-up. Second, the participants were a convenience sample of young adults from an out-patient facility and thus may not be representative of all patients with chronic non-specific cervical spine complaints. Third, the outcome measures we used to verify if correction of thoracic kyphosis alignment improves sensori-motor control, pain, and disability may not be the only or the ideal assessments for CNSNP outcomes. Fourth, we measured the thoracic kyphosis using an external posture assessment device and this does not provide the same quantitative data as radiographic or other advanced imaging methods for measurement of thoracic kyphosis.

Finally, both groups received the same time and number of sessions for the multimodal treatments. However, the participants in the intervention group received an extra intervention (and time) using the Denneroll™ thoracic extension traction device. We attempted to provide the same time of attention equivalence in each group provided by the treating therapist during the intervention sessions. However, as attention and interpersonal interactions alone may influence pain, and other health outcomes, this is a limitation to the study design in as much as the groups did not receive equal interventions. Importantly though, previously, it has been identified that when a placebo device is added to the control groups' interventions to mimic the time and number of sessions on the Denneroll™ in the cervical spine, that the placebo device did not influence the outcomes of neck pain and disability [49]. Still, this is something that should be addressed in future projects.

6. Conclusions

Notwithstanding the study limitations, the unique contribution of the current investigation is that we determined thoracic hyper-kyphosis reduction plays a significant role in improving both the short and long-term outcomes in patients suffering from chronic nonspecific neck pain. In these relevant populations, it would seem of value to rehabilitate thoracic hyper-kyphosis abnormalities towards normal alignment as a primary management strategy. The DTTO investigated in this study is a simple orthotic that can be prescribed for home use or utilized under the supervision of a treating clinician as used in this investigation.

Author Contributions: I.M.M., T.M.S. and D.E.H. conceived the research idea and participated in its design; I.M.M., T.M.S., L.M.W., V.R. and D.E.H. all contributed to the statistical analysis; I.M.M., T.M.S., L.M.W. and V.R. participated in the data collection and study supervision; I.M.M., T.M.S., L.M.W., V.R. and D.E.H. all contributed to the interpretation of the results and wrote the original and final drafts. All authors have read and agreed to the published version of the manuscript.

Funding: The thoracic Dennerolls used in this study were funded by Denneroll Industries, International P/L of Wheeler Heights, NSW 2097, Australia. CBP NonProfit funded author travel and conference fees to present this abstract at combined sections meeting of the Academy of Orthopaedic Physical Therapy, Denver, CO, 2020.

Institutional Review Board Statement: The study was conducted in accordance with the Declaration of Helsinki, and approved by the Ethics Committee of the Faculty of Physical Therapy, Cairo University with the ethical approval No. Cairo -6-2018-11M.S. Following Ethics Committee approval, participant recruitment began in September 2018. The participants were followed up for 1 year (till October 2019); all participants signed informed consent prior to data collection. The reason behind the retrospective registration was that legislation in Egypt only requires local registration for clinical trials and this what was completed at the outset by prospectively registering in a non-WHO-approved registry.

Informed Consent Statement: Written informed consent was not obtained for the person depicted in Figure 2 as this is a photo from a model production shoot and the copyright holder is an author (DEH) on the manuscript and has provided consent for this image to be reproduced.

Data Availability Statement: The datasets analyzed in the current study are available from the corresponding author on reasonable request.

Conflicts of Interest: D.E.H. teaches rehabilitation methods and sells the Denneroll™ products to physicians for patient care as used in this manuscript. D.E.H. is not a patent holder for the Denneroll™ products. All the other authors declare that they have no competing interest.

References

1. Cohen, S.P. Epidemiology, Diagnosis, and Treatment of Neck Pain. *Mayo Clin. Proc.* **2015**, *90*, 284–299. [CrossRef] [PubMed]
2. Oxland, T.R. Fundamental biomechanics of the spine—What we have learned in the past 25 years and future directions. *J. Biomech.* **2015**, *49*, 817–832. [CrossRef] [PubMed]
3. Lau, K.T.; Cheung, K.Y.; Chan, K.B.; Chan, M.H.; Lo, K.Y.; Chiu, T.T.W. Relationships between sagittal postures of thoracic and cervical spine, presence of neck pain, neck pain severity and disability. *Man. Ther.* **2010**, *15*, 457–462. [CrossRef]

4. Bergmann, T.F.; Peterson, D.H. *Chiropractic Technique Principles and Procedures*; Mosby: Maryland Heights, MO, USA, 2011.
5. Norlander, S.; Gustavsson, B.A.; Lindell, J.; Nordgren, B. Reduced mobility in the cervico-thoracic motion segment: A risk factor for musculoskeletal neck-shoulder pain: A two-year prospective follow-up study. *Scand. J. Rehabil. Med.* **1997**, *29*, 167–174. [PubMed]
6. Norlander, S.; Aste-Norlander, U.; Nordgren, B.; Sahlstedt, B. Mobility in the cervico-thoracic motion segment: An indicative factor of musculo-skeletal neck-shoulder pain. *Scand. J. Rehabil. Med.* **1996**, *28*, 183–192. [PubMed]
7. Fernández-De-Las-Peñas, C.; Fernández-Carnero, J.; Fernández, A.P.; Lomas-Vega, R.; Miangolarra-Page, J.C. Dorsal Manipulation in Whiplash Injury Treatment. *J. Whiplash Relat. Disord.* **2004**, *3*, 55–72. [CrossRef]
8. Cleland, J.; Selleck, B.; Stowell, T.; Browne, L.; Alberini, S.; Cyr, H.S.; Caron, T. Short-Term Effects of Thoracic Manipulation on Lower Trapezius Muscle Strength. *J. Man. Manip. Ther.* **2004**, *12*, 82–90. [CrossRef]
9. Jull, G.A.; O'Leary, S.P.; Falla, D.L. Clinical Assessment of the Deep Cervical Flexor Muscles: The Craniocervical Flexion Test. *J. Manip. Physiol. Ther.* **2008**, *31*, 525–533. [CrossRef]
10. Quek, J.; Pua, Y.-H.; Clark, R.A.; Bryant, A.L. Effects of thoracic kyphosis and forward head posture on cervical range of motion in older adults. *Man. Ther.* **2013**, *18*, 65–71. [CrossRef]
11. Kaya, D.; Çelenay, T. An investigation of sagittal thoracic spinal curvature and mobility in subjects with and without chronic neck pain: Cut-off points and pain relationship. *Turk. J. Med. Sci.* **2017**, *47*, 891–896. [CrossRef]
12. Falla, D.; Gizzi, L.; Parsa, H.; Dieterich, A.; Petzke, F. People with Chronic Neck Pain Walk with a Stiffer Spine. *J. Orthop. Sports Phys. Ther.* **2017**, *47*, 268–277. [CrossRef] [PubMed]
13. Joshi, S.; Balthillaya, G.; Neelapala, Y.V.R. Thoracic Posture and Mobility in Mechanical Neck Pain Population: A Review of the Literature. *Asian Spine J.* **2019**, *13*, 849–860. [CrossRef] [PubMed]
14. Costello, M. Treatment of a Patient with Cervical Radiculopathy Using Thoracic Spine Thrust Manipulation, Soft Tissue Mobilization, and Exercise. *J. Man. Manip. Ther.* **2008**, *16*, 129–135. [CrossRef] [PubMed]
15. Oakly, P.A.; Harrison, D.E. Reducing thoracic hyperkyphosis subluxation deformity: A systematic review of chiropractic biophysics® methods employed in its structural improvement. *J. Contemp. Chiropr.* **2018**, *1*, 59–66.
16. Oakley, P.A.; Ehsani, N.N.; Moustafa, I.M.; Harrison, D.E. Restoring lumbar lordosis: A systematic review of controlled trials utilizing Chiropractic Bio Physics® (CBP®) non-surgical approach to increasing lumbar lordosis in the treatment of low back disorders. *J. Phys. Ther. Sci.* **2020**, *32*, 601–610. [CrossRef]
17. Oakley, P.A.; Ehsani, N.N.; Moustafa, I.M.; Harrison, D.E. Restoring cervical lordosis by cervical extension traction methods in the treatment of cervical spine disorders: A systematic review of controlled trials. *J. Phys. Ther. Sci.* **2021**, *33*, 784–794. [CrossRef]
18. Shanahan, C.; Ward, A.R.; Robertson, V.J. Comparison of the analgesic efficacy of interferential therapy and transcutaneous electrical nerve stimulation. *Physiotherapy* **2006**, *92*, 247–253. [CrossRef]
19. Vasudevan, J.M.; Plastaras, C.; Becker, S. Cervical radiculopathy. In *Therapeutic Programs for Musculoskeletal Disorders*, 1st ed.; Wyss, J.F., Patel, A.D., Eds.; Demos Medical: New York, NY, USA, 2013; pp. 279–288.
20. Harman, K.; Hubley-Kozey, C.; Butler, H. Effectiveness of an Exercise Program to Improve Forward Head Posture in Normal Adults: A Randomized, Controlled 10-Week Trial. *J. Man. Manip. Ther.* **2005**, *13*, 163–176. [CrossRef]
21. Flynn, T.W. *The Thoracic Spine and Rib Cage: Musculoskeletal Evaluation and Treatment*; Butterworth-Heinemann: Boston, MA, USA, 1994; pp. 171–201.
22. Betsch, M.; Wild, M.; Jungbluth, P.; Hakimi, M.; Windolf, J.; Haex, B.; Horstmann, T.; Rapp, W. Reliability and validity of 4D rasterstereography under dynamic conditions. *Comput. Biol. Med.* **2011**, *41*, 308–312. [CrossRef]
23. Frerich, J.M.; Hertzler, K.; Knott, P.; Mardjetko, S. Comparison of Radiographic and Surface Topography Measurements in Adolescents with Idiopathic Scoliosis. *Open Orthop. J.* **2012**, *6*, 261–265. [CrossRef]
24. Harrison, D.E.; Janik, T.J.; Harrison, D.D.; Cailliet, R.; Harmon, S.F. Can the Thoracic Kyphosis Be Modeled With a Simple Geometric Shape? *J. Spinal Disord. Tech.* **2002**, *15*, 213–220. [CrossRef] [PubMed]
25. MacDermid, J.C.; Walton, D.M.; Avery, S.; Blanchard, A.; Etruw, E.; McAlpine, C.; Goldsmith, C.H. Measurement Properties of the Neck Disability Index: A Systematic Review. *J. Orthop. Sports Phys. Ther.* **2009**, *39*, 400–417. [CrossRef]
26. Lundeberg, T.; Lund, I.; Dahlin, L.; Borg, E.; Gustafsson, C.; Sandin, L.; Rosén, A.; Kowalski, J.; Eriksson, S.V. Reliability and responsiveness of three different pain assessments. *J. Rehabil. Med.* **2001**, *33*, 279–283. [CrossRef] [PubMed]
27. Bijur, P.E.; Latimer, C.T.; Gallagher, E.J. Validation of a verbally administered numerical rating scale of acute pain for use in the emergency department. *Acad. Emerg. Med.* **2003**, *10*, 390–392. [CrossRef]
28. Wibault, J.; Vaillant, J.; Vuillerme, N.; Dedering, A.; Peolsson, A. Using the cervical range of motion (CROM) device to assess head repositioning accuracy in individuals with cervical radiculopathy in comparison to neck- healthy individuals. *Man. Ther.* **2013**, *18*, 403–409. [CrossRef] [PubMed]
29. Loudon, J.K.; Ruhl, M.; Field-Fote, E. Ability to Reproduce Head Position after Whiplash Injury. *Spine* **1997**, *22*, 865–868. [CrossRef] [PubMed]
30. Treleaven, J.; Jull, G.; Sterling, M. Dizziness and unsteadiness following whiplash injury: Characteristic features and relationship with cervical joint position error. *J. Rehabil. Med.* **2003**, *35*, 36–43. [CrossRef]
31. Jia, Y.; Tyler, C.W. Measurement of saccadic eye movements by electrooculography for simultaneous EEG recording. *Behav. Res. Methods* **2019**, *51*, 2139–2151. [CrossRef]
32. Tjell, C.; Rosenhall, U. Smooth pursuit neck torsion test: A specific test for cervical dizziness. *Am. J. Otol.* **1998**, *19*, 76–81.

33. Schmitz, R.; Arnold, B. Intertester and Intratester Reliability of a Dynamic Balance Protocol Using the Biodex Stability System. *J. Sport Rehabil.* **1998**, *7*, 95–101. [CrossRef]
34. Parraca, J.; Olivares, P.; Carbonell-baeza, A.; Aparicio, V.; Adsuar, J.; Gusi, N. Test-Retest Reliability of Biodex Balance SD on Physically Active Old People. *J Hum. Sport Exerc.* **2011**, *8*, 444–451. [CrossRef]
35. Dawson, N.; Dzurino, D.; Karleskint, M.; Tucker, J. Examining the reliability, correlation, and validity of commonly used as-sessment tools to measure balance. *Health Sci. Rep.* **2018**, *1*, e98. [CrossRef]
36. Hinman, M.R. Factors Affecting Reliability of the Biodex Balance System: A Summary of Four Studies. *J. Sport Rehabil.* **2000**, *9*, 240–252. [CrossRef]
37. Cohen, J. *Statistical Power Analysis for the Behavioral Sciences*; Academic Press: Cambridge, MA, USA, 1977.
38. Rubin, D.B. *Multiple Imputation for Nonresponse in Surveys*; John Wiley & Sons: New York, NY, USA, 2004; Volume 81.
39. Pellise, F.; Vila-Casademunt, A.; Ferrer, M.; Domingo-Sabat, M.; Bago, J.; Perez-Grueso, F.J.; Alanay, A.; Mannion, A.F.; Acaroglu, E.; European Spine Study Group, ESSG. Impact on health related quality of life of adult spine deformity (ASD) compared with other chronic conditions. *Eur. Spine J.* **2015**, *24*, 3–11. [CrossRef] [PubMed]
40. Bess, S.; Line, B.; Fu, K.M.; McCarthy, I.; Lafage, V.; Schwab, F.; Shaffrey, C.; Ames, C.; Akbarnia, B.; Jo, H.; et al. The Health Impact of Symptomatic Adult Spi-nal Deformity: Comparison of Deformity Types to United States Population Norms and Chronic Diseases. *Spine* **2016**, *41*, 224–233. [CrossRef]
41. Bess, S.; Protopsaltis, T.S.; Lafage, V.; Lafage, R.; Ames, C.P.; Errico, T.; Smith, J.S.; International Spine Study Group. Clinical and Radiographic Evaluation of Adult Spinal Deformity. *Clin. Spine Surg.* **2016**, *29*, 6–16. [CrossRef]
42. Petcharaporn, M.; Pawelek, J.; Bastrom, T.; Lonner, B.; Newton, P.O. The Relationship between Thoracic Hyperkyphosis and the Scoliosis Research Society Outcomes Instrument. *Spine* **2007**, *32*, 2226–2231. [CrossRef]
43. Nissinen, M.; Heliövaara, M.; Seitsamo, J.; Poussa, M. Left Handedness and Risk of Thoracic Hyperkyphosis in Prepubertal Schoolchildren. *Int. J. Epidemiol.* **1995**, *24*, 1178–1181. [CrossRef]
44. González-Gálvez, N.; Gea-García, G.M.; Marcos-Pardo, P.J. Effects of exercise programs on kyphosis and lordosis angle: A systematic review and meta-analysis. *PLoS ONE* **2019**, *14*, e0216180. [CrossRef] [PubMed]
45. Pizzutillo, P.D. Nonsurgical treatment of kyphosis. *Instr. Course Lect.* **2004**, *53*, 485–491.
46. Bezalel, T.; Carmeli, E.; Levi, D.; Kalichman, L. The Effect of Schroth Therapy on Thoracic Kyphotic Curve and Quality of Life in Scheuermann's Patients: A Randomized Controlled Trial. *Asian Spine J.* **2019**, *13*, 490–499. [CrossRef] [PubMed]
47. Hunter, D.J.; Rivett, D.A.; McKiernan, S.; Weerasekara, I.; Snodgrass, S.J. Is the inclinometer a valid measure of thoracic kyphosis? A cross-sectional study. *Braz. J. Phys. Ther.* **2018**, *22*, 310–317. [CrossRef]
48. Moustafa, I.M.; Youssef, A.; Ahbouch, A.; Tamim, M.; Harrison, D.E. Is forward head posture relevant to autonomic nervous system function and cervical sensorimotor control? Cross sectional study. *Gait Posture* **2020**, *77*, 29–35. [CrossRef] [PubMed]
49. Moustafa, I.M.; Diab, A.A.; Harrison, D.E. The effect of normalizing the sagittal cervical configuration on dizziness, neck pain, and cervicocephalic kinesthetic sensibility: A 1-year randomized controlled study. *Eur. J. Phys. Rehabil. Med.* **2017**, *53*, 57–71. [CrossRef] [PubMed]

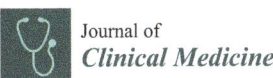

Article

Post-Traumatic Atlanto-Axial Instability: A Combined Clinical and Radiological Approach for the Diagnosis of Pathological Rotational Movement in the Upper Cervical Spine

Bertel Rune Kaale [1,*], Tony J. McArthur [1], Maria H. Barbosa [1] and Michael D. Freeman [2]

1. Firda Medical Center AS, 6823 Sandane, Norway
2. CAPHRI School for Public Health and Primary Care, Faculty of Health, Medicine, and Life Sciences, Maastricht University, 6211 LM Maastricht, The Netherlands
* Correspondence: bertel.kaale@enivest.net

Abstract: Post-traumatic rotational instability at the atlanto-axial (C1-2) joint is difficult to assess, much less quantify, due to the orientation and motion plane of the joint. Prior investigations have demonstrated that a dynamic axial CT scan, during which the patient maximally rotates the head right and left, can be used to evaluate and quantify the amount of residual overlap between the inferior articulating facet of C1 and the superior facet of C2, as an index of ligamentous laxity at the joint. We have previously demonstrated that a novel orthopedic test of rotational instability, the atlas-axis rotational test (A-ART), may have utility in identifying patients with imaging evidence of upper cervical ligament injury. In the present investigation, we assessed the correlation between a positive A-ART and a CT scan assessment of the relative quantity of residual C1-2 overlap, as a percent of the superior articulating facet surface area of C2. A retrospective review was conducted of the records of consecutive patients presenting to a physical therapy and rehabilitation clinic, over a 5-year period (2015–20) for chronic head and neck pain after whiplash trauma. The primary inclusion criteria were that the patient had undergone both a clinical evaluation with A-ART and a dynamic axial CT to evaluate for C1-2 residual facet overlap at maximum rotation. The records for a total of 57 patients (44 female/13 male) were identified who fit the selection criteria, and among these, there were 43 with a positive A-ART (i.e., "cases") and 14 with a negative A-ART (i.e., "controls"). The analysis demonstrated that a positive A-ART was highly predictive of decreased residual C1-2 facet overlap: the average overlap area among the cases was approximately one-third that of the control group (on the left, 10.7% versus 29.1%, and 13.6% versus 31.0% on the right). These results suggest that a positive A-ART is a reliable indicator of underlying rotational instability at C1-2 in patients with chronic head and neck symptoms following whiplash trauma.

Keywords: upper cervical instability; atlas-axis rotational test (A-ART); CT scan; whiplash trauma

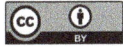

1. Introduction

Intervertebral instability secondary to intervertebral ligamentous injury is a relatively common finding among patients with whiplash trauma-related chronic neck pain [1]. The clinical presentation can be particularly complicated when the instability is in the upper cervical spine (i.e., between the occiput, atlas, and axis [C0-2]), as patients may suffer from nonspecific symptoms of headache, vertigo, and neck pain, the origin of which can be difficult to pinpoint [2].

The diagnosis of symptomatic spinal instability requires a combination of symptoms consistent with the condition, and radiographic evidence of extra-physiologic movement at the joint in the relevant plane and direction, which may or may not be accompanied by MRI evidence of ligamentous disruption. A diagnosis of anterior or posterior instability of the sub-axial spine (C2–C7) may be made via flexion and extension radiographs, or more involved evaluations of wider range of movements can be accomplished via fluoroscopic examination [1]. In contrast, the evaluation and diagnosis of instability in the upper cervical spine is made more difficult by the anatomical complexity and predominant type of movement of the joints, which is rotation about the vertical axis [3]. Thus, while lateral flexion instability of C1 on C2 can be evaluated dynamically with anterior to posterior open mouth radiographs, excessive rotational movement can only be evaluated via imaging in an axial (up to down) orientation.

There are two prior studies that have described the use of CT scanning to assess the degree of rotational movement at C1 on C2 by quantifying the loss of facet joint surface overlap at maximum voluntary head rotation. The first study, from 1999, evaluated an uninjured population of 10 children, and described a maximal joint contact loss of 74 to 85% [4]. The second study, published 10 years later, evaluated the percent decrease of joint overlap in a healthy group of 40 adults at maximal head rotation, finding an average loss of 70% of joint overlap (range 42–86%), thus leaving an average residual overlap area of 30% [5]. No other publications describing an investigation of the technique in either healthy or injured populations were identified, following a search of the literature using key terms.

In 2008, Kaale and colleagues described a novel clinical examination protocol for evaluating upper cervical rotational instability (UCRI) called the "atlas-axis rotational test," abbreviated as "A-ART" henceforth [6]. The orthopedic test is performed on a passive seated patient, by palpating and stabilizing the transverse process of C2 while rotating the patient's head and palpating the degree of end play of the lateral mass of C1 at maximal tolerable rotation, see Figure 1. Instability of C1 on C2 is graded 0–3 based on the perceived degree of abnormality of end play. The authors compared the A-ART results of 122 patients to MRI evaluation of the integrity of the upper cervical ligaments (alar and transverse) and tectorial and posterior atlanto-occipital membranes. When the clinical test results were dichotomized as either normal (0–1) or abnormal (2–3), there was good to excellent agreement (i.e., kappa coefficient of 0.7–0.9) between the ability of the A-ART rotational test to detect abnormal joint end play and the MRI confirmation of ligamentous abnormality. Although these results were encouraging, they could not confirm that the instability inferred from the dynamic clinical examination was in fact correlated with actual instability, as the MRI evaluations were performed in a neutral position, and thus cannot be considered a "gold standard" test of rotational instability of C1 on C2. The validation of A-ART for the detection of UCRI would have utility in the medicolegal investigation of the pain source in patients with chronic symptoms suggestive of upper cervical instability following whiplash trauma, as the test could help identify patients with a higher likelihood of positive objective imaging indicative of traumatic injury.

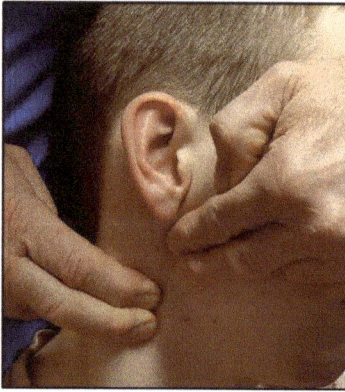

Figure 1. Examiner hand position during the atlas-axis rotational test (A-ART). While standing behind the seated patient, the examiner places both hands on the occipito-cervical junction, opposite the side of head rotation. With the 2nd and 3rd fingers, the examiner's lower hand (right, in the

photograph) is used to stabilize and traction posteriorly against the transverse process of C2. The 2nd and 3rd fingers of the other hand (left, in the photograph) contact the mastoid process of the occiput and lateral mass of the atlas, respectively. The test is then performed with varying angles of cervical rotation, to locate the position that yields maximal movement between C1 and C2, and graded by the amount of C1 versus C2 movement described in the text. For the purposes of the present study, a grade of 0–1 equates to little perceived relative rotational motion between the transverse processes of C1 and C2 (subjectively gauged, less than ~5 mm), and 2 or more exceeds this threshold.

In this study we present the results of an investigation of the correlation between the results of a dynamic orthopedic test for UCRI (the A-ART) and a dynamic imaging analysis of UCRI, via residual C1-C2 facet overlap analysis. The purpose of the investigation is to assess the diagnostic accuracy of the A-ART using a direct radiographic measure of excessive joint excursion and instability.

2. Methods

2.1. Inclusion Criteria

The data used for the analysis were retrospectively abstracted from medical records and imaging files for patients who had been referred by their general practitioner (GP) to a single physiotherapy and rehabilitation practice for evaluation and treatment of chronic post-traumatic neck pain (range 4 to 8 years after injury), from 2015 through 2020. The primary inclusion criteria for the study were that (1) there was a relatively high clinical suspicion of UCRI based on the clinical presentation, and (2) both the A-ART and a dynamic rotational CT scan were performed on the patient.

The clinical suspicion of UCRI was based on the presence of chronic (i.e., >6 months duration) neck pain complaints combined with symptoms potentially of a craniocervical origin, including dizziness, headache, and a sense of head pressure, including a worsening of the symptoms with head rotation, including during normal activities. The provoked symptoms in some cases would persist for hours to days. The A-ART was performed on the patients by 2 blinded clinicians, and graded 0 to 3. and the patient was subsequently referred to an outpatient imaging center for a CT scan of the upper cervical spine which included a dynamic rotational stress protocol. As noted above, prior to the CT scan, all of the patients had a cervical MRI study in order to rule out significant CNS or musculoskeletal pathology.

A total of 57 patients (44 female/13 male) were identified for study, after the exclusion of one patient with a suspected connective tissue disorder. For the purposes of the study, most accurately described as a prospective cohort design, patients were dichotomized into 2 groups by A-ART grade, following the same protocol described by Kaale et al. [6], in which a result of 2–3 was deemed "abnormal" or positive for UCRI (little to no stop feeling of C1 lateral mass at the end of rotation), and 0–1 was deemed "normal" and negative for UCRI (solid or soft stop feeling during rotation). See Figure 1. Two physiotherapist examiners, both experienced with application of the A-ART, had to agree that the A-ART grade was 2 or 3 for the patient to be categorized in the "abnormal" group. As these data were gathered retrospectively, no protocol was in place to blind the second examiner to the first examiner's finding, and thus the level of inter-examiner agreement between initial findings could not be reconstructed. For further analysis, the patients with an abnormal A-ART result were deemed as "cases" and the patients with a normal A-ART test were deemed "controls".

2.2. CT Scan Protocol

Referral for the CT scan was provided by the referring GP, and was based on either a high degree of suspicion of UCRI among the 43 patients with a positive A-ART, or to rule out other cervical spine pathology (including UCRI) in the 14 A-ART negative patients. The CT scan was performed on the same day (and at the same facility) as a cervical MRI study, which was ordered at the same time at the CT scan. All patients were provided with information regarding the risks of the procedure, and given the alternative to opt out of the diagnostic study as part of the procedures, alternatives, and risk (PAR) conference. The scans were obtained from just above the base of the skull to the T1/T2 level, and performed on a Toshiba Aquilion ONE CT scanner, using 80 kVp and 80 mAs, with a 0.5 s scan time. Bone and soft tissue target algorithms were used, and the scans were performed without gantry angulation. The scans were 0.5 mm thick and were obtained in one single volume of 160 mm and reconstructed as 0.5mm axial slices every 0.25 mm, yielding a total of 320 × 0.25 mm axial slices. The 2 rotational scan sequences were each approximately 4 min in duration.

The entire cervical spine scan was performed with the patient's head in a neutral position, and then upper cervical images were obtained with the head in maximal tolerable rotation, so as to reproduce the conditions of the A-ART in a supine position, using previously described upper cervical imaging protocol [7,8]. 3D Volumetric CT scans were reviewed on a Vitrea (Vital Images) workstation using both 3D and cross-sectional imaging techniques. The total scan dose was 2.2 mSv (millisieverts). For reference, the doses of an abdominal CT scan and single chest X-ray are 10 and 0.02 mSv, respectively [9].

2.3. CT Scan Interpretation

The neutral position scans were first evaluated for significant pathology, which were negative for all patients. To evaluate the atlas-axis facet coverage at maximal rotation, the axial slices that optimized the view of the cortical rim around the facets was used. The joint surface of the superior facet of C2 was then identified, and the online software program GeoGebra Classic (http://www.geogebra.org/) was used to delineate the anatomical perimeter of the articulating surface, as well as quantify the area [10]. Next, the posteromedial margin of only the part of the inferior articulating surface of C1 that was overlapping with the C2 superior facet surface was outlined, and the area of overlap was calculated by the software as a percentage of the area of the C2 joint surface, see Figure 2a–c.

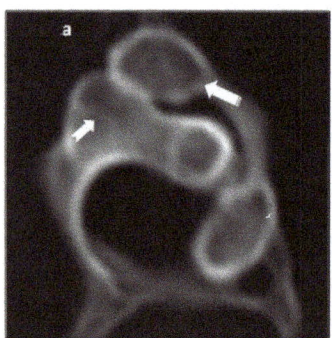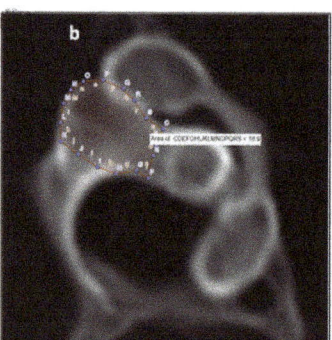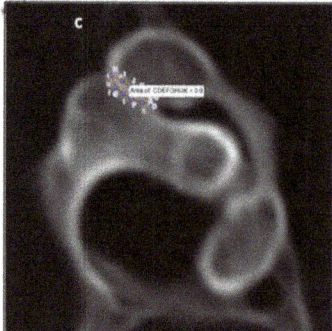

Figure 2. (a) CT scan, axial view, with the patient's head rotated maximally to the left. The notched arrow points to the right superior articulating facet of C2, and the striped arrow points to the right inferior articulating facet of C1. (b) The same scan as in Figure 2a, with the outer margin of the right superior articulating facet of C2 outlined using the GeoGebra software, resulting in an area of 18.9 cm^2. (c) The same scan as depicted in Figure 2a and b, but with the residual overlapping area of C1 and C2 outlined using the GeoGebra software, resulting in an area of 0.9 cm^2. The area of residual overlap, as a percent of the total area of the superior articulating facet of C2, is calculated as (0.9/18.9 × 100%), and is thus 4.8%. (R—right, L—left, A—anterior, P—posterior).

2.4. Statistical Analysis

Welch's Two-Sample t-test was used to analyze the differences in the mean values of right and left overlap percentage, as well as the distribution of age between the case and control groups. The multivariate relationships between right and left overlap and age between the 2 groups were analyzed using generalized linear modeling. The Kolmogorov–Smirnov (K-S) test of normality was used to assess the distribution of the ages in each group. A *p*-value of 0.05 or lower was considered statistically significant for all analyses, which were performed using RStudio, version 2022.020 + 443 (RStudio Team: Integrated Development for R. RStudio, PBC, Boston, MA, USA).

2.5. Consent

All patients were contacted and asked for consent for their anonymized archived medical information to be used for the present investigation. All patients gave consent. This study was exempted from ethics review because of the use of archived medical information, which was described collectively, rather than individually.

3. Results

Both right and left overlap percentages were significantly lower among the patients with an abnormal A-ART, versus the patients with normal tests (see Table 1). The average percentage of overlap among the cases was approximately one-third of the average in the control group (10.7% versus 29.1% on the left, and 13.6% versus 31.0% on the right). Although the right side values were slightly higher than the left side values in both groups, the difference was not significant. While normally distributed in both groups (i.e., K-S was not significant), age was significantly lower in the patient group; on average, the cases were 8.1 years younger than the control group, with a range of ages among the cases of 15 to 70, and 28 to 77 for the controls. There was a nominal disparity in sex distribution between cases and controls, with 10/43 (23%) males in the former, and 3/14 (21%) males in the latter. Multivariate linear regression was used to examine the role of age and sex as a predictor of overlap; however, no significant associations were discerned.

Table 1. Mean Values (Standard Deviations, SD) of percent of atlanto-axial residual facet overlap at the extreme of right and left rotation, and average difference between the 2 groups (95% confidence intervals [CI]), and age distribution among 43 cases and 14 controls.

		Mean Values (SD)			
	N	Female/Male	R Overlap	L Overlap	Age (Years)
Cases	43	33/10	13.6% (5.81)	10.7% (5.06)	39.8 (12.27) Range 15–70
Controls	14	11/3	31.0% (10.11)	29.1% (11.15)	47.9 (12.83) Range 28–77
p-value			<0.001	<0.001	0.0499
Mean difference			17.4%	18.4%	8.1 years
(95% CI)			(11.5, 23.3)	(12.0, 24.8)	(0.02, 16.2)

4. Discussion

The results of the present investigation are noteworthy in two respects; they demonstrate the potential utility of axial CT scanning for the objective evaluation of rotational instability in patients with symptoms consistent with upper cervical instability, and they provide quantitative objective evidence of the clinical utility of the A-ART for identifying rotational ligamentous instability at C1-2. Both findings are unique in the literature. Prior investigations of upper cervical rotational instability have primarily focused on the evaluation of injury to the alar ligaments.

Despite the fact that the 14 subjects in the control group were seeking treatment for persisting craniocervical symptoms following a cervical spine trauma (i.e., whiplash trauma), the average residual atlanto-axial overlap in the control group of approximately 29 to 31% (left and right, respectively) fell well within the range described by Mönckeberg and colleagues in an asymptomatic population of 40 adults (30%) [5]. In contrast, the residual overlap among the cases in the present investigation fell outside the range observed in the prior asymptomatic population study, in which the lowest residual overlap of any of the subjects was 14.3%, versus the 10.7% and 13.6% (left and right, respectively) average among the cases.

Aside from significantly lower residual overlap at C1-2, the distinguishing feature among the cases, versus the controls, was an abnormal A-ART. It is thus reasonable to infer from these findings that the A-ART is a relatively accurate test for atlanto-axial rotational instability, although the degree of accuracy cannot be quantified from these data, as there is no gold standard threshold or cut point to measure the individual findings against. While the findings may also be attributable to an unexamined confounding factor related both to instability and the A-ART (aside from sex and age, which were not found to be correlated in the analysis), this explanation is unlikely, given that the pathomechanics resulting in the decreased C1-2 facet overlap would also reasonably result in a palpable alteration in joint end play (and abnormal A-ART result). The authors have not observed any negative effects during administration of the A-ART; however, we advise a slow and cautious approach any time maximal head rotation is assessed in the patient with suspected ligamentous instability in the upper cervical spine, keeping in mind the proximity of the bony structures to the upper cervical spinal cord.

As noted in Section 2, all of the patients underwent an upper cervical CT scan on the same day that they underwent a cervical MRI study. A look back at the MRI images revealed that the majority did not include the C1-2 levels, and thus the correlation between the CT scan evidence of instability with possible MRI evidence of ligamentous integrity was not feasible given the limitations of the available data. This may be a fertile avenue of future investigation, however. Based on the results of the present study, it is reasonable that for the patient with persistent symptoms of upper cervical instability and a positive (i.e., Grade 2+) A-ART, that the next step in evaluating the source of the ongoing symptoms would include both a cervical MRI and the CT scan of upper cervical rotation.

Prior investigations of upper cervical ligamentous injury have largely focused on non-dynamic imaging of morphological changes in the upper cervical ligaments, with particular focus on the alar and transverse ligaments, with the head in a neutral position [11,12]. The degree of association between such imaging findings and patient outcomes, if any, is uncertain, however [13]. Dynamic CT evaluations of the upper cervical spine have been described in the evaluation of instability secondary to rheumatoid arthritis or healing odontoid fractures, but few describe the technique for the evaluation of ligamentous integrity following traumatic injury [14,15]. In one such study, authors used CT scanning to quantify rotational instability in 47 patients with chronic symptoms after whiplash trauma, in comparison with 26 uninjured controls, by quantifying the relative segmental rotation at each level versus total cervical rotation [16]. The authors found excessive rotation at C0-C1 in the injured group, but not at C1-2. In contrast with the present study, however, no prior research has evaluated residual overlap at C1-2 in an injured population.

There are several potential weaknesses of the present investigation which prompts caution in interpreting the results: the foremost is that the A-ART evaluation was performed by two examiners with substantial experience with the test, and thus, the reliability of the test when performed by other clinicians cannot be established with these results. Further, there are no established norms for the amount of palpable rotational movement between C1 and C2 that would fall into the negative (Grade 0–1) versus positive (Grade 2–3) A-ART result, and the ~5 mm threshold described for the test is an unmeasured approximation. Additionally, the average and range of values for the residual facet overlap evaluation in healthy adults was only found in a single prior publication; thus the technique is relatively novel and has not been validated on a more diverse population. The results of the present study are the first to describe residual facet overlap in a symptomatic population with a history of traumatic injury, however.

For patients with rotational instability at C1-2, therapeutic options are minimal, and results uncertain. Some, but not all of the patients in the current study had positive results from rehabilitation and physical therapy modalities. For patients with refractory symptoms, surgical fusion of C1-C2 is a viable option, although outcomes and complication rates are not well established.

We cautiously interpret these results to suggest that the atlas-axis rotational test (A-ART) is a potentially useful physical examination tool for identifying the pathological source of persisting cervicocranial symptoms consistent with upper cervical rotational instability. As such, the test offers potential benefits in the medicolegal investigation of the pain generator in patients with persisting unexplained upper cervicocranial symptoms after whiplash trauma, in that the patients most likely to have objective imaging evidence of rotational instability at C1-2 can be identified with greater accuracy, thus providing legally admissible proof of the location and extent of injury. Further investigation is warranted to evaluate the practicality and diagnostic accuracy of the A-ART in larger patient populations.

5. Conclusions

An accurate diagnosis can be elusive for the patient with persisting whiplash trauma-related craniocervical symptoms, in part because injury that results in rotational instability can be difficult to identify or quantify. The use of the atlas-axis rotational (A-ART) orthopedic test may provide reliable evidence for the presence of upper cervical instability, and should be considered as a useful initial test for differential diagnosis of the source of persisting head and neck symptoms in patients with chronic pain following whiplash trauma. For patients with a positive A-ART, an axial CT scan will provide a definitive diagnosis, as well as quantification, of rotational instability.

Supplementary Materials: The following supporting information can be downloaded at: https://www.mdpi.com/article/10.3390/jcm12041469/s1.

Author Contributions: B.R.K., T.J.M., M.H.B. and M.D.F. all participated in the study conception, design, analysis, and drafting of the manuscript, and all authors have approved the submitted version of the manuscript and have agreed both to be personally accountable for their own contributions and to ensure that questions related to the accuracy or integrity of any part of the work are appropriately investigated, resolved, and the resolution documented in the literature. All authors have read and agreed to the published version of the manuscript.

Funding: No outside funding was used for the study.

Informed Consent Statement: All of the study subjects consented to the procedures as part of clinically indicated routine diagnostic procedures. The anonymized retrospective record review protocol was exempt from ethics review.

Data Availability Statement: The data that served as the source material for the analysis are provided in a supplemental file.

Conflicts of Interest: M.D.F. provides expert medicolegal consultation. No conflicts are declared for the remaining authors.

Abbreviations

UCRI—upper cervical instability test; A-ART—atlas-axis rotational test; CT—computed tomography.

References

1. Freeman, M.D.; Katz, E.A.; Rosa, S.L.; Gatterman, B.G.; Strömmer, E.M.F.; Leith, W.M. Diagnostic Accuracy of Videofluoroscopy for Symptomatic Cervical Spine Injury Following Whiplash Trauma. *Int. J. Environ. Res. Public Health* **2020**, *17*, 1693. [CrossRef] [PubMed]
2. Steilen, D.; Hauser, R.; Woldin, B.; Sawyer, S. Chronic Neck Pain: Making the Connection between Capsular Ligament Laxity and Cervical Instability. *Open Orthop. J.* **2014**, *8*, 326–345. [CrossRef]
3. Dumas, J.L.; Sainte Rose, M.; Dreyfus, P.; Goldlust, D.; Chevrel, J.P. Rotation of the Cervical Spinal Column: A Computed Tomography in Vivo Study. *Surg. Radiol. Anat.* **1993**, *15*, 333–339. [CrossRef] [PubMed]
4. Villas, C.; Arriagada, C.; Zubieta, J.L. Preliminary CT Study of C1-C2 Rotational Mobility in Normal Subjects. *Eur. Spine J.* **1999**, *8*, 223–228. [CrossRef] [PubMed]

5. Mönckeberg, J.E.; Tomé, C.V.; Matías, A.; Alonso, A.; Vásquez, J.; Zubieta, J.L. CT Scan Study of Atlantoaxial Rotatory Mobility in Asymptomatic Adult Subjects: A Basis for Better Understanding C1-C2 Rotatory Fixation and Subluxation. *Spine* **2009**, *34*, 1292–1295. [CrossRef] [PubMed]
6. Kaale, B.R.; Krakenes, J.; Albrektsen, G.; Wester, K. Clinical Assessment Techniques for Detecting Ligament and Membrane Injuries in the Upper Cervical Spine Region–a Comparison with MRI Results. *Man. Ther.* **2008**, *13*, 397–403. [CrossRef] [PubMed]
7. Zhai, X.; Kang, J.; Chen, X.; Dong, J.; Qiu, X.-W.; Ding, X.-A.; Liu, J.; He, X.-J. [In vivo measurement of three-dimensional motion of the upper cervical spine using CT three-dimensional reconstruction]. *Zhongguo Gu Shang* **2019**, *32*, 658–665. [CrossRef]
8. Kang, J.; Chen, G.; Zhai, X.; He, X. In Vivo Three-Dimensional Kinematics of the Cervical Spine during Maximal Active Head Rotation. *PLoS ONE* **2019**, *14*, e0215357. [CrossRef] [PubMed]
9. Lee, R.K.L.; Chu, W.C.W.; Graham, C.A.; Rainer, T.H.; Ahuja, A.T. Knowledge of Radiation Exposure in Common Radiological Investigations: A Comparison between Radiologists and Non-Radiologists. *Emerg. Med. J.* **2012**, *29*, 306–308. [CrossRef] [PubMed]
10. GeoGebra. Available online: https://www.geogebra.org (accessed on 9 February 2023).
11. Krakenes, J.; Kaale, B.; Moen, G.; Nordli, H.; Gilhus, N.; Rorvik, J. MRI Assessment of the Alar Ligaments in the Late Stage of Whiplash Injury—A Study of Structural Abnormalities and Observer Agreement. *Neuroradiology* **2002**, *44*, 617–624. [CrossRef] [PubMed]
12. Krakenes, J.; Kaale, B.R. Magnetic Resonance Imaging Assessment of Craniovertebral Ligaments and Membranes After Whiplash Trauma. *Spine* **2006**, *31*, 2820–2826. [CrossRef] [PubMed]
13. Vetti, N.; Kråkenes, J.; Eide, G.E.; Rørvik, J.; Gilhus, N.E.; Espeland, A. Are MRI High-Signal Changes of Alar and Transverse Ligaments in Acute Whiplash Injury Related to Outcome? *BMC Musculoskelet. Disord.* **2010**, *11*, 260. [CrossRef]
14. Söderman, T.; Olerud, C.; Shalabi, A.; Alavi, K.; Sundin, A. Static and Dynamic CT Imaging of the Cervical Spine in Patients with Rheumatoid Arthritis. *Skelet. Radiol.* **2015**, *44*, 241–248. [CrossRef] [PubMed]
15. Lofrese, G.; Musio, A.; De Iure, F.; Cultrera, F.; Martucci, A.; Iaccarino, C.; Essayed, W.I.; Ghadirpour, R.; Servadei, F.; Cavallo, M.A.; et al. Type II Odontoid Fracture in Elderly Patients Treated Conservatively: Is Fracture Healing the Goal? *Eur. Spine J.* **2019**, *28*, 1064–1071. [CrossRef] [PubMed]
16. Patijn, J.; Wilmink, J.; ter Linden, F.H.; Kingma, H. CT Study of Craniovertebral Rotation in Whiplash Injury. *Eur. Spine J.* **2001**, *10*, 38–43. [CrossRef] [PubMed]

Disclaimer/Publisher's Note: The statements, opinions and data contained in all publications are solely those of the individual author(s) and contributor(s) and not of MDPI and/or the editor(s). MDPI and/or the editor(s) disclaim responsibility for any injury to people or property resulting from any ideas, methods, instructions or products referred to in the content.

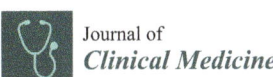

Article

Non-Surgical Management of Upper Cervical Instability via Improved Cervical Lordosis: A Case Series of Adult Patients

Evan A. Katz [1], Seana B. Katz [1] and Michael D. Freeman [2,*]

1. Independent Researcher, Boulder, CO 80302, USA
2. Faculty of Health Medicine and Life Sciences, Maastricht University, 6229 ER Maastricht, The Netherlands
* Correspondence: m.freeman@maastrichtuniversity.nl

Abstract: Injury to the head and neck resulting from whiplash trauma can result in upper cervical instability (UCIS), in which excessive movement at C1 on C2 is observed radiologically. In some cases of UCIS there is also a loss of normal cervical lordosis. We postulate that improvement or restoration of the normal mid to lower cervical lordosis in patients with UCIS can improve the biomechanical function of the upper cervical spine, and thus potentially improve symptoms and radiographic findings associated with UCIS. Nine patients with both radiographically confirmed UCIS and loss of cervical lordosis underwent a chiropractic treatment regimen directed primarily at the restoration of the normal cervical lordotic curve. In all nine cases, significant improvements in radiographic indicators of both cervical lordosis and UCIS were observed, along with symptomatic and functional improvement. Statistical analysis of the radiographic data revealed a significant correlation ($R^2 = 0.46$, $p = 0.04$) between improved cervical lordosis and reduction in measurable instability, determined by C1 lateral mass overhang on C2 with lateral flexion. These observations suggest that enhancing cervical lordosis can contribute to improvement in signs and symptoms of upper cervical instability secondary to traumatic injury.

Keywords: cervical lordosis; motor vehicle crash; digital motion X-ray; upper cervical instability

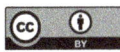

1. Introduction

Whiplash is an injury mechanism most typically associated with the rapid flexion/extension, compression and rotation of the cervical spine that can occur in a motor-vehicle crash [1]. Injuries resulting from whiplash trauma are common; it is estimated that there are approximately 2.9 million cases of whiplash trauma-associated injury that occur annually in the US [2]. The constellation of chronic symptoms, largely affecting the head and neck, that can result from acute injury after whiplash trauma can present a complex problem for both patients and clinicians [3]. Chronic symptoms associated with "late whiplash" can include headaches, dizziness, neck and upper back pain, as well as widespread pain [4]. Cervical spine pathology associated with whiplash trauma includes facet derangement, disk injury, and spinal ligament strain and rupture, often in the upper cervical spine [5].

Whiplash trauma can also result in upper cervical instability (UCIS), a condition in which excessive movement is observed at the C1–2 levels in combination with a wide constellation of head and neck somatic signs and symptoms [6,7].

UCIS is typically identified and diagnosed by comparing radiographic findings in patients with clinical complaints to accepted normal radiographic values (Figure 1). Radiographic evidence of UCIS includes anterior translation of C1 on C2 such that the atlanto-dental interspace exceeds 3.5 mm (as observed on lateral flexion radiographs), [8] and lateral translation of C1 on C2 such that there is more than 2.0 mm of lateral overhang of the lateral mass of C1 on the superior articulating facet of C2 (as observed in anterior to posterior (AP) open-mouth radiographs with lateral bending movements), in combination with asymmetry of the peri-odontoid space. While the 2.0 mm overhang threshold has only moderate sensitivity and positive predictive value (PPV) for upper cervical injury in the whiplash-injured population with chronic symptoms (64% and 75%, respectively), and the more subjective asymmetry assessment has low sensitivity (29%) but high PPV (95%), in combination the two findings have a PPV of 100% [9].

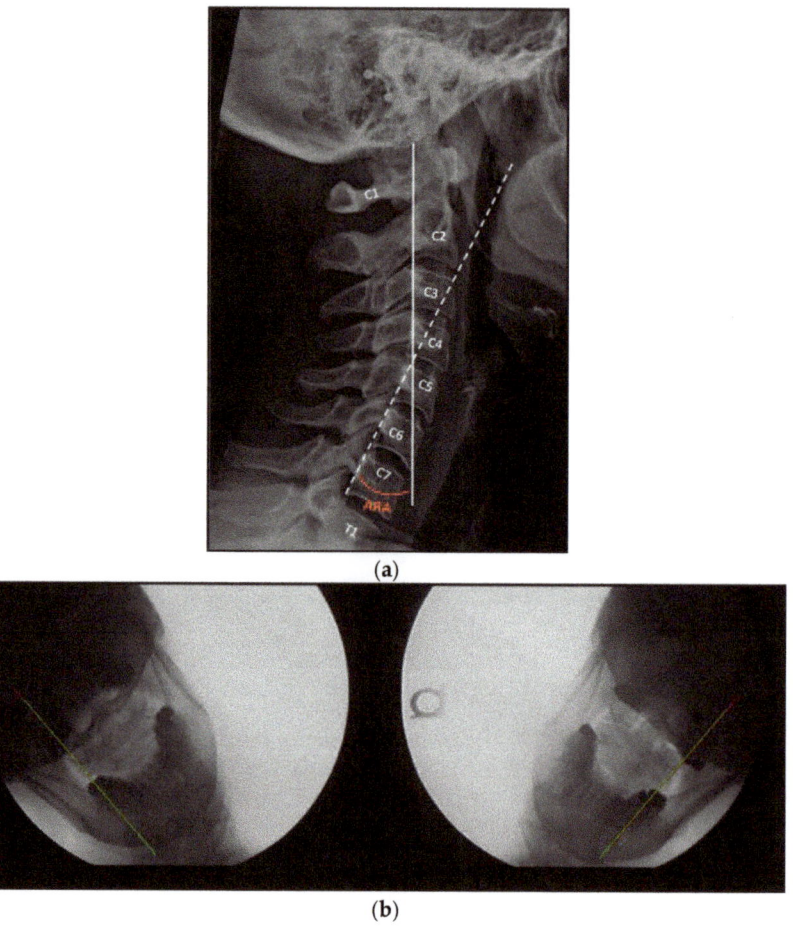

Figure 1. (a) Actual rotational angles (ARA) measurement in a patient with a normal cervical lordosis. The ARA (in red) indicates the angle between the posterior body margins of C2 (solid white line) and C7 (dashed white line). (b) AP open mouth lateral bending still shots from the DMX study (left and right lateral flexion on the left and right, respectively), with the green line indicating the lateral mass margin of C1, and the red line indicating the lateral body margin of C2. The lines overlap, indicating no overhang of C1 on C2.

The presence of instability is generally assumed to result from ligamentous and facet capsule damage resulting from the incipient trauma [10]. The loss of ligamentous integrity in the upper cervical spine in turn raises the concern of increased risk of future injury in the unfortunate event of a subsequent trauma [11]. Patients with symptomatic UCIS may complain of symptoms with varying degrees of specificity to the pathology—ranging from seemingly high specificity (i.e., difficulty holding the head up without support, intolerance to prolonged static postures, persisting sensation of suboccipital clicking) to nonspecific (i.e., head, neck, and shoulder pain) [12,13].

For UCIS patients with refractory symptoms, surgical fusion of the C1–C2 vertebrae is a viable, albeit under-investigated therapeutic option, as success and complication rates for the relatively rare procedure are not reliably established in the literature. Like all spinal fusion surgeries, fusion for C1–2 instability is expensive, invasive, and carries some degree of risk [14]. In addition to the immediate risks associated with surgery such as blood loss and neurological injury, intermediate (i.e., infection, graft subsidence) and long-term risks (adjacent segment pathology) are also potential complications of spinal fusion surgery [15]. In spite of the risks, upper cervical fusion is often the only option presented to the patient with refractory symptoms and demonstrable UCIS.

Loss of the normal cervical lordotic curve is a common radiographic finding in patients with chronic pain after whiplash [16], although there is no general consensus in the literature as to whether the finding indicates true pathology or a normal variant [17–20]. It is well established, however, that the normal cervical lordosis is the biomechanically ideal posture of the cervical spine, as mechanical stresses in the spine are most evenly balanced between the intervertebral disk and zygapophyseal joints when the "C"-shaped curve of the neck is maintained [21]. The clinical benefits of a lordotic cervical curve have been demonstrated in multiple studies. As an example, in a study of 300 neck pain patients under the age of 40, Gao and colleagues found an increased degree of disk herniation in the patients with straight and kyphotic cervical spines, in comparison with the lordotic necks [22]. They also reported an improvement in disk height and a decrease in disk herniation severity and associated spinal cord compression in the patients who had an improvement in lordosis. A recent systematic review of controlled clinical trials of lordosis restoration therapy for neck pain patients demonstrated that when treatment included extension traction directed at improvement of the lordotic curve, symptomatic improvements were maintained for more than 1 year after cessation of therapy [23]. In comparison, control treatment groups without extension traction were more likely to relapse after cessation of therapy.

A therapeutic model directed at methods of restoring the normal cervical curve is called Chiropractic Biophysics^{TM} (CBP). CBP relies on a combination of common chiropractic modalities (e.g., manipulation), Mirror Image® exercises, and spinal extension traction (Figure 2) [24]. There is evidence that suggests that CBP therapy is effective for restoring cervical lordosis [25].

While it is the mid to lower cervical spine that benefits most from the restoration of normal lordosis, there is evidence that the upper cervical spine can also benefit from a normal cervical curve, as a straight or kyphotic cervical spine is compensated at the C0-1-2 level by excessive craniocervical extension in an effort to keep the eyes level with the horizon [26,27].

In the present investigation, we describe nine cases of radiographically confirmed and symptomatically congruent UCIS in patients with chronic symptoms following whiplash trauma. In all nine cases, the patients were also found to have a reduction in normal cervical lordosis, and thus treatment was directed at restoring the lordotic curve via the CBP® approach. Baseline and post-treatment radiographic parameters of both UCIS and cervical lordosis are described, as well as subjective response to treatment.

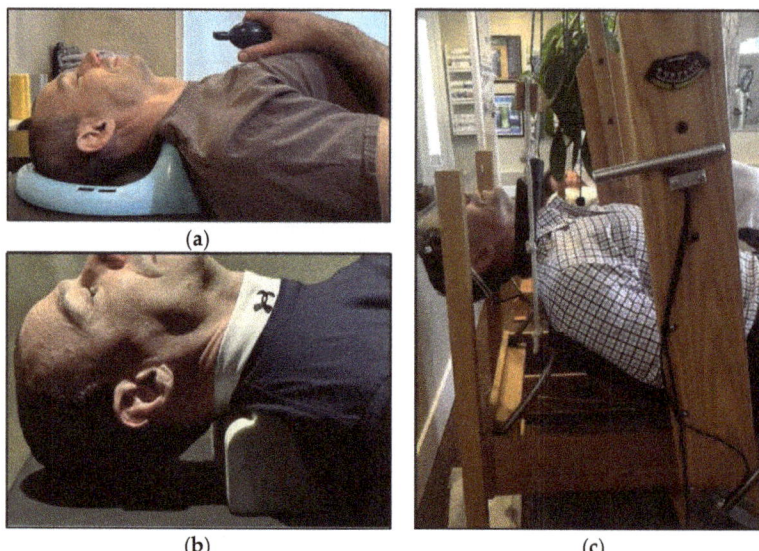

Figure 2. (a) Cervical posture pump® demonstration. (b) Denneroll™ demonstration. (c) 2-way extension traction demonstration. Note: the model in all figures is author EAK.

2. Materials and Methods

This case series includes nine patients (2 male, 7 female), ranging in age from 28 to 52 years with an average age of 39 years (Table 1). Each patient presented to the same chiropractic practice (authors EK and SK) for evaluation of acute or chronic symptoms consistent with upper cervical instability. The majority of the patients had undergone evaluation with other clinicians, including neurosurgeons or orthopedic spine surgeons, or had been previously treated with physical therapy or chiropractic manipulation. The inclusion criterion for the cases was all consecutive patients presenting with radiographic evidence of both UCIS and loss of cervical lordosis, following a history of traumatic injury of the neck (primarily whiplash trauma). A finding of fracture, dislocation, or myelopathy or other concerning neurological manifestation of the instability was an exclusion criterion, as such patients would be uniformly referred for urgent neurosurgical or orthopedic evaluation as part of the clinic protocol. The patient histories and treatment course varied widely, and the median time between baseline and follow-up radiographic examination was 16 weeks (with an interquartile range of 32 weeks).

Table 1. Patient characteristics.

Patient Number	Gender (M/F)	Age	Duration [a] (Weeks)	Symptoms [b]
1	F	46	7	Neck pain and weakness, dizziness.
2	F	36	10	Neck pain, headaches.
3	M	37	12	Pain at the base of the skull, clicking sensation dizziness.
4	F	52	16	Head and neck pain, blurred vision.
5	F	34	16	Head and neck pain, blurred vision, arm tingling, clicking sensation, sleep disruption.
6	M	28	19	Head and neck pain, occipital spasms, blurred vision, dizziness.

Table 1. *Cont.*

Patient Number	Gender (M/F)	Age	Duration [a] (Weeks)	Symptoms [b]
7	F	35	44	Head and neck pain, arm tingling.
8	F	53	52	Head and neck pain, head pressure, pain behind left eye, sleep disruption
9	F	30	68	Debilitating Headaches, neck pain.

[a] Duration indicates the period of time between baseline radiographic measurement and follow-up evaluation.
[b] Symptoms listed are only those consistent with UCIS. Patients may have had other less UCIS-specific symptoms.

2.1. Radiographic Analysis

Video-Fluoroscopic (VF) examination of the cervical spine was performed using digital motion X-ray (DMX). This imaging protocol allows for continuous examination of movement within the cervical spine. DMX records 30 images per second of continuous X-ray and captures an active range of motion allowing dynamic four-dimensional visualization of the integrity of the ligaments of the upper cervical spine. DMX imaging, therefore, provides the opportunity to assess both static and dynamic parameters of vertebral alignment [28,29].

Two DMX views were used to assess the degree of lordotic curvature and to identify and quantify findings consistent with UCIS; a neutral lateral cervical (NLC) and anterior to posterior open-mouth lateral cervical bending (APOM-LCB). Both examinations were performed at the baseline and prior to initiation of therapy, and then repeated no less than 72 h after therapy was concluded, as the goal was to avoid imaging of any temporary cervical curve improvement directly following extension traction. In order to produce images that were consistent with each other, the patient was positioned in the same fashion in both studies, each conducted by the same author, (either EAK or SBK), with the central ray at C5, back or shoulder touching the image intensifier (depending on view), and with a 20 mm marker on the patient's skin for calibration of the PostureRay® measuring software.

Actual Rotational Angles (ARA) were calculated from sagittal NLC images using PostureRay® software (PostureCo, Inc., Trinity, FL, USA) for Computerized Radiographic Mensuration Analysis (see Figure 1a). The cervical ARA is the angular measurement between the posterior vertebral body margins of C2 and C7, and the average ARA for a maintained cervical lordosis is $-34°$ [30]. All images include a standard X-ray marker for calibration prior to each measurement in order to avoid magnification error.

The ARA was used to quantify the deviation of the segmental rotational angles from C2–C7 from normal cervical lordosis values. Static images of right and left APOM-LCB were taken as frames from DMX videos at the extremes of comfortable lateral flexion. The images were analyzed using the PostureRay® software to quantify the amount of C1–C2 lateral mass overhang margin at maximum right and left lateral cervical bending (Figure 1b). An overhang margin of >3 mm was used as the threshold for the study inclusion criterion of potential C1 on C2 instability, in combination with asymmetry of the peri-odontoid space. As noted above, at this threshold of combined findings, the sensitivity (i.e., true positive rate) and positive predictive value (i.e., true positive rate/all positives) for traumatic injury is 100% [9].

Along with findings consistent with UCIS, included patients also demonstrated a loss of lordosis, defined as an increase from the average normal lordotic ARA of $-34°$ (see Table 2), resulting in an appearance of straightening or reversal (i.e., kyphosis) of the normal lordotic curve. Combined with an initial evaluation indicating symptomatic instability, the radiological examination confirmed a diagnosis of both loss of normal cervical lordosis and upper cervical instability for each of the nine patients included for study, as well as some degree of presumed injury to the upper cervical ligaments, including the alar, transverse, and other stabilizing ligaments [31].

Table 2. Radiographic measurements, pre and post intervention.

	Time of X-ray, Relative to Intervention [a]	ARA [b] C2–C7	C1–2 Lateral Overhang Margin [c]	
			Left	Right
Patient 1	Baseline	−14.1°	8.8 mm	6.1 mm
	Post intervention	−30.4°	6.3 mm	2.1 mm
Patient 2	Baseline	−4.1°	7.5 mm	1.8 mm
	Post intervention	−23.6°	2.3 mm	1.6 mm
Patient 3	Baseline	−2.8°	5.2 mm	2.4 mm
	Post Intervention	−4.6°	1.3 mm	1.8 mm
Patient 4	Baseline	3.0°	3.6 mm	1.2 mm
	Post intervention	−17.9°	1.1 mm	0.5 mm
Patient 5	Baseline	−8.8°	8.8 mm	6.1 mm
	Post intervention	−18.2°	6.3 mm	2.1 mm
Patient 6	Baseline	−19.9°	3.2 mm	3.0 mm
	Post intervention	−29.6°	2.2 mm	0.5 mm
Patient 7	Baseline	−11.2°	7.0 mm	1.9 mm
	Post intervention	−17.0°	2.5 mm	1.2 mm
Patient 8	Baseline	−12.0°	5.5 mm	3.5 mm
	Post intervention	−14.8°	2.8 mm	2.9 mm
Patient 9	Baseline	−19.7°	4.6 mm	2.0 mm
	Post intervention	−29.0°	2.0 mm	1.3 mm

[a] During the period of time between the first and follow-up X-rays (the 'treatment duration'), patients underwent treatment according to the intervention protocol. [b] ARA: Absolute Rotational Angle. Normal value is −34.0° or less. [c] Normal value 2 mm or less.

2.2. Intervention

Patients were treated twice per week on average for the indicated durations of treatment between radiographic evaluations (Table 1). Treatments incorporated full spine chiropractic adjustments, as well as Mirror Image® adjustments using a drop-piece table. Mirror Image® adjustments involve placing the cervical spine into an extended, overcorrected position during the chiropractic adjustment in order to achieve optimal progression toward proper spinal alignment [32]. The manipulations were solely directed at hypomobile spinal segments in the mid and lower cervical spine, as manipulation at the unstable upper cervical spine would be contraindicated. Several forms of cervical extension traction to restore or improve the cervical lordosis were also administered. These consisted of the following:

(1) Use of a Cervical posture pump® (Posture Pro, Inc., Huntington Beach, CA, USA), a self-controlled device with an inflatable airbladder that is applied to the supine mid-cervical spine. See Figure 2a.
(2) Home use of a cervical Denneroll™ (Denneroll Industries International Pty Ltd., Sydney, Australia), used like a pillow while the patient is supine, and positioned at the mid to lower cervical spine. See Figure 2b.
(3) Once tolerance to the previous two devices was established, the patient was progressed into a form of 2-way extension traction performed in office [33]. This therapy is applied while the patient lies supine on a specially designed chair, that employs a forehead harness to fix the head in a slightly extended position. A second strap is used to apply anterior tension to the mid to lower cervical spine, along the plane of the mid cervical spinal disks. See Figure 2c.

2.3. Statistical Analysis

Average treatment effect was assessed via the difference between the pre- and post-treatment radiographic measurements of ARA and lateral mass overhang using the Student's t-test for normally distributed differences and the signed rank test for non-normally distributed differences. Linear regression was used to assess the correlation between the percent change in ARA and the average of the left and right percent changes in C1–C2 overhang measurement (percent change = [post-measurement − pre-measurement]/pre-measurement; average overhang percent change = [left percent change + right percent change]/2). Normality of each difference and the average overhang percent change was assessed using the Shapiro-Wilk test. p-values < 0.05 were considered significant. All analyses were performed using SAS Software, version 9.4 (SAS Institute, Inc., Cary, NC, USA).

3. Results

Following the intervention period, clinical evaluations and radiographic analyses of each patient were repeated. After the intervention, each patient described marked improvements in overall pain scores, cervical range of motion, and quality of life. Patients who reported symptoms most closely associated with UCIS, including dizziness and blurred vision (patients one, two, five, and six), reported cessation that they are no longer experiencing those symptoms as of the end of this study. Additionally, those patients who had been managing their pain with prescription pain medications were no longer doing so. Furthermore, each patient described in this report has been able to resume activities which had been precluded by their neck pain and symptoms relating to instability. Patient three was able to resume participation in martial arts, and patients four and five also reported improved function. Patients seven, eight and nine reported a decrease or cessation of chronic and frequent headaches.

Radiographic re-evaluations, performed at least 72 h after the most recent therapy, revealed substantially improved cervical lordosis (i.e., progress toward the ideal ARA of $-34°$) in all of the patients. Mean ARA value at baseline was $-10°$, compared to $-21°$ after the intervention ($p = 0.002$, see Table 3). Three of the patients (one, six, and nine) had ARA values at or approaching $-30°$ (see Table 2). There was an average reduction in C1–C2 lateral mass overhang from 6.0 mm to 3.0 mm on the left (p = <0.001), and from 3.1 mm to 1.6 mm on the right ($p = 0.004$) (see Table 3). The average percent change in C1–2 overhang was normally distributed ($p = 0.91$). The percent change in ARA and average percent change in C1–2 overhang were moderately correlated (see Figure 3, $R^2 = 0.46$, $p = 0.04$).

Table 3. Differences between post- and pre-treatment measurements (negative values denote improvement).

Patient	ARA	Left Overhang	Right Overhang
1	−16.3	−2.5	−4.0
2	−19.5	−5.2	−0.2
3	−1.8	−3.9	−0.6
4	−20.9	−2.5	−0.7
5	−9.4	−2.5	−4.0
6	−9.7	−1.0	−2.5
7	−5.8	−4.5	−0.7
8	−2.8	−2.7	−0.6
9	−9.3	−2.6	−0.7
Shapiro-Wilk test of normality p-value [a]	0.4	0.29	0.004
Mean difference (standard deviation)	−10.6 (6.9)	−3.0 (1.27)	−1.6 (1.5)
Mean difference 95% CI	[−15.9, −5.3]	[−4.0, −2.1]	[−2.7, −0.4]
Test statistic [b]	−4.6	−7.2	−22.5
Degrees of freedom (df)	8	8	NA
p-value	0.0018	<0.0001	0.0039

[a] For sample sizes < 2000, Shapiro-Wilk is the appropriate test of normality. [b] Paired t-test for ARA and left overhang; signed rank test for right overhang.

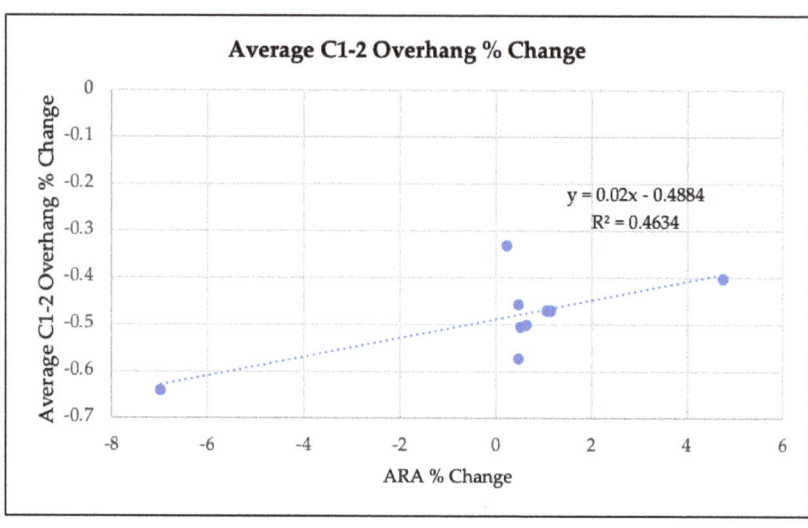

Figure 3. Linear regression analysis of average % change in C1-2 overhang versus the % change in ARA.

4. Discussion

There are several plausible explanations for the observed association between symptomatic improvement, improved cervical lordosis, and decreased C1–2 instability in the described cases. One explanation is that the symptoms resolved spontaneously, and that the improvements were unrelated to the treatment or radiographic changes. While plausible, this explanation defies logic and convention. The patients had been symptomatic for months to years and had all tried other treatments without success prior to initiating the cervical lordosis correction therapy. The positive changes observed in the imaging are thus much more likely to be explained by the therapy, rather than the natural course of the condition, which had reached a static level in all of the patients.

The remaining explanations are that the therapy directed at improving cervical lordosis improved the lordosis, the symptoms, and the C1–2 instability, or that the symptoms and instability improved for some reason unrelated to the alteration of the lordosis. We favor the former explanation. The upper cervical instability (and associated symptoms indicative of UCIS) is the result of upper cervical ligament injury and associated laxity. Loss of normal cervical lordosis produces a relatively flexed posture of the upper cervical spine, requiring extension accommodation at the head to keep the neutral gaze level with the horizon [34,35]. It makes sense that a persistently abnormal posture of the upper cervical spine would likely put a higher degree of strain on the upper cervical ligaments during normal activity, relative to having the head in a neutral position relative to C1–2, as occurs with normal extension at the craniocervical junction. We hypothesize that improvement of the cervical lordosis results in improved biomechanics of the upper cervical spine, and that this in turn allows for improvement of the integrity of the ligaments responsible for craniocervical stability. This hypothesis is an extension of the findings of prior authors, who have described a correlation between increased angle of the upper cervical (C0–2) spine and increased risk of cervical kyphosis [27]. Ours is the first study to demonstrate a relationship between loss of normal cervical curve and symptomatic instability, however.

Because the design of the present study was conceived of only after the association between cervical curve improvement and decreased upper cervical instability was noted, the evidence for symptomatic improvement was derived from narrative histories, rather than consistently used metrics. Future investigation would thus benefit from an a priori design with standardized objective measurements of the non-radiographic changes described in this study (e.g., Neck Disability Index, etc.), as well as the inclusion of a comparison group of patients who did not improve radiographically in either cervical curve or upper cervical instability. Moreover, the ability to generalize from this small sample of highly selected patients is limited, and thus another goal for future investigation is to increase the number of study subjects.

Author Contributions: Conceptualization, E.A.K., S.B.K. and M.D.F.; methodology, E.A.K., S.B.K. and M.D.F.; formal analysis, M.D.F.; investigation, E.A.K., S.B.K. and M.D.F.; resources, E.A.K. and S.B.K.; writing—original draft preparation, M.D.F.; writing—review and editing, E.A.K., S.B.K. and M.D.F. All authors have read and agreed to the published version of the manuscript.

Funding: This research received no external funding.

Informed Consent Statement: Informed consent was obtained from all subjects involved in the study. As the data were gathered retrospectively from anonymized files of patients who were treated under standard clinical protocol, the study was exempt from institutional review board oversight.

Data Availability Statement: All data were provided in the manuscript.

Acknowledgments: The authors thank Wendy Leith MPH MS for assistance with the data analysis, and Deed Harrison for his many helpful suggestions and encouragement.

Conflicts of Interest: The authors declare no conflict of interest.

References

1. Yadla, S.; Ratliff, J.K.; Harrop, J.S. Whiplash: Diagnosis, Treatment, and Associated Injuries. *Curr. Rev. Musculoskelet. Med.* **2008**, *1*, 65–68. [CrossRef] [PubMed]
2. Freeman, M.D.; Croft, A.C.; Rossignol, A.M.; Weaver, D.S.; Reiser, M. A Review and Methodologic Critique of the Literature Refuting Whiplash Syndrome. *Spine* **1999**, *24*, 86–96. [CrossRef] [PubMed]
3. Pastakia, K.; Kumar, S. Acute Whiplash Associated Disorders (WAD). *Open Access Emerg. Med.* **2011**, *3*, 29–32. [CrossRef] [PubMed]
4. Berglund, A.; Alfredsson, L.; Cassidy, J.D.; Jensen, I.; Nygren, A. The Association between Exposure to a Rear-End Collision and Future Neck or Shoulder Pain: A Cohort Study. *J. Clin. Epidemiol.* **2000**, *53*, 1089–1094. [CrossRef] [PubMed]
5. Freeman, M.D.; Centeno, C.J.; Katz, E. Magnetic Resonance Imaging of Whiplash Injury in the Upper Cervical Spine: Controversy or Confounding? *Spine J.* **2009**, *9*, 789–790. [CrossRef]
6. Derrick, L.J.; Chesworth, B.M. Post-Motor Vehicle Accident Alar Ligament Laxity. *J. Orthop. Sports Phys. Ther.* **1992**, *16*, 6–11. [CrossRef]
7. Grauer, J.N.; Panjabi, M.M.; Cholewicki, J.; Nibu, K.; Dvorak, J. Whiplash Produces an S-Shaped Curvature of the Neck with Hyperextension at Lower Levels. *Spine* **1997**, *22*, 2489–2494. [CrossRef]
8. Yang, S.Y.; Boniello, A.J.; Poorman, C.E.; Chang, A.L.; Wang, S.; Passias, P.G. A Review of the Diagnosis and Treatment of Atlantoaxial Dislocations. *Glob. Spine J.* **2014**, *4*, 197–210. [CrossRef]
9. Freeman, M.D.; Katz, E.A.; Rosa, S.L.; Gatterman, B.G.; Strömmer, E.M.F.; Leith, W.M. Diagnostic Accuracy of Videofluoroscopy for Symptomatic Cervical Spine Injury Following Whiplash Trauma. *Int. J. Environ. Res. Public Health* **2020**, *17*, 1693. [CrossRef]
10. Evaniew, N.; Yarascavitch, B.; Madden, K.; Ghert, M.; Drew, B.; Bhandari, M.; Kwok, D. Atlantoaxial Instability in Acute Odontoid Fractures Is Associated with Nonunion and Mortality. *Spine J.* **2015**, *15*, 910–917. [CrossRef]
11. Maiman, D.J.; Yoganandan, N.; Pintar, F.A. Preinjury Cervical Alignment Affecting Spinal Trauma. *J. Neurosurg.* **2002**, *97*, 57–62. [CrossRef] [PubMed]
12. Cook, C.; Brismée, J.-M.; Fleming, R.; Sizer, P.S.J. Identifiers Suggestive of Clinical Cervical Spine Instability: A Delphi Study of Physical Therapists. *Phys. Ther.* **2005**, *85*, 895–906. [CrossRef] [PubMed]
13. Olson, K.A.; Joder, D. Diagnosis and Treatment of Cervical Spine Clinical Instability. *J. Orthop. Sports Phys. Ther.* **2001**, *31*, 194–206. [CrossRef] [PubMed]
14. Jacobson, M.E.; Khan, S.N.; An, H.S. C1-C2 Posterior Fixation: Indications, Technique, and Results. *Orthop. Clin. N. Am.* **2012**, *43*, 11–18, vii. [CrossRef]
15. Smith, M.D.; Phillips, W.A.; Hensinger, R.N. Complications of Fusion to the Upper Cervical Spine. *Spine* **1991**, *16*, 702–705. [CrossRef]
16. Griffiths, H.J.; Olson, P.N.; Everson, L.I.; Winemiller, M. Hyperextension Strain or "Whiplash" Injuries to the Cervical Spine. *Skeletal. Radiol.* **1995**, *24*, 263–266. [CrossRef]
17. Marshall, D.L.; Tuchin, P.J. Correlation of Cervical Lordosis Measurement with Incidence of Motor Vehicle Accidents. *Australas. Chiropr. Osteopat.* **1996**, *5*, 79–85.
18. Lippa, L.; Lippa, L.; Cacciola, F. Loss of Cervical Lordosis: What Is the Prognosis? *J. Craniovertebral Junction Spine* **2017**, *8*, 9–14. [CrossRef]

19. Kristjansson, E.; Jónsson, H.J. Is the Sagittal Configuration of the Cervical Spine Changed in Women with Chronic Whiplash Syndrome? A Comparative Computer-Assisted Radiographic Assessment. *J. Manip. Physiol. Ther.* **2002**, *25*, 550–555. [CrossRef]
20. Matsumoto, M.; Fujimura, Y.; Suzuki, N.; Toyama, Y.; Shiga, H. Cervical Curvature in Acute Whiplash Injuries: Prospective Comparative Study with Asymptomatic Subjects. *Injury* **1998**, *29*, 775–778. [CrossRef]
21. Scheer, J.K.; Tang, J.A.; Smith, J.S.; Acosta, F.L.J.; Protopsaltis, T.S.; Blondel, B.; Bess, S.; Shaffrey, C.I.; Deviren, V.; Lafage, V.; et al. Cervical Spine Alignment, Sagittal Deformity, and Clinical Implications: A Review. *J. Neurosurg. Spine* **2013**, *19*, 141–159. [CrossRef] [PubMed]
22. Gao, K.; Zhang, J.; Lai, J.; Liu, W.; Lyu, H.; Wu, Y.; Lin, Z.; Cao, Y. Correlation between Cervical Lordosis and Cervical Disc Herniation in Young Patients with Neck Pain. *Medicine* **2019**, *98*, e16545. [CrossRef] [PubMed]
23. Oakley, P.A.; Ehsani, N.N.; Moustafa, I.M.; Harrison, D.E. Restoring Cervical Lordosis by Cervical Extension Traction Methods in the Treatment of Cervical Spine Disorders: A Systematic Review of Controlled Trials. *J. Phys. Ther. Sci.* **2021**, *33*, 784–794. [CrossRef]
24. Oakley, P.A.; Harrison, D.D.; Harrison, D.E.; Haas, J.W. Evidence-Based Protocol for Structural Rehabilitation of the Spine and Posture: Review of Clinical Biomechanics of Posture (CBP) Publications. *J. Can. Chiropr. Assoc.* **2005**, *49*, 270–296. [PubMed]
25. Moustafa, I.M.; Diab, A.A.; Harrison, D.E. The Effect of Normalizing the Sagittal Cervical Configuration on Dizziness, Neck Pain, and Cervicocephalic Kinesthetic Sensibility: A 1-Year Randomized Controlled Study. *Eur. J. Phys. Rehabil. Med.* **2017**, *53*, 57–71. [CrossRef] [PubMed]
26. Patwardhan, A.G.; Havey, R.M.; Khayatzadeh, S.; Muriuki, M.G.; Voronov, L.I.; Carandang, G.; Nguyen, N.-L.; Ghanayem, A.J.; Schuit, D.; Patel, A.A.; et al. Postural Consequences of Cervical Sagittal Imbalance: A Novel Laboratory Model. *Spine* **2015**, *40*, 783–792. [CrossRef]
27. Paholpak, P.; Vega, A.; Formanek, B.; Tamai, K.; Wang, J.C.; Buser, Z. Impact of Cervical Sagittal Balance and Cervical Spine Alignment on Craniocervical Junction Motion: An Analysis Using Upright Multi-Positional MRI. *Eur. Spine J.* **2021**, *30*, 444–453. [CrossRef]
28. Buonocore, E.; Hartman, J.T.; Nelson, C.L. Cineradiograms of Cervical Spine in Diagnosis of Soft-Tissue Injuries. *JAMA* **1966**, *198*, 143–147. [CrossRef]
29. Hino, H.; Abumi, K.; Kanayama, M.; Kaneda, K. Dynamic Motion Analysis of Normal and Unstable Cervical Spines Using Cineradiography. An in Vivo Study. *Spine* **1999**, *24*, 163–168. [CrossRef]
30. Harrison, D.D.; Janik, T.J.; Troyanovich, S.J.; Holland, B. Comparisons of Lordotic Cervical Spine Curvatures to a Theoretical Ideal Model of the Static Sagittal Cervical Spine. *Spine* **1996**, *21*, 667–675. [CrossRef]
31. Krakenes, J.; Kaale, B.; Moen, G.; Nordli, H.; Gilhus, N.; Rorvik, J. MRI Assessment of the Alar Ligaments in the Late Stage of Whiplash Injury—A Study of Structural Abnormalities and Observer Agreement. *Neuroradiology* **2002**, *44*, 617–624. [CrossRef] [PubMed]
32. Harrison, D.D.; Janik, T.J.; Harrison, G.R.; Troyanovich, S.; Harrison, D.E.; Harrison, S.O. Chiropractic Biophysics Technique: A Linear Algebra Approach to Posture in Chiropractic. *J. Manip. Physiol. Ther.* **1996**, *19*, 525–535.
33. Harrison, D.E.; Cailliet, R.; Harrison, D.D.; Janik, T.J.; Holland, B. A New 3-Point Bending Traction Method for Restoring Cervical Lordosis and Cervical Manipulation: A Nonrandomized Clinical Controlled Trial. *Arch. Phys. Med. Rehabil.* **2002**, *83*, 447–453. [CrossRef] [PubMed]
34. Mesfar, W.; Moglo, K. Effect of the Transverse Ligament Rupture on the Biomechanics of the Cervical Spine under a Compressive Loading. *Clin. Biomech.* **2013**, *28*, 846–852. [CrossRef]
35. Miyamoto, H.; Hashimoto, K.; Ikeda, T.; Akagi, M. Effect of Correction Surgery for Cervical Kyphosis on Compensatory Mechanisms in Overall Spinopelvic Sagittal Alignment. *Eur. Spine J.* **2017**, *26*, 2380–2385. [CrossRef]

Disclaimer/Publisher's Note: The statements, opinions and data contained in all publications are solely those of the individual author(s) and contributor(s) and not of MDPI and/or the editor(s). MDPI and/or the editor(s) disclaim responsibility for any injury to people or property resulting from any ideas, methods, instructions or products referred to in the content.

MDPI
St. Alban-Anlage 66
4052 Basel
Switzerland
www.mdpi.com

Journal of Clinical Medicine Editorial Office
E-mail: jcm@mdpi.com
www.mdpi.com/journal/jcm

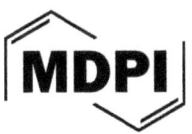

Disclaimer/Publisher's Note: The statements, opinions and data contained in all publications are solely those of the individual author(s) and contributor(s) and not of MDPI and/or the editor(s). MDPI and/or the editor(s) disclaim responsibility for any injury to people or property resulting from any ideas, methods, instructions or products referred to in the content.

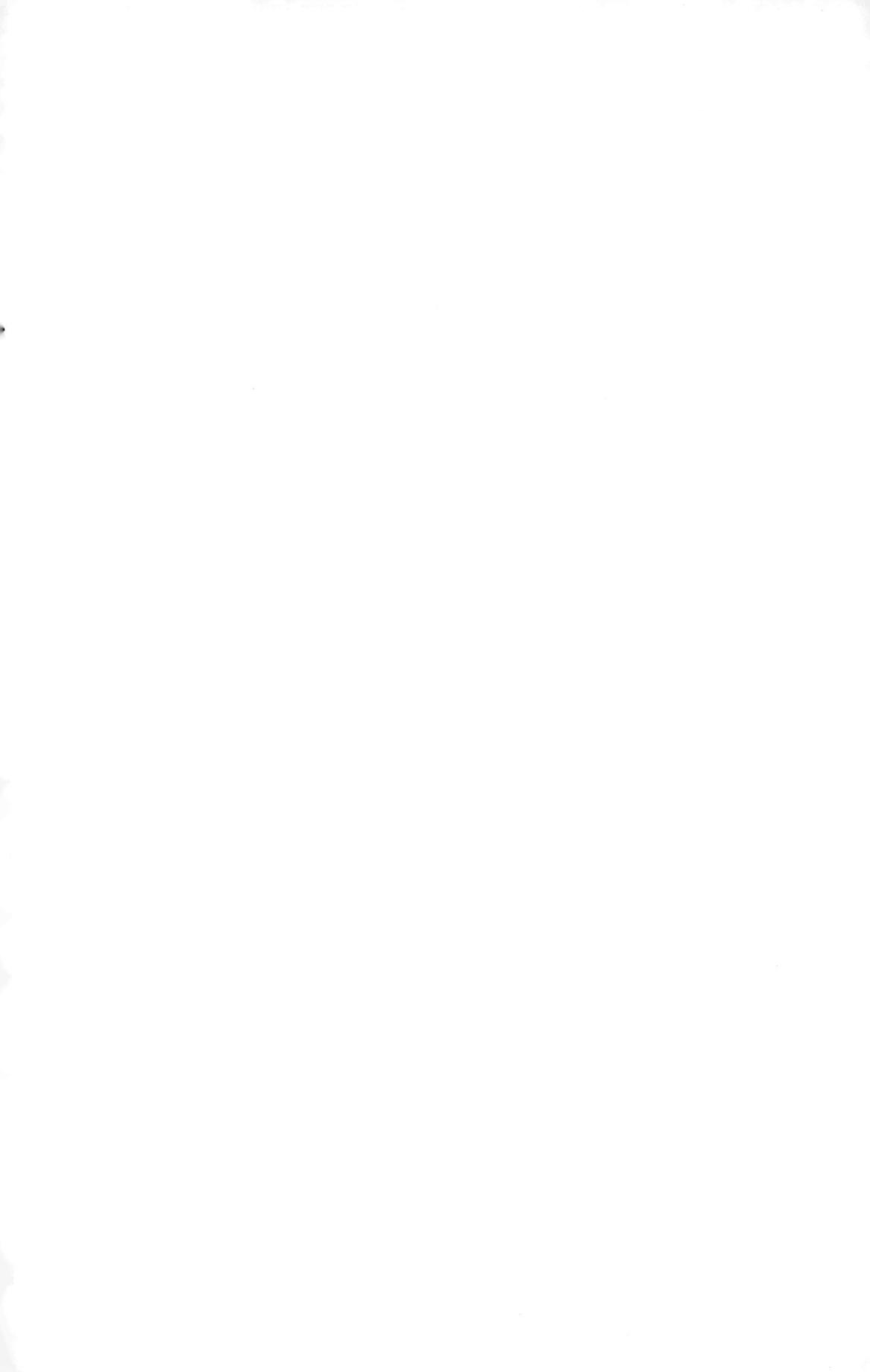

www.ingramcontent.com/pod-product-compliance
Lightning Source LLC
LaVergne TN
LVHW070507100526
838202LV00014B/1809